An Atlas of Interpretative Radiographic Anatomy of the Dog & Cat

An Atlas of Interpretative Radiographic Anatomy of the Dog & Cat

ARLENE COULSON B.Vet.Med. D.V.R. M.R.C.V.S.

with

NOREEN LEWIS B.Sc. D.V.R. M.R.C.V.S.

Blackwell
Science

© 2002 by Blackwell Science Ltd, a Blackwell Publishing Company
Editorial Offices:
Blackwell Science Ltd, 9600 Garsington Rd, OX4 2DQ, UK
  Tel: +44 (0)1865 776868
Blackwell Publishing Professional, 2121 State Avenue, Ames, Iowa 50014-8300, USA
  Tel: +1 515 292 0140
Blackwell Science Asia Pty Ltd, 54 University Street, Carlton, Victoria 3053, Australia
  Tel: +61 (0)3 9347 0300

First published 2002
2   2006

Library of Congress Cataloging-in-Publication Data

Coulson, Arlene.
  An atlas of interpretative radiographic anatomy of the dog and cat / Arlene Coulson,
Noreen D. Lewis.
   p. cm.
  Includes bibliographical references (p.).
  ISBN 0-632-04078-5
   1. Dogs–Anatomy–Atlases. 2. Cats–Anatomy–Atlases.
  3. Veterinary radiography–Atlases.
  I. Lewis, Noreen D. II. Title.

SF767.D6 C68 2001
636.7′089607572–dc21   00-068009

ISBN 0-632-04078-5

A catalogue record for this title is available from the British Library

Set in Times by Gray Publishing, Tunbridge Wells, Kent
Printed and bound in Denmark by
Narayana Press, Odder

For further information on Blackwell Publishing, visit our website:
www.blackwellpublishing.com

Contents

Introduction

Aim of the book

The primary aim of this book is to provide a detailed reference for the basic radiographic anatomy of the dog and cat. This is achieved by the inclusion of both radiographs and drawings.

The immature animal and, where relevant, a spectrum of breeds have been included.

A selection of anatomical variants and a few of the more common radiographic 'pitfalls' are also to be found following the 'normal' radiograph.

Following the anatomical sections of plain radiography is a series of the more commonly employed contrast studies. Confusion can occur when trying to interpret such techniques, and many anatomical features can only be seen with the aid of contrast agents. Hence these have been included, hoping they aid evaluation of the studies performed more regularly in general practice. In addition a few of the less common studies are found for anatomical understanding.

From personal experience in teaching and examining veterinary surgeons for post-graduate radiology certification it is clear that a good basic knowledge of radiographic anatomy is essential. Unfortunately, all too often 'normality' is not recognised, especially where breed variation has to be considered.

A short bibliography is in the last few pages of this book. The list includes only books and publications consulted, and relevant, for the figures and text of this manuscript. No individual references are cited in the text.

No index has been included as the atlas is intended to be used as a visual reference for normality. To facilitate this a comprehensive contents list, divided into anatomical regions for plain and contrast radiography, is provided.

Although initially it would appear that the book is mainly for the benefit of veterinary surgeons wanting to obtain additional radiology qualifications, basic radiographic anatomy will be of value to both undergraduates and veterinary surgeons in general practice. It is hoped that this atlas will become a useful and well used reference book for both the specialising and non-specialising veterinary audience.

Drawings

The drawings follow tracings of the radiographs. Only shadows seen in the radiograph have been traced, even if anatomically more detail should have been present. Each drawing has a detailed key.

It is hoped that the radiographic reproduction is of a sufficient standard to allow recognition of all the radiographic shadows that have been traced.

Where the shadows are complex, as in the skull, a number of drawings have been made to avoid interpretative confusion of numerous lines within small regions.

Every effort has been made not to overdraw or over-label the drawings correlating to the radiographs. In this way it is hoped that the reader will quickly recognise the important shadows and become familiar with radiographic anatomy.

Separate line drawings have also been included of soft tissue structures surrounding bony shadows. These structures are often overlooked when attention is focused on the more obvious opaque shadows. Much valuable information can be gained from the soft tissue surrounding, for example, the stifle joint.

In addition to the line drawings, schematic drawings of many projections have been made to familiarise the reader with anatomical features not visible on the radiograph. In this way the reader will be more able to make logical diagnosis/differential diagnosis when faced with radiographs demonstrating abnormal features.

Animals

Most of the radiographs in this book are original and for the exclusive use of the authors. The remainder have been given to the authors by generous colleagues.

The radiographs have been obtained over a period of five to six years and a brief summary of their source follows.

The 'normal' dog radiographs are mainly from a group of Beagle Hounds while the 'normal' cat radiographs are from a number of individual British Domestic Short Haired cats.

In both cases the radiographs were obtained specifically for the book, radiography taking place in conjunction with routine surgery or dentistry requiring general anaesthesia.

The different breeds, anatomical variants and radiographic 'pitfall' radiographs were either obtained primarily for this book or were taken from veterinary college files. This was probably one of the most difficult sections to complete for publication as radiographs falling into 'variant' or 'pitfall' are not usually recorded.

The dog juvenile section was commissioned for this book and radiography was performed on the same dog (Samoyed Crossbred entire male) from 1 month to 15 months of age at intervals of one month. This is probably the ideal situation for a juvenile study as individual, feeding and housing variations are all under control.

The study was based at University of Guelph in Ontario Canada under the watchful eye of Professor Sumner-Smith.

The cat juvenile section usually involved a different cat at each monthly age. Individuals from a breeding group were radiographed specifically for this book, during studies on clinical anaesthesia based in Newcastle, England.

Although this is not ideal as some individual variation is present, variations with feeding and housing were eliminated. The significant advantage of undertaking the work in this manner has been to ensure consistent anaesthetic and radiographic techniques in producing the final radiographs. Radiography was from four weeks to 96 weeks of age at four-weekly intervals.

All cats were entire and it was interesting to see the differences in bone size between male and female cats. The latter is especially relevant with the skull section.

The contrast study section radiographs were obtained from college files spanning over 20 years from 1975 to 1995. It was not thought to be ethical to introduce contrast medium, of any type, into a normal animal for the sole purpose of this book.

Radiography

All radiography performed in England, specifically for this book, was under the Ionising Radiation Regulations of 1985.

Every effort has been made to include only radiographs of a high radiographic quality.

As a variety of X-ray machines and accessory equipment have been used, no specific details of the equipment, nor exposure details are included in this book.

A comprehensive description of radiographic positioning of the animal has purposely been excluded as there are a number of excellent books on this subject. In addition it is not the main objective of this atlas to teach positioning.

Instead a line drawing, from a photograph of the live 'normal' dog being radiographed, is to be found below the relevant radiograph. Positioning for the 'normal' cat will be similar.

The centre point for the primary beam has been indicated on each drawing by a symbol varying with the photographic exposure angle.

Normality

The quest for radiographs showing classic and completely 'normal' radiographic anatomy proved to be very difficult in a number of skeletal regions. So much so that it was decided to include some radiographs which demonstrated normal radiographic shadows of the bones which were to be detailed in the keys but had evidence of degenerative signs elsewhere.

In every case the bony degenerative changes were causing no clinical signs. The reader is reminded that during radiological analysis of clinical cases, over interpretation of obvious chronic bony degeneration can result in failure to observe active bony changes elsewhere. In their early stages acute skeletal lesions are soft tissue alterations followed by subtle bony changes.

In the case of the stifle joint of the cat the absence of a bony shadow for the medial fabella of the m.gastrocnemius was commonplace. A craniocaudal shadow of the femur has been included for the sole purpose of showing this medial sesamoid bone.

With regards to the soft tissue radiographs of particular note is the cat thorax which showed considerable cardiac shadow variation. As it proved to be such a frequent finding a number of these 'anomalies' have been included in the thoracic section.

In addition to the cardiac shadow abnormal lung opacities were commonly seen, especially affecting the right middle lung lobe.

Radiographs of these lung opacities have not been included in the book as it was considered to be too close to disease patterns, but unexpected radiographic findings in seemingly clinically normal animals are something of which the reader should be aware.

Care has been taken to indicate variation of 'normal' radiographic anatomy, plus bony degenerative changes. Also a full range of what would be expected as 'normal' is included in the book.

An Atlas of Interpretative Radiographic Anatomy of the Dog and Cat

Acknowledgements

This book could not have been possible without the support of a vast number of people.

An enormous thank you to Dr Ray Ashdown, East Sussex, UK, our anatomical and terminological consultant, for his vast knowledge which has made such a vital and valuable contribution to this book and which has been offered so patiently during the preparation of this material.

Mr Jonathan Clayton-Jones, London, UK, has prepared the numerous drawings, line and schematic, based on the original tracings prepared by the authors. These represent the culmination of many drafts and re-drafts to reproduce satisfactorily for publication. Without his skill and patience the interpretation of many of the radiographs to the satisfaction of the authors would not have been possible.

Janet Butler at the Animal Health Trust, Newmarket, UK has provided her expertise in preparing photographs from many of the original radiographs.

Mr David Gunn at the Royal Veterinary College, London, UK has kindly allowed line drawings to be prepared from photographs of radiographic positioning prepared at the College.

Our special thanks are extended to a number of veterinary surgeons in general practice and academia who at the time persevered with obtaining normal radiographs to fill the gaps for the book.

Academic colleagues from:

- University of Bristol School of Veterinary Science, Department of Clinical Veterinary Science, Bristol, UK, in particular Dr Christine Gibbs
- University of Edinburgh, Royal (Dick) School of Veterinary Studies, Department of Veterinary Clinical Studies, Edinburgh, UK, in particular Mr Andrew Burnie.
- University of London, The Royal Veterinary College, Department of Small Animal Medicine and Surgery, London, UK, in particular Dr Gary England and Carol France.
- The Medical School, University of Newcastl, Newcastle, UK, in particular Dr Paul Flecknell.
- University of Guelph, Ontario Veterinary College, Department of Clinical Studies, Guelph, Canada, in particular Professor Sumner-Smith.

Practitioner colleagues from:

- The Well House Veterinary Clinic, Crowborough, East Sussex, UK, in particular Mark and Teresa Johnston.
- Castle Veterinary Centre, Nottingham, UK, in particular Brin and Ewan McNeill.
- Highlands Surgery, Tenterden, Kent, UK, in particular Gary Clayton-Jones.
- Eton Veterinary Hospital, Tonbridge, Kent, UK, in particular Rodney Noble and Juliette Winchurst.
- Culverden Veterinary Group, Tunbridge Wells, Kent, UK, in particular Hilary Egan.
- Grove Lodge Veterinary Hospital, Worthing, West Sussex, UK, in particular Jo Arthur and Peter Fry.

Companies for providing copious quantities of radiographic film: 3M, UK and Fuji UK.

This atlas is dedicated to Odette Rebecca Coulson,
Arlene's young daughter who died in April 2001.
Her good humour, artistic suggestions and flexibility
in demands on her mother's time were as
invaluable as the encouragement of
her husband Andrew.

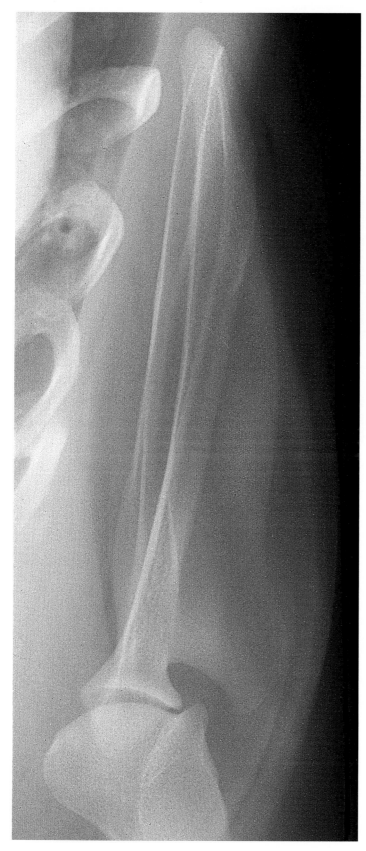

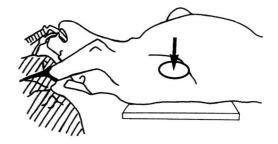

Figure 2 Line drawing of photograph representing radiographic positioning for Figure 1.

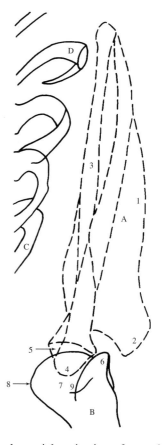

Figure 3 Caudocranial projection of scapula.

A Scapula
    1 Spine
    2 Acromion
    3 Subscapular fossa
    4 Supraglenoid tubercle
    5 Glenoid cavity

B Humerus
    6 Greater tubercle
    7 Head
    8 Lesser tubercle
    9 Intertubercular groove

C 1st. rib

D 4th. rib

Figure 1 Caudocranial projection of scapula. Beagle dog 2.5 years old, entire male.

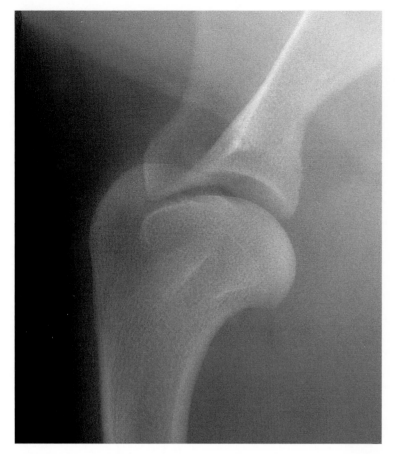

Figure 4   Mediolateral projection of shoulder joint. Beagle dog 2.5 years old, entire male.

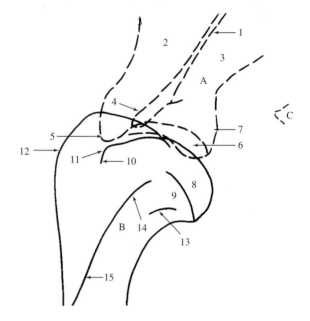

Figure 6   Mediolateral projection of shoulder joint.

A Scapula
  1 Spine
  2 Supraspinous fossa
  3 Infraspinous fossa
  4 Acromion
  5 Supraglenoid tubercle
  6 Glenoid cavity
  7 Infraglenoid tuberosity

B Humerus
  8 Head
  9 Neck
  10 Lesser tubercle
  11 Intertubercular groove
  12 Greater tubercle
  13 Crest of the lesser tubercle
  14 Tricipital line
  15 Deltoid tuberosity

C Manubrium of sternum

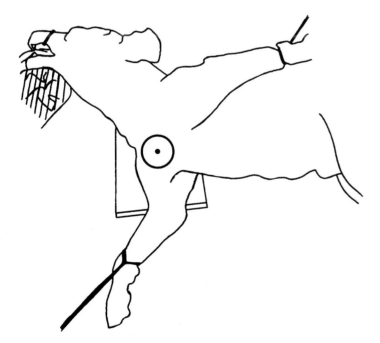

Figure 5   Line drawing of photograph representing radiographic positioning for Figure 4.

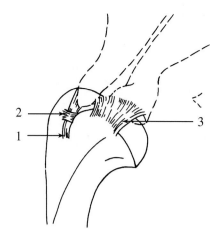

Figure 8 Schematic drawing of mediolateral projection of shoulder joint to demonstrate the ligaments and biceps brachii tendon.

1 = Biceps brachii tendon (found on medial aspect of joint)

2 = Transverse humeral ligament (found on medial aspect of joint)

3 = Thickening of inner surface of joint capsule forming the medial and lateral glenohumeral ligaments

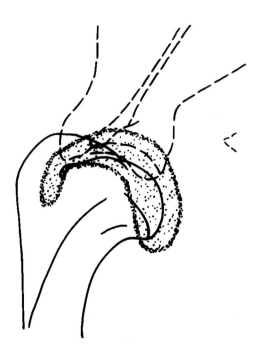

Figure 7 Schematic drawing of mediolateral projection of shoulder joint to demonstrate the extent of joint capsule.

= Joint capsule

= Synovial space

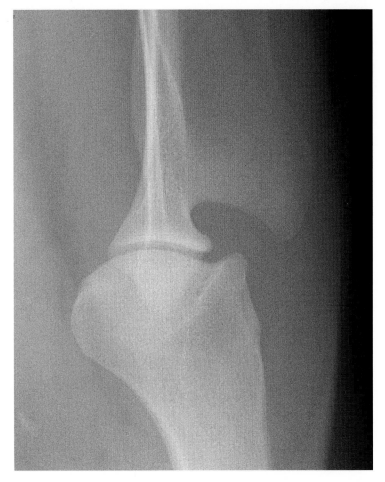

Figure 9 Caudocranial projection of shoulder joint. Beagle dog 2.5 years old, entire male.

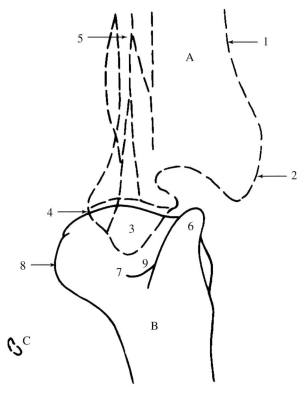

Figure 11 Caudocranial projection of shoulder joint.

A Scapula
  1 Spine
  2 Acromion
  3 Supraglenoid tubercle including coracoid process medially
  4 Glenoid cavity
  5 Subscapular fossa

B Humerus
  6 Greater tubercle
  7 Head
  8 Lesser tubercle
  9 Intertubercular groove

C Clavicle. Often seen in this projection.

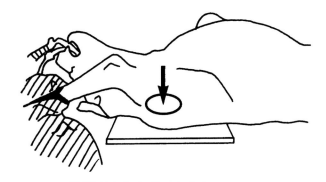

Figure 10 Line drawing of photograph representing radiographic positioning for Figure 9.

An Atlas of Interpretative Radiographic Anatomy of the Dog and Cat

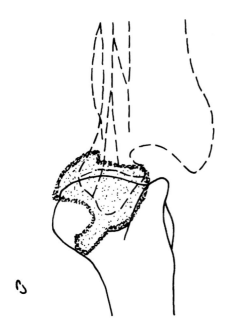

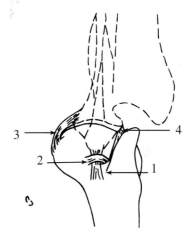

Figure 12 Schematic drawing of caudocranial projection of shoulder joint to demonstrate extent of joint capsule.

= Joint capsule

= Synovial space

Figure 13 Schematic drawing of caudocranial projection of shoulder joint to demonstrate ligaments and biceps brachii tendon.

1 = Biceps brachii tendon

2 = Transverse humeral ligament

3 = Medial glenohumeral ligament

4 = Lateral glenohumeral ligament

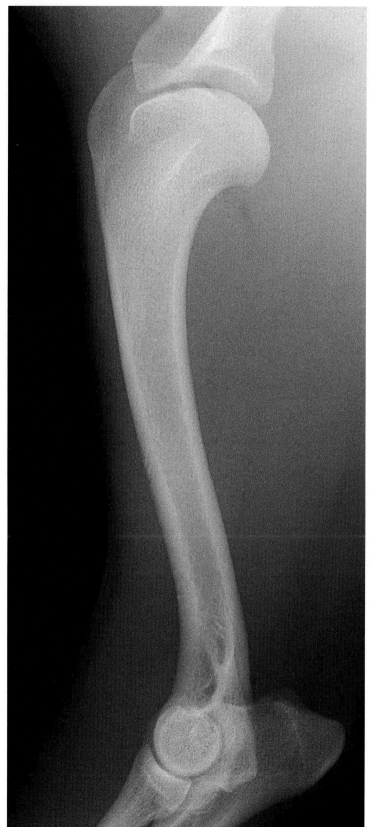

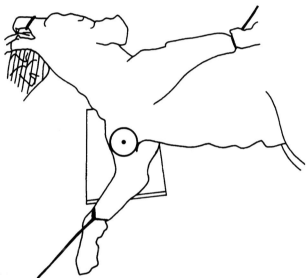

Figure 15 Line drawing of photograph representing radiographic positioning for Figure 14.

Figure 14 Mediolateral projection of humerus. Beagle dog 2.5 years old, entire male.

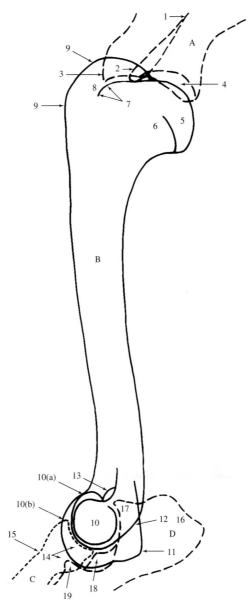

Figure 16   Mediolateral projection of humerus.

A   Scapula
  1   Spine
  2   Acromion
  3   Supraglenoid tubercle
  4   Glenoid cavity

B   Humerus
  5   Head
  6   Neck
  7   Lesser tubercle
  8   Intertubercular groove
  9   Greater tubercle
 10   Condyle. Anatomically only one condyle is present in the dog but frequently the terms lateral and medial condyle are used.
    10(a)   Capitulum (lateral aspect)

    10(b)   Trochlea (medial aspect)
 11   Medial epicondyle
 12   Lateral epicondyle
 13   Supratrochlear foramen. This foramen lies between the radial fossa and the olecranon fossa which houses the anconeal process of the ulna.

C   Radius
 14   Head
 15   Neck

D   Ulna
 16   Olecranon
 17   Anconeal process
 18   Lateral coronoid process
 19   Medial coronoid process

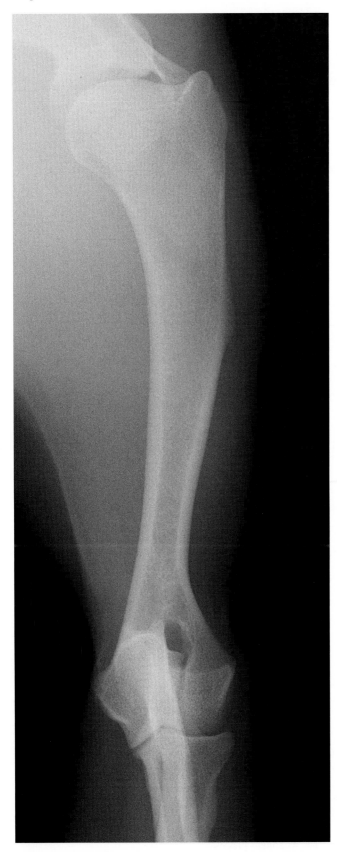

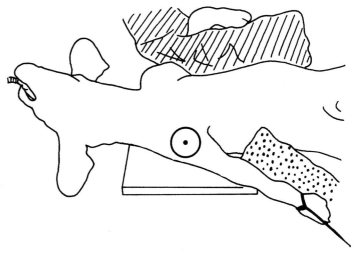

Figure 18 Line drawing of photograph representing radiographic positioning for Figure 17.

Figure 17 Craniocaudal projection of humerus. Beagle dog 2.5 years old, entire male.

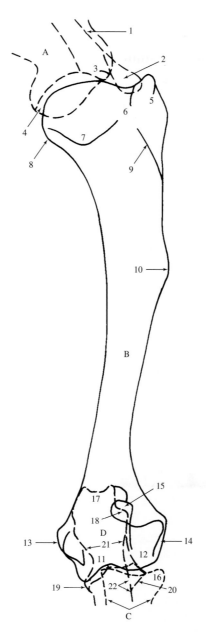

Figure 19 Craniocaudal projection of humerus.

A Scapula
  1 Spine
  2 Acromion
  3 Supraglenoid tubercle
  4 Glenoid cavity

B Humerus
  5 Greater tubercle
  6 Intertubercular groove
  7 Head
  8 Lesser tubercle
  9 Tricipital line
  10 Deltoid tuberosity
  11 Trochlea. Medial aspect of the dog's single condyle.
  12 Capitulum. Lateral aspect of the dog's single condyle.

13 Medial epicondyle
14 Lateral epicondyle
15 Supratrochlear foramen

C Radius
  16 Head

D Ulna
  17 Olecranon
  18 Anconeal process
  19 Medial coronoid process
  20 Lateral coronoid process
  21 Trochlear notch
  22 Lateral cortical margin

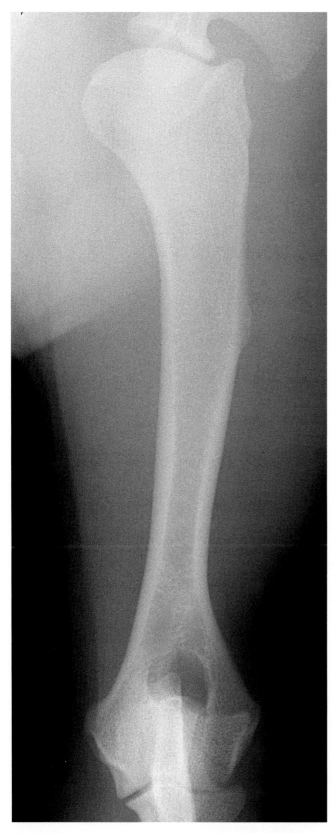

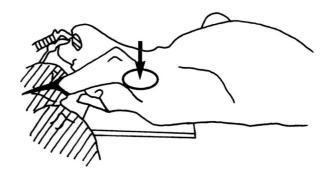

Figure 21   Line drawing of photograph representing radiographic positioning for Figure 20.

Figure 20   Caudocranial projection of humerus. Beagle dog 2.5 years old, entire male (same dog as in craniocaudal projection of humerus, Figure 17).

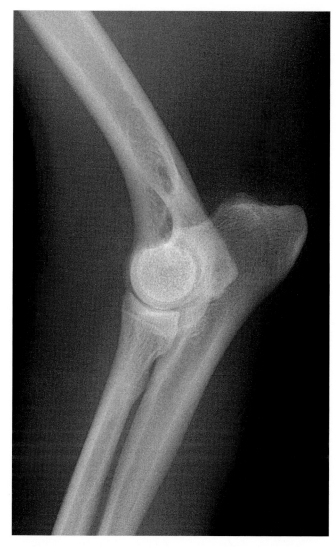

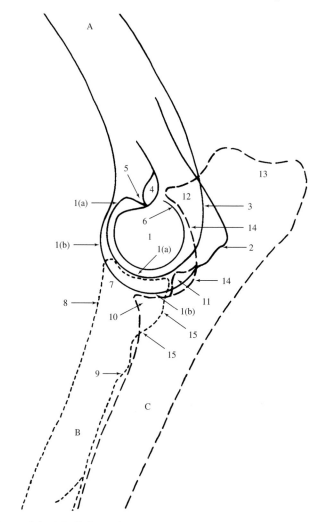

Figure 24 Mediolateral projection of extended elbow joint.

A Humerus
1 Condyle. Only one condyle is present.
1(a) Capitulum. Lateral aspect.
1(b) Trochlea. Medial aspect.
2 Medial epicondyle
3 Lateral epicondyle
4 Supratrochlear foramen
5 Radial fossa
6 Olecranon fossa

B Radius
7 Head
8 Neck
9 Eminence for attachment of lateral collateral ligament of the elbow joint

C Ulna
10 Medial coronoid process
11 Lateral coronoid process
12 Anconeal process
13 Olecranon
14 Trochlear notch
15 Proximal articulation of radius and ulna

Figure 22 Mediolateral projection of the extended elbow joint. Beagle dog 2.5 years old, entire male.

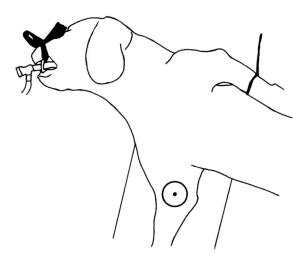

Figure 23 Line drawing of photograph representing radiographic positioning for Figure 22.

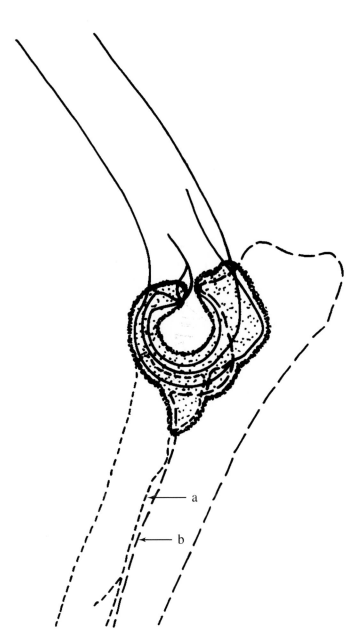

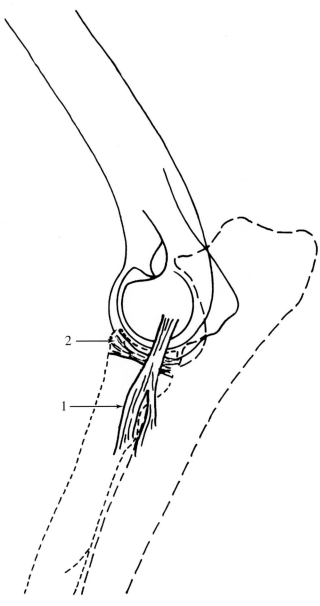

Figure 25 Schematic drawing of mediolateral projection of the extended elbow joint to demonstrate extent of joint capsule.

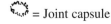 = Joint capsule

= Synovial space

Additional soft tissue shadows relating to interosseous area
a = Interosseous membrane
b = Interosseous ligament. Irregular cortical radial and ulnar margins are often seen in this region, sometimes involving extensive periosteal new bone creating cortical thickening with smoothly undulating cortical bone margins.

Figure 26 Schematic drawing of mediolateral projection of the extended elbow joint to demonstrate ligaments at joint capsule.

1 = Lateral and medial collateral ligaments. Both distally divide into two crura to attach to the radius and ulna and on a lateral projection are almost superimposed. Cranial crus attaches to the radial tuberosity medially and radial eminence laterally.

2 = Annular ligament of the radius. Lies under collateral ligaments. Attached to lateral and medial aspects of the radial notch of the ulna, it forms a 'loop' in which the head of the radius can rotate around its long axis.

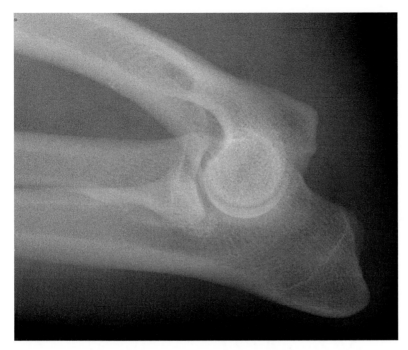

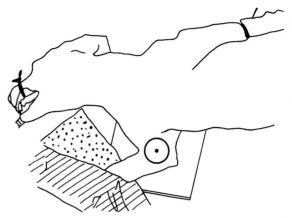

Figure 28 Line drawing of photograph representing radiographic positioning for Figure 27.

Figure 27 Mediolateral projection of the flexed elbow joint. Beagle dog 2.5 years old, entire male.

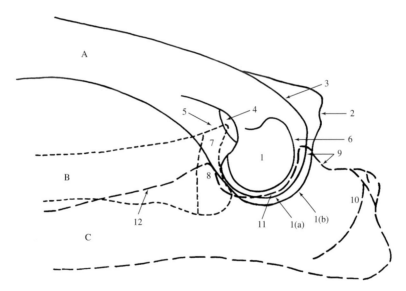

Figure 29 Mediolateral projection of the flexed elbow joint.

A Humerus
  1 Condyle. Only one condyle is present.
    1(a) Capitulum. Lateral aspect.
    1(b) Trochlea. Medial aspect.
  2 Medial epicondyle
  3 Lateral epicondyle
  4 Supratrochlear foramen
  5 Radial fossa
  6 Olecranon fossa

B Radius
  7 Head

C Ulna
  8 Medial coronoid process. Note that in this projection the lateral coronoid process cannot be seen as a distinct shadow. The extended mediolateral projection of the elbow joint does show the lateral coronoid process.
  9 Anconeal process
  10 Olecranon
  11 Trochlear notch
  12 Cranial cortical margin

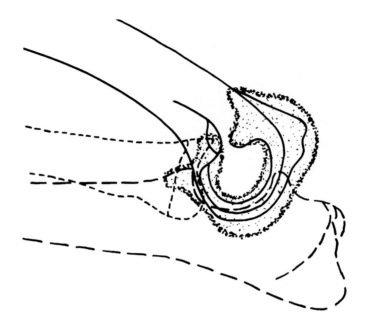

Figure 30   Schematic drawing of mediolateral projection of the flexed elbow joint to demonstrate the extent of joint capsule.

⌇ = Joint capsule

⠿ = Synovial space. There is a voluminous sac of synovial cavity in the cranial and caudal parts of this joint but these do not communicate through the supratrochlear foramen. On the lateral and medial aspects the joint capsule is taut with no sac formation.

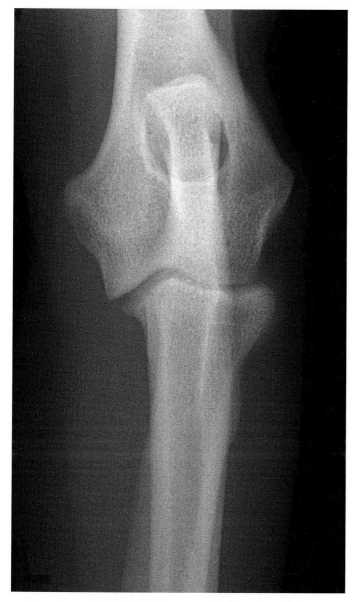

Figure 31 Craniocaudal projection of elbow joint. Beagle dog 2.5 years old, entire male.

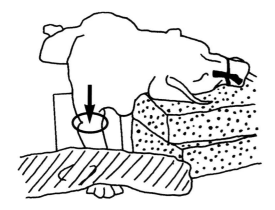

Figure 32 Line drawing of photograph representing radiographic positioning for Figure 31.

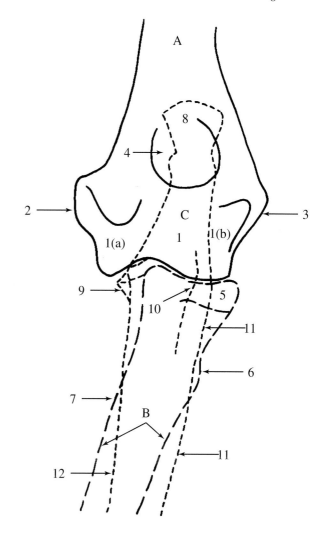

Figure 33 Craniocaudal projection of elbow joint.

A Humerus
    1 Condyle. Only one condyle is present.
      1(a) Trochlea. Medial aspect.
      1(b) Capitulum. Lateral aspect.
    2 Medial epicondyle
    3 Lateral epicondyle
    4 Supratrochlear foramen

B Radius
    5 Head
    6 Lateral eminence
    7 Position of radial tuberosity

Numbers 6 and 7 are landmarks for collateral ligaments

C Ulna
    8 Olecranon
    9 Medial coronoid process
    10 Lateral coronoid process
    11 Lateral cortical margin
    12 Medial cortical margin

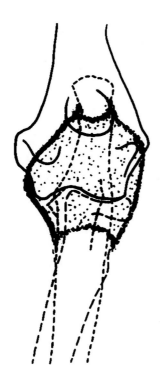

Figure 34 Schematic drawing of craniocaudal projection of elbow joint to demonstrate extent of joint capsule.

= Joint capsule

= Synovial space

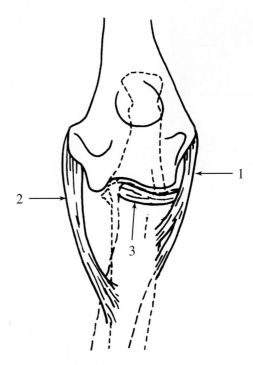

Figure 35 Schematic drawing of craniocaudal projection of elbow joint to demonstrate ligaments at joint capsule.

1 = Lateral collateral ligament

2 = Medial collateral ligament

3 = Annular ligament of the radius

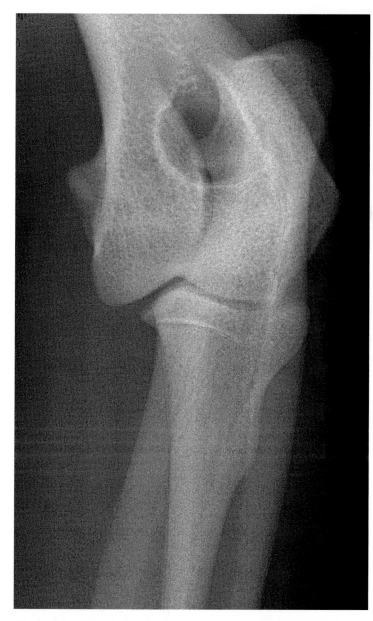

Figure 36 Craniolateral–caudomedial oblique projection of elbow joint. Beagle dog 2.5 years old, entire male.

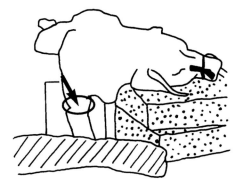

Figure 37 Line drawing of photograph representing radiographic positioning for Figure 36.

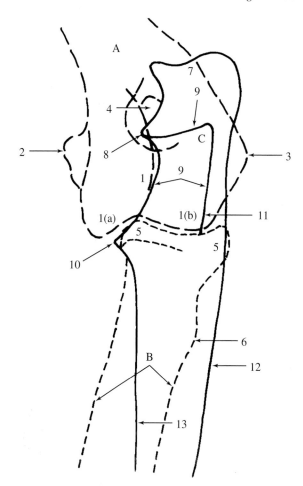

Figure 38 Craniolateral–caudomedial oblique projection of elbow joint.

A Humerus
  1 Condyle. Only one condyle is present.
    1(a) Trochlea. Medial aspect.
    1(b) Capitulum. Lateral aspect.
  2 Medial epicondyle
  3 Lateral epicondyle
  4 Supratrochlear foramen

B Radius
  5 Head
  6 Lateral eminence for attachment of lateral collateral ligament

C Ulna
  7 Olecranon
  8 Anconeal process
  9 Trochlear notch
  10 Medial coronoid process
  11 Lateral coronoid process (seen as a very opaque linear shadow on the lateral edge of the trochlear notch)
  12 Lateral cortical margin
  13 Medial cortical margin

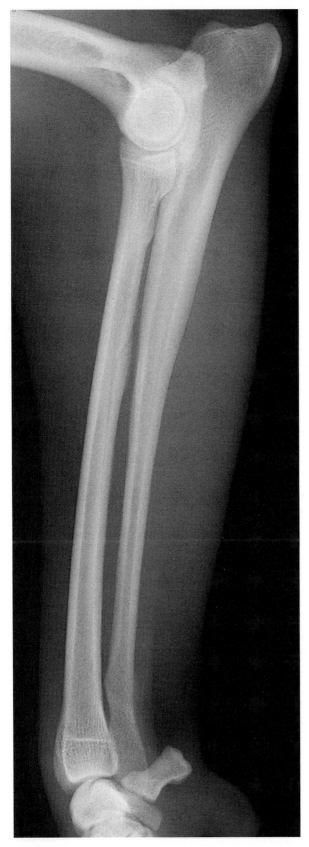

Figure 39 Mediolateral projection of radius and ulna. Beagle dog 2.5 years old, entire male.

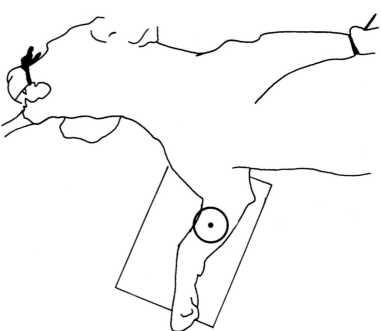

Figure 40 Line drawing of photograph representing radiographic positioning for Figure 39.

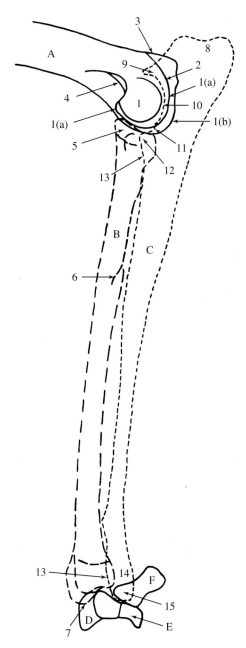

Figure 41 Mediolateral projection of radius and ulna.

A Humerus
   1 Condyle. Only one condyle is present.
      1(a) Capitulum. Lateral aspect.
      1(b) Trochlea. Medial aspect.
   2 Lateral epicondyle
   3 Medial epicondyle
   4 Supratrochlear foramen

B Radius
   5 Head
   6 Nutrient foramen
   7 Medial styloid process

   Both proximal and distal growth plate 'scars' are visible

C Ulna
   8 Olecranon
   9 Anconeal process
  10 Trochlear notch
  11 Lateral coronoid process
  12 Medial coronoid process
  13 Cranial cortical margin
  14 Head
  15 Lateral styloid process

D Radial carpal bone

E Ulnar carpal bone

F Accessory carpal bone

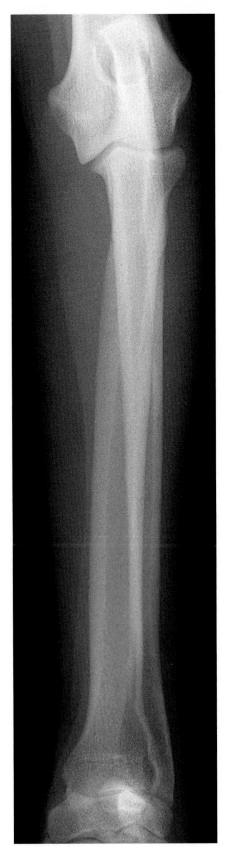

Figure 42 Craniocaudal projection of radius and ulna. Beagle dog 2.5 years old, entire male.

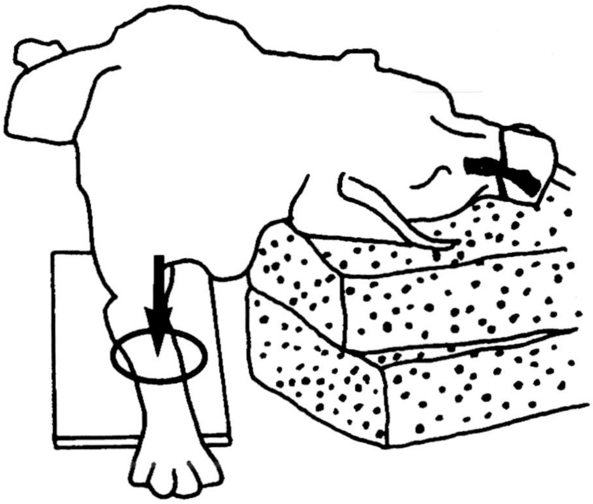

Figure 43 Line drawing of photograph representing radiographic positioning for Figure 42.

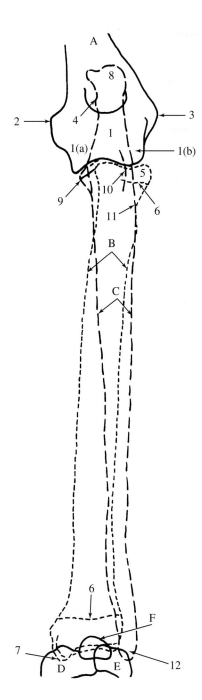

Figure 44   Craniocaudal projection of radius and ulna.

A Humerus
    1 Condyle. Only one condyle is present.
       1(a) Trochlea. Medial aspect.
       1(b) Capitulum. Lateral aspect.
    2 Medial epicondyle
    3 Lateral epicondyle
    4 Supratrochlear foramen

B Radius
    5 Head
    6 Growth plate scars
    7 Medial styloid process

C Ulna
    8 Olecranon
    9 Medial coronoid process
   10 Lateral coronoid process
   11 Lateral cortical margin
   12 Lateral styloid process

D Radial carpal bone

E Ulnar carpal bone

F Accessory carpal bone

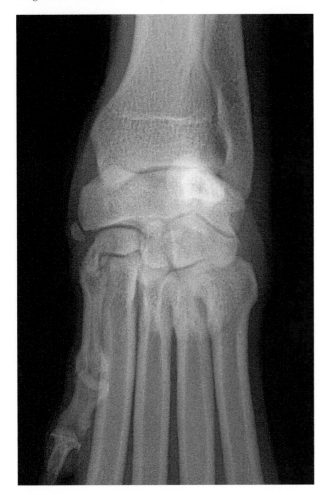

Figure 45 Dorsopalmar projection of carpus. Beagle dog 2.5 years old, entire male.

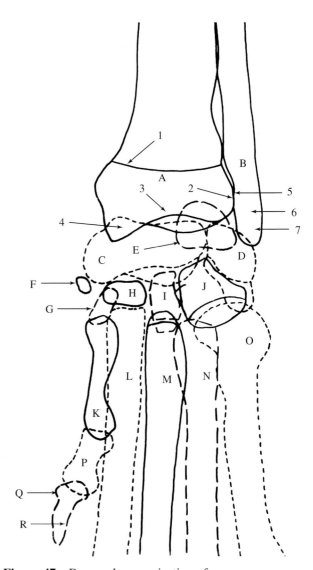

Figure 47 Dorsopalmar projection of carpus.

A Radius
  1 Growth plate scar
  2 Ulnar notch
  3 Carpal articular surface
  4 Medial styloid process

B Ulna
  5 Distal articular facet for the radius
  6 Head
  7 Lateral styloid process

C Radial carpal bone

D Ulnar carpal bone

E Accessory carpal bone

F Sesamoid bone in the tendon of m.abductor pollicis longus

G Carpal bone 1

H Carpal bone 2

I Carpal bone 3

J Carpal bone 4

K Metacarpal bone 1

L Metacarpal bone 2

M Metacarpal bone 3

N Metacarpal bone 4

O Metacarpal bone 5

P Proximal phalanx

Q Distal phalanx

R Ungual process

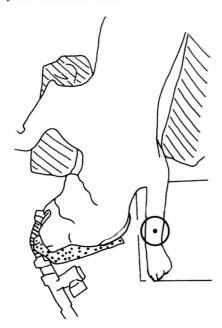

Figure 46 Line drawing of photograph representing radiographic positioning for Figure 45.

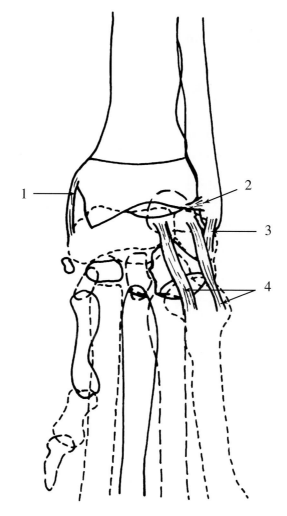

Figure 48 Schematic drawing of dorsopalmar projection of carpus to demonstrate some clinically important ligaments of the carpus.

1 = Short radial collateral ligament. On medial surface.

2 = Radioulnar ligament. On dorsal surface.

3 = Short ulnar collateral ligament. On lateral surface.

4 = Accessoro-metacarpal ligaments. On palmar surface.

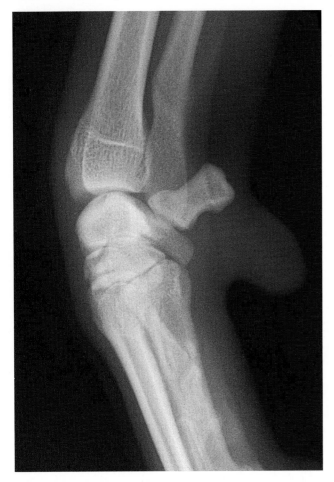

Figure 49 Mediolateral projection of carpus. Beagle dog 2.5 years old, entire male.

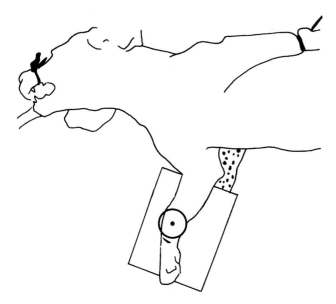

Figure 50 Line drawing of photograph representing radiographic positioning for Figure 49.

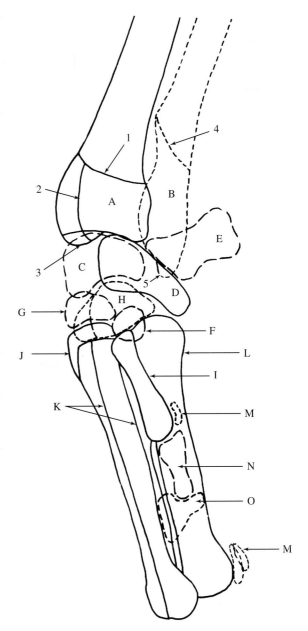

Figure 51 Mediolateral projection of carpus.

A Radius
  1 Growth plate scar
  2 Groove for the m.extensor carpi radialis
  3 Medial styloid process

B Ulna
  4 Growth plate scar
  5 Lateral styloid process

C Radial carpal bone

D Ulnar carpal bone

E Accessory carpal bone

F Carpal bone 1

G Carpal bone 2

H Carpal bones 3 and 4 (superimposed shadows)

I Metacarpal bone 1

J Metacarpal bone 2

K Metacarpal bones 3 and 4 (superimposed shadows)

L Metacarpal bone 5

M Proximal sesamoid bones

N Proximal phalanx of digit 1

O Distal phalanx of digit 1

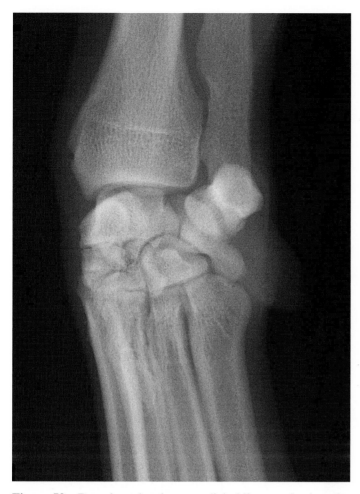

Figure 52 Dorsolateral–palmaromedial oblique projection of carpus. Samoyed dog 6 years old, entire female.

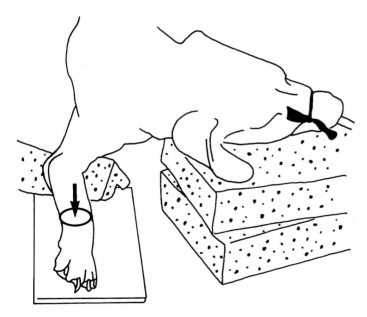

Figure 53 Line drawing of photograph representing radiographic positioning for Figure 52.

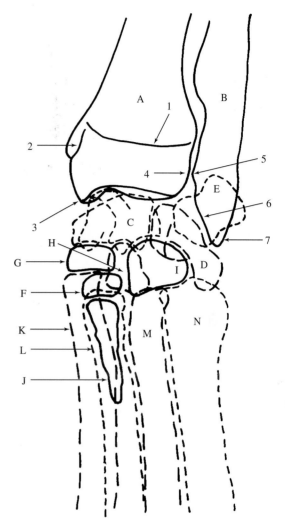

Figure 54 Dorsolateral–palmaromedial oblique projection of carpus.

A Radius
  1 Growth plate scar
  2 Groove for the tendon of m.abductor pollicis longus
  3 Medial styloid process
  4 Ulnar notch

B Ulna
  5 Distal radial articular surface
  6 Articular surface for ulnar carpal bone
  7 Lateral styloid process

C Radial carpal bone

D Ulnar carpal bone

E Accessory carpal bone

F Carpal bone 1

G Carpal bone 2

H Carpal bone 3

I Carpal bone 4

J Metacarpal bone 1

K Metacarpal bone 2

L Metacarpal bone 3

M Metacarpal bone 4

N Metacarpal bone 5

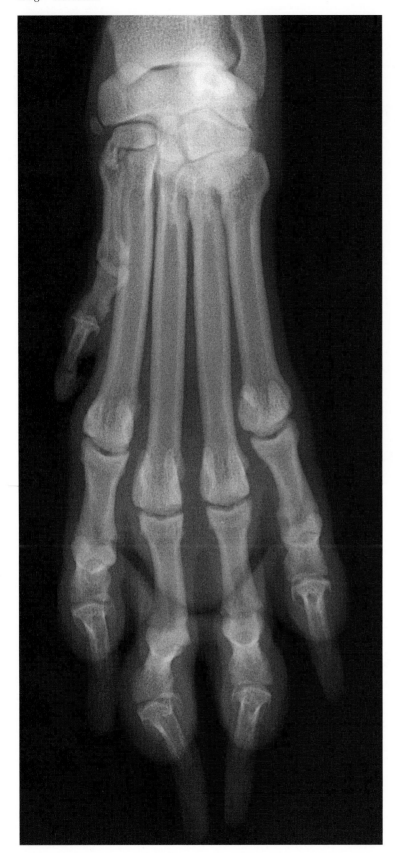

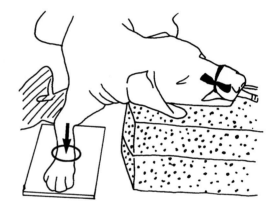

Figure 56 Line drawing of photograph representing radiographic positioning for Figure 55.

Figure 55 Dorsopalmar projection of manus. Beagle dog 2.5 years old, entire male.

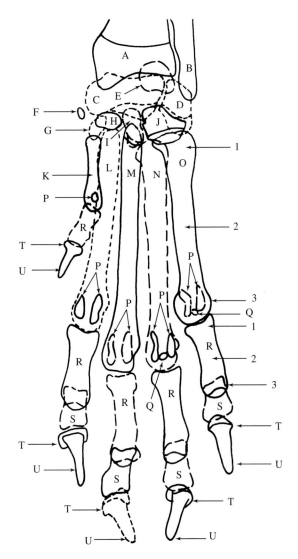

Figure 57 Dorsopalmar projection of manus.

A Radius

B Ulna

C Radial carpal bone

D Ulnar carpal bone

E Accessory carpal bone

F Sesamoid bone in the tendon of the m.abductor pollicis longus

G Carpal bone 1

H Carpal bone 2

I Carpal bone 3

J Carpal bone 4

K Metacarpal bone 1

L Metacarpal bone 2

M Metacarpal bone 3

N Metacarpal bone 4

O Metacarpal bone 5

P Proximal sesamoid bones. These are present on palmar aspect of metacarpophalangeal joints in tendons of mm.interossei (2 to 5) and m.flexor pollicis brevis. Only one at digit 1 and two at digits 2 to 5.

Q Dorsal sesamoid bones. These are present on dorsal aspect of distal metacarpal bones 2 to 5 and lie within the metacarpophalangeal joint capsules.

R Proximal phalanges

S Middle phalanges

T Distal phalanges

U Ungual processes

Metacarpal bones, proximal and middle phalanges divided into

   1 Base

   2 Body

   3 Head

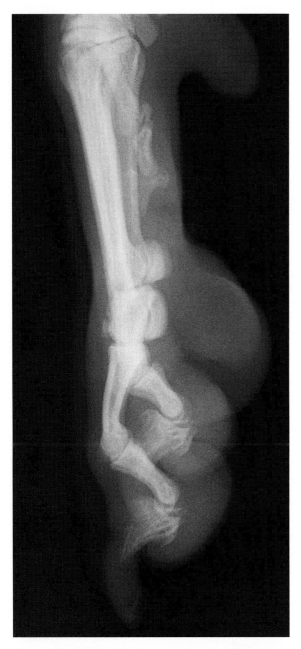

Figure 58 Mediolateral projection of manus. Beagle dog 2.5 years old, entire male.

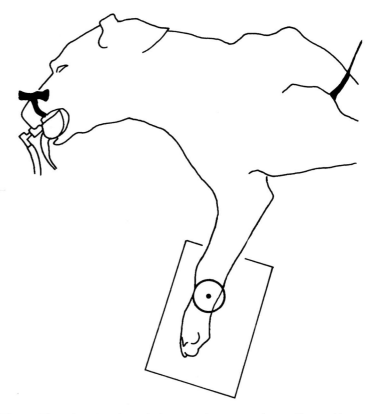

Figure 59 Line drawing of photograph representing radiographic positioning for Figure 58.

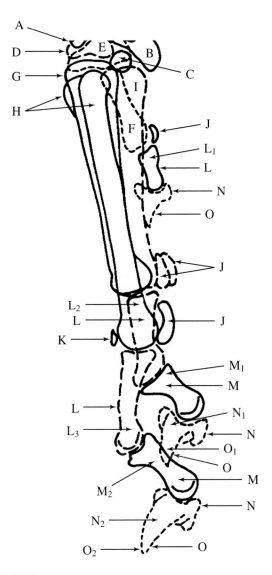

Figure 60 Mediolateral projection of manus.

A Radial carpal bone

B Ulnar carpal bone

C Carpal bone 1

D Carpal bone 2

E Carpal bones 2 and 4 (superimposed shadows)

F Metacarpal bone 1

G Metacarpal bone 2

H Metacarpal bones 3 and 4 (superimposed shadows. The dorsal protuberance seen is metacarpal bone 3.)

I Metacarpal bone 5

J Proximal sesamoid bones. Two are present in the tendons of mm.interossei at palmar aspect of metacarpophalangeal joints 2 to 5. Only one is present in metacarpophalangeal joint 1.

K Dorsal sesamoid bone. These are present in joint capsules at dorsal aspect of distal metacarpal bones 2 to 5.

L Proximal phalanges
L_1 Digit 1
L_2 Digits 2 and 5 (superimposed shadows)
L_3 Digits 3 and 4 (superimposed shadows)

M Middle phalanges
M_1 Digits 2 and 5 (superimposed shadows)
M_2 Digits 3 and 4 (superimposed shadows)

N Distal phalanges
N_1 Digits 2 and 5 (superimposed shadows)
N_2 Digits 3 and 4 (superimposed shadows)

O Ungual processes
O_1 Digits 2 and 5 (superimposed shadows)
O_2 Digits 3 and 4 (superimposed shadows)

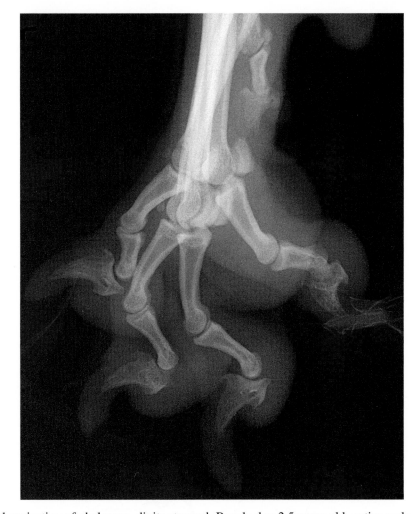

Figure 61   Mediolateral projection of phalanges, digits stressed. Beagle dog 2.5 years old, entire male.

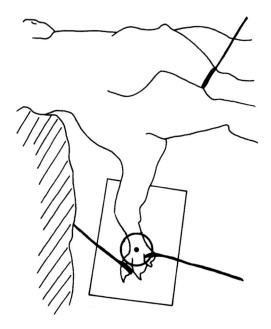

Figure 62   Line drawing of photograph representing radiographic positioning for Figure 61.

An Atlas of Interpretative Radiographic Anatomy of the Dog and Cat

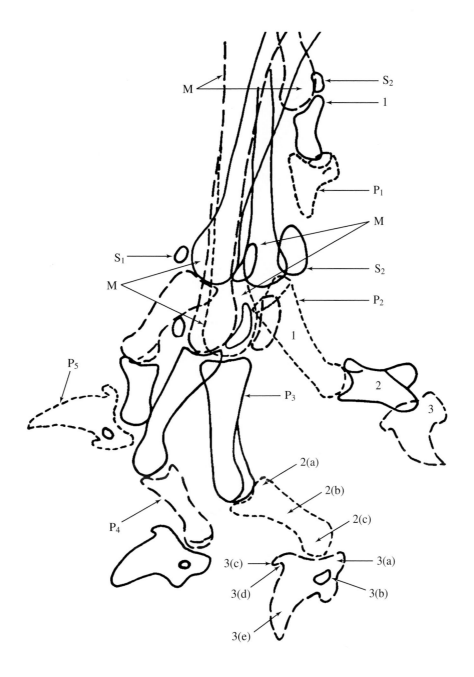

Figure 63   Mediolateral projection of phalanges. digits stressed.

M   Metacarpal bones
   P_1 Digit 1
   P_2 Digit 2
   P_3 Digit 3
   P_4 Digit 4
   P_5 Digit 5

   Bones of digits
  1   Proximal phalanx
  2   Middle phalanx
    2(a)   Base
    2(b)   Body
    2(c)   Head

3   Distal phalanx
   3(a)   Flexor tubercle
   3(b)   Solar foramen
   3(c)   Ungual crest
   3(d)   Ungual sulcus
   3(e)   Ungual process

S_1 Dorsal sesamoid bone. These are present in dorsal aspect of metacarpophalangeal joint capsules 2 to 5.

S_2 Proximal sesamoid bone. Two are present in tendons of mm.interossei at palmar aspect of metacarpophalangeal joints 2 to 5. Metacarpophalangeal joint 1 has one sesamoid bone in the tendon of m.flexor pollicis brevis.

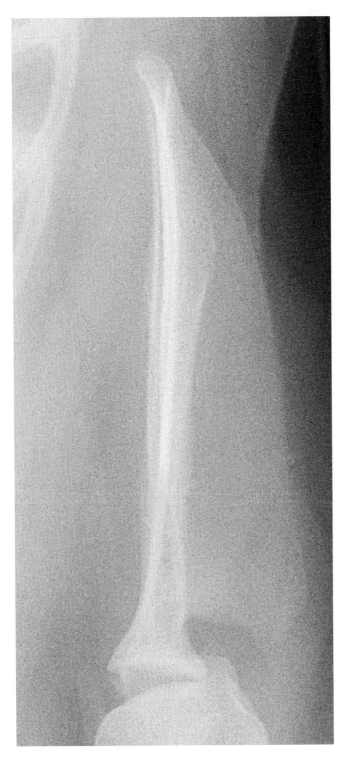

Figure 64 Caudocranial projection of scapula.
Chondrodystrophic breed of dog. Miniature Dachshund
dog 6 years old, neutered female.

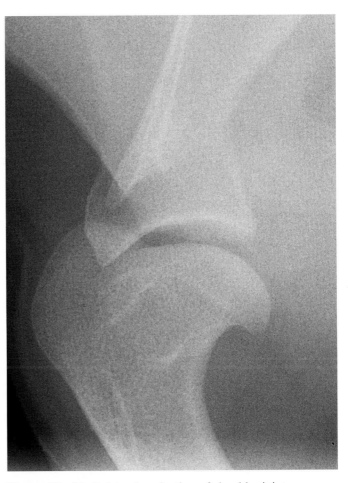

Figure 65 Mediolateral projection of shoulder joint.
Chondrodystrophic breed of dog. Miniature Dachshund dog
6 years old, neutered female.

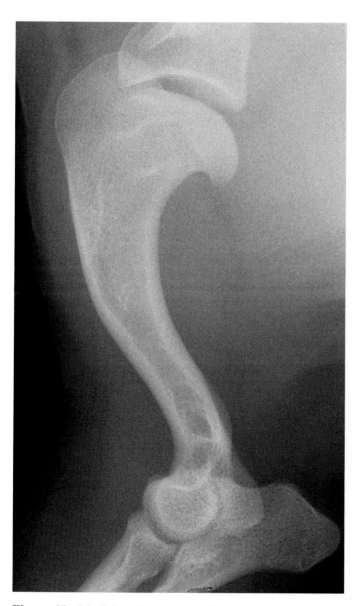

Figure 66   Mediolateral projection of humerus.
Chondrodystrophic breed of dog. Miniature Dachshund dog
6 years old, neutered female.

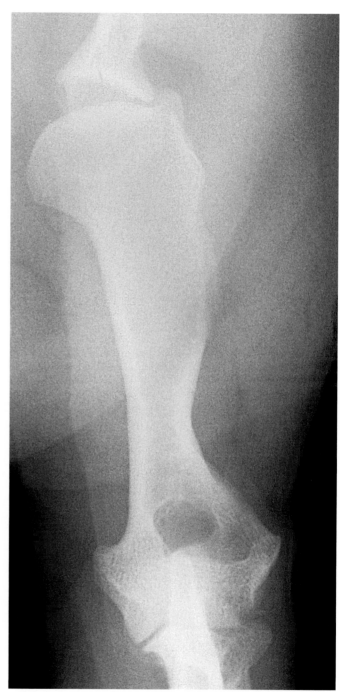

Figure 67   Caudocranial projection of humerus.
Chondrodystrophic breed of dog. Miniature Dachshund dog
6 years old, neutered female.

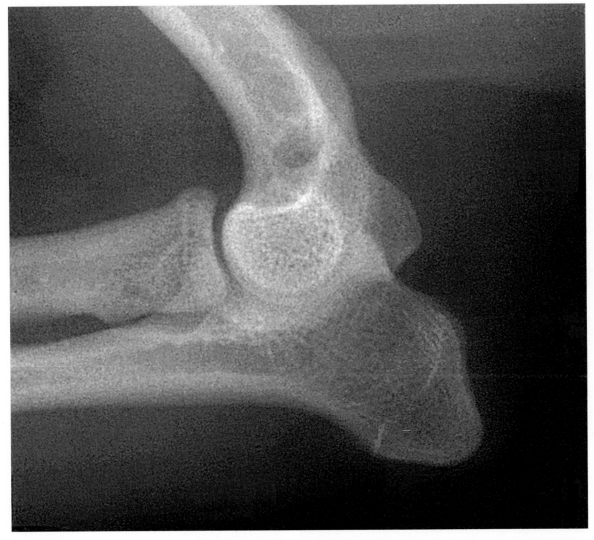

Figure 68 Flexed mediolateral projection of elbow joint. Chondrodystrophic breed of dog. Miniature Dachshund dog 6 years old, neutered female.

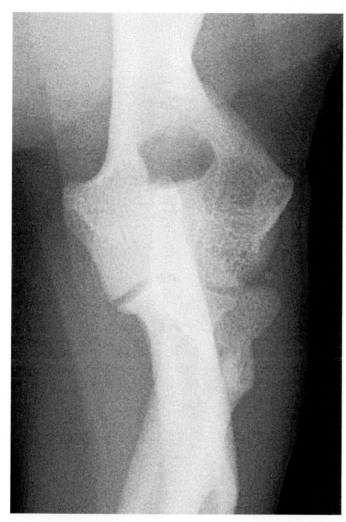

Caudocranial projection of elbow joint. Chondrodystrophic breed of dog. Miniature Dachshund dog 6 years old, neutered female.

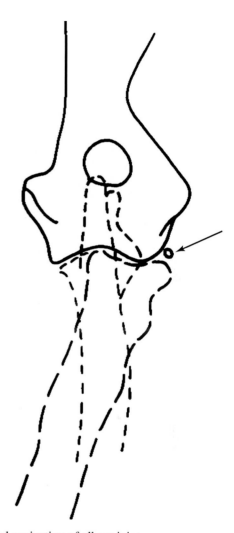

Caudocranial projection of elbow joint.

Figure 69   Caudocranial projection of elbow joint. The drawing has been included to indicate the presence of a lateral sesamoid bone (arrow) in the elbow joint. The sesamoid bone is more frequently seen on the lateral aspect and is thought to be within the tendon of the m.supinator. Occasionally a medial sesamoid bone is observed in the collateral ligament and joint capsule.

Although both the lateral and medial sesamoid bones have been cited as a cause of lameness by some authors, by most authorities they are not clinically significant. Indeed sesamoid cartilage is often present but non-mineralised, and hence cannot be seen in a radiograph. In this particular dog there was no forelimb lameness.

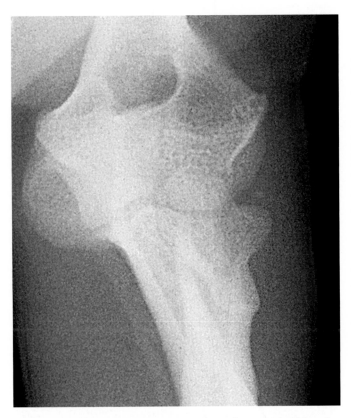

Figure 70   Caudolateral-craniomedial oblique projection of elbow joint. Chondrodystrophic breed of dog. Miniature Dachshund dog 6 years old, neutered female.

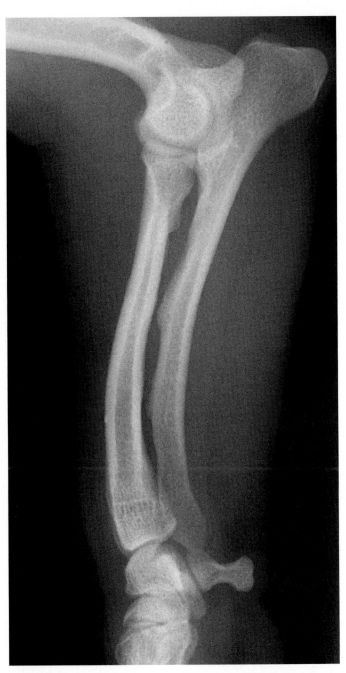

Figure 71   Mediolateral projection of radius and ulna. Chondrodystrophic breed of dog. Miniature Dachshund dog 6 years old, neutered female.

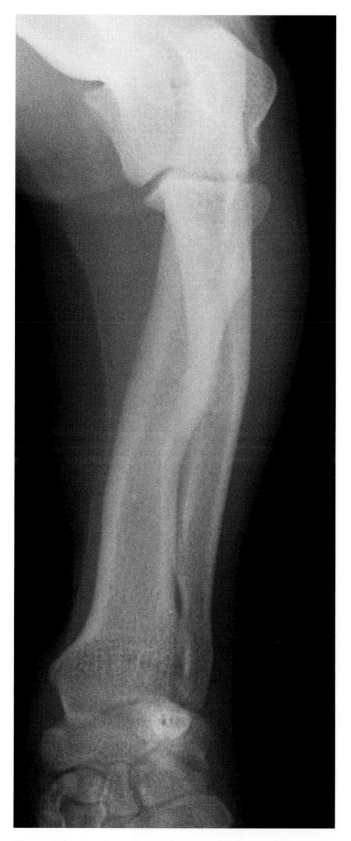

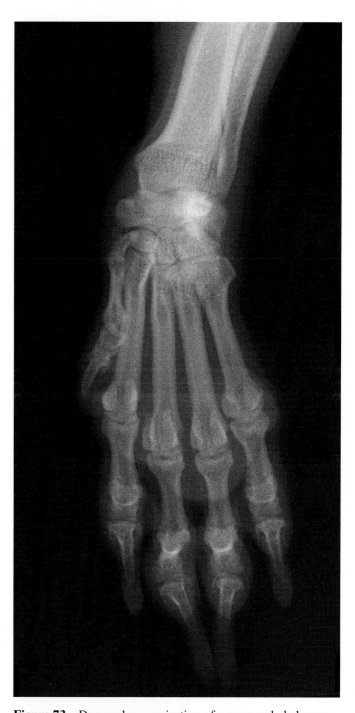

Figure 73 Dorsopalmar projection of carpus and phalanges. Chondrodystrophic breed of dog. Miniature Dachshund dog 6 years old, neutered female.

Figure 72 Craniocaudal projection of radius and ulna. Chondrodystrophic breed of dog. Miniature Dachshund dog 6 years old, neutered female.

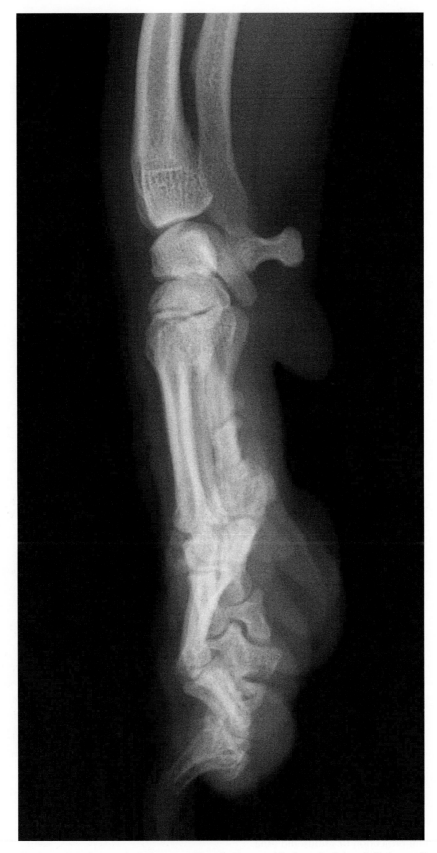

Figure 74 Mediolateral projection of carpus and phalanges. Chondrodystrophic breed of dog. Miniature Dachshund dog 6 years old, neutered female.

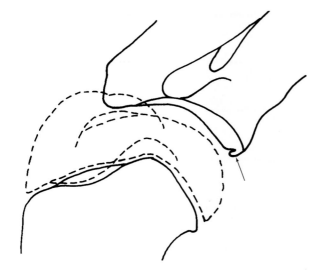

Figure 75 Mediolateral projection of shoulder joint. Glenoid cavity variant. (Corresponds to radiograph not included in book.) Great Dane German Shepherd crossbred dog 5 months old, entire male.

The drawing demonstrates a separate ossification centre for the glenoid cavity (arrow). As the dog matures the centre often forms a separate bony shadow parallel to the glenoid cavity. This must not be mistaken for an osteochondrosis fragment.

The variant seen here is most commonly found in the giant breed of dog, in particular the Irish Wolfhound.

A similar, separate ossification centre may occasionally be seen at the acetabulum. Here the variant forms a separate bony shadow parallel to the cranial effective acetabular rim.

Care must be taken not to confuse this shadow with a fracture fragment or ossicle. The smooth cortical outline of the bony variant together with a normal acetabular shadow enables differentiation from abnormality.

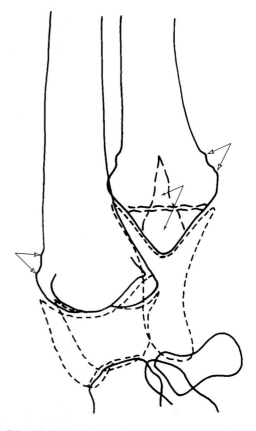

Figure 76 Mediolateral projection of distal radius and ulna. Retained cartilaginous core. (Corresponds to radiograph not included in book.) Great Dane German Shepherd crossbred dog 5 months old, entire male.

The drawing shows a retained cartilaginous core (closed arrows) in the distal ulna metaphyseal region. The core is typically seen at this 5-month age, especially in the Great Dane, although other large and giant breeds can be affected.

Although at one time it was thought to retard growth its presence alone is not significant and the core will disappear as the dog matures. Note the normal growth plates in this dog with the core.

Also present on the drawing is the typical irregular cortical outline of the metaphyseal regions (open arrows). The latter is invariably seen in large and giant breeds of immature dogs. This, together with a relatively opaque appearance of the metaphyseal regions, seen in all immature dogs, must not be mistaken for a bony metabolic abnormality such as rickets. Examination of the bony cortical opacity, and thickness, is required to establish normality in the immature animal.

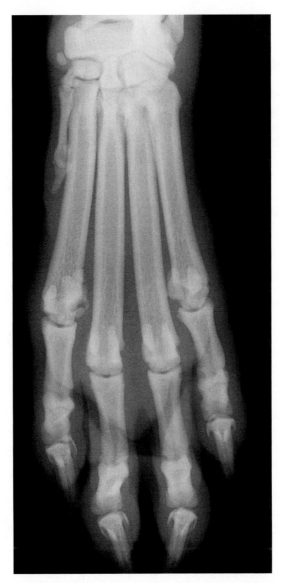

Figure 77 Dorsopalmar projection of manus. Multipartite sesamoid bones. Rottweiler dog 2 years old, entire male.

The radiograph shows the characteristic multiple bony shadows associated with multipartite sesamoid bones. The proximal sesamoid bones of the 2nd. and 5th. digits are affected in this dog, numbers 2 and 7, these also being the most commonly affected digits.

Multipartite sesamoid bones in the digits of immature, and young, large breeds of dogs, in particular the Rottweiler, have been reported to be involved with lameness. Such a lameness has been called sesamoid disease but the exact role of multipartite sesamoid bones remains unclear. In a number of these cases attributed to abnormal sesamoid bones, recovery was spontaneous and in others concurrent skeletal abnormalities, known to be a cause of lameness, were often present.

Reports of multipartite sesamoid bones affecting the proximal sesamoid bones of the feet conclude that the Rottweiler breed is commonly predisposed but other large breeds, such as the Labrador, can be affected.

Multipartite sesamoid bones are also found in the proximal sesamoid bones of the hind foot. The variant is often bilateral.

From the radiograph the smooth bony outline of the multipartite sesamoid bones can be seen. This together with the presence of a number of opaque bodies of irregular shape allows differentiation from fractures as seen in racing Greyhounds. Fractures of the 2nd. and 7th. proximal sesamoid bones are well recognised in racing Greyhounds.

Diagnosis of lameness due to proximal sesamoid bone abnormality, be it multipartite with degenerative changes or fractures, must be made with great caution. It is generally accepted that the multipartite condition is a normal variant of ossification and not clinically significant. In addition, even in fractures with racing Greyhounds it has been shown to be unassociated with lameness.

Multipartite sesamoid bones can also be seen in the stifle joint. The medial fabella of m.gastrocnemius, fabella of m.popliteus and the patella have all been reported to show multiple bony shadows replacing single sesamoid bodies.

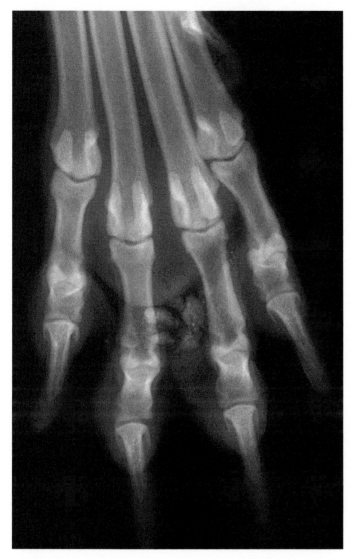

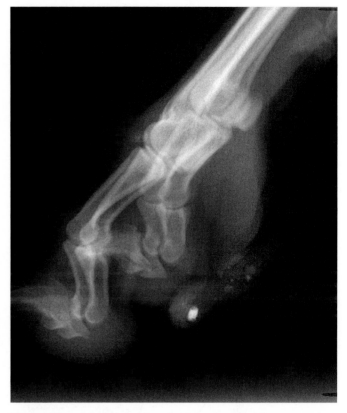

Figure 78 Dorsopalmar projection of manus. Presence of foreign material on the palmar surface. Collie crossbred dog 10 years old, neutered male (same dog as in Figure 78a).

The irregular, well-defined radiopacities caused by dirt between the metacarpal and digital pads, plus between individual digital pads, in this foot show how important patient preparation is.

Although the lumps of dirt in this case are large and unlikely to be over looked during radiography of the foot, traces of dirt between the pads may easily be missed on a routine inspection of the animal prior to radiography.

Wherever there are unusual shadows in the region of the pads, careful examination of the skin's surface must be undertaken. This also applies to any contamination of the hair by solid or liquid material.

Figure 78a Mediolateral projection of manus. Presence of foreign material on the palmar surface. Collie crossbred dog 10 years old, neutered male (same dog as in Figure 78).

The corresponding mediolateral projection to Figure 78 has been included to show that the obvious, extremely radiopaque metallic fragment within the dirt on the palmar surface of the foot was not clearly seen in the dorsopalmar projection.

Such a finding demonstrates the value of two projections of the same region, even though one may appear to suffice for diagnosis.

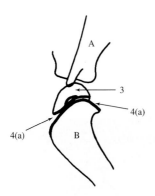

Figure 79

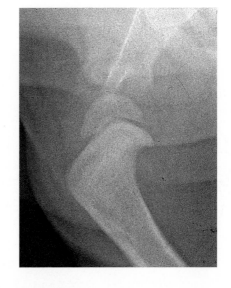

Figure 79 Age 4 weeks.

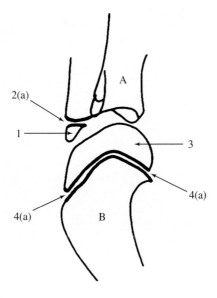

Figure 80

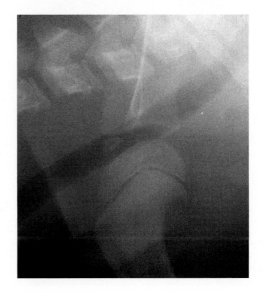

Figure 80 Age 8 weeks.

Figures 79, 80, 81, 82, 83, 84, 85, 86 Mediolateral projection of shoulder joint. Samoyed crossbred dog-entire male, at 4, 8, 13, 17, 25, 30, 43 and 56 weeks of age.

A Scapula
   1 Epiphysis of supraglenoid tubercle
   2 Growth plate
      2(a) Open
      2(b) Closing

B Humerus
   3 Proximal epiphysis of humerus
   4 Proximal growth plate
      4(a) Open
      4(b) Closing
      4(c) Remnant
   5 Greater tubercle

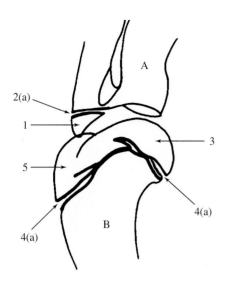

Figure 81

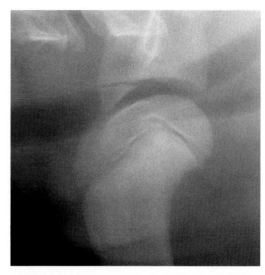

Figure 81   Age 13 weeks.

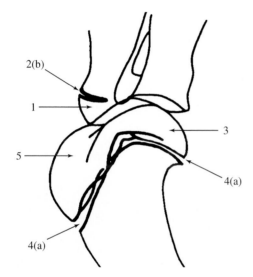

Figure 82

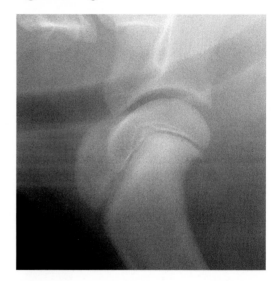

Figure 82   Age 17 weeks.

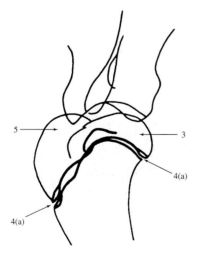

Figure 83

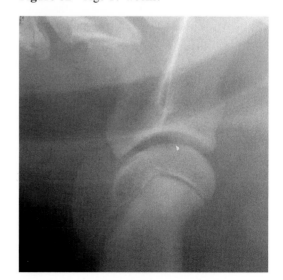

Figure 83   Age 25 weeks.

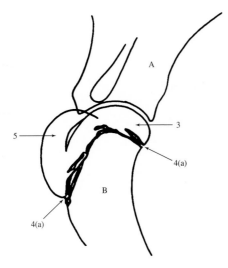

Figure 84

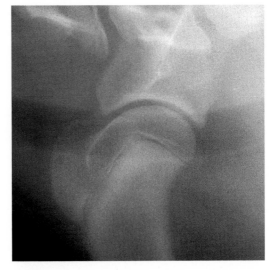

Figure 84 Age 30 weeks.

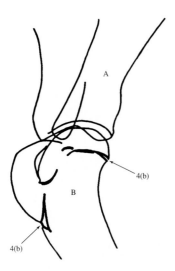

Figure 85

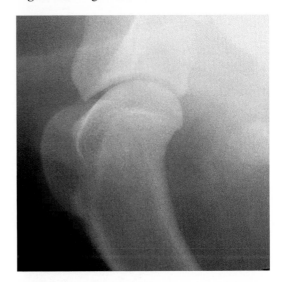

Figure 85 Age 43 weeks.

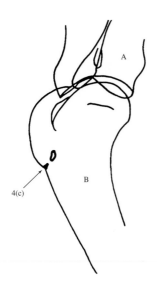

Figure 86

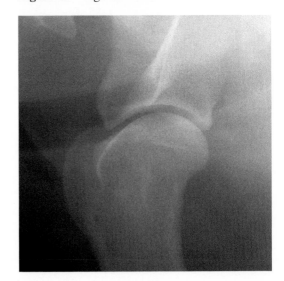

Figure 86 Age 56 weeks.

An Atlas of Interpretative Radiographic Anatomy of the Dog and Cat

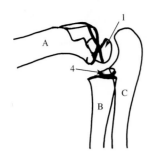

Figure 87

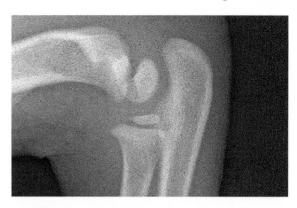

Figure 87   Age 4 weeks.

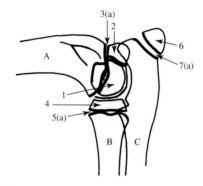

Figure 88

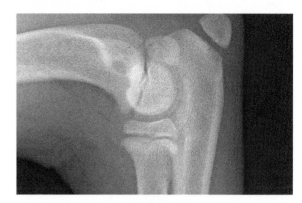

Figure 88   Age 8 weeks.

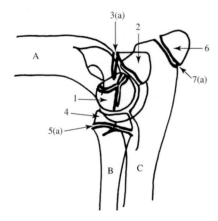

Figure 89

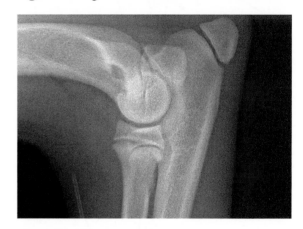

Figure 89   Age 13 weeks.

Figures 87, 88, 89, 90, 91, 92   Mediolateral projection of elbow joint. Samoyed crossbred dog, entire male, at 4, 8, 13, 17, 25 and 34 weeks of age.

A Humerus
   1   Distal epiphysis
   2   Epiphysis of medial epicondyle
   3   Distal growth plate and medial epicondyle growth
      plate
      3(a) Open
      3(b) Closing
      3(c) Remnant

B Radius
   4   Proximal epiphysis

   5   Proximal growth plate
      5(a) Open
      5(c) Remnant

C Ulna
   6   Proximal epiphysis
   7   Proximal growth plate
      7(a) Open
      7(b) Closing
      7(c) Remnant

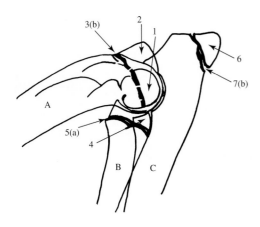

Figure 90

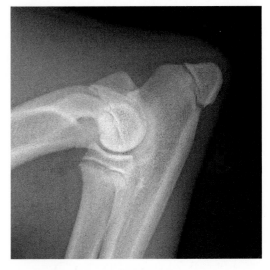

Figure 90   Age 17 weeks.

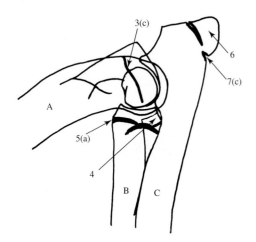

Figure 91

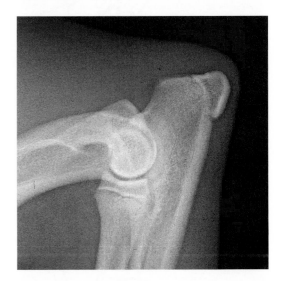

Figure 91   Age 25 weeks.

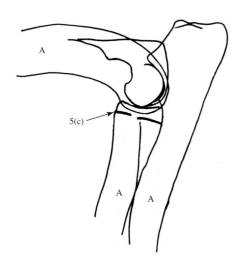

Figure 92

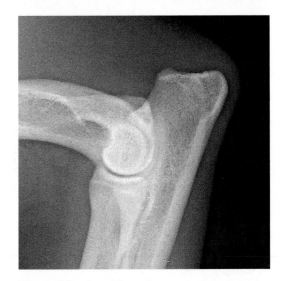

Figure 92   Age 34 weeks.

An Atlas of Interpretative Radiographic Anatomy of the Dog and Cat

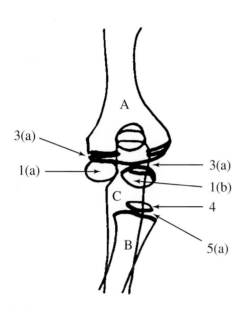

Figure 93

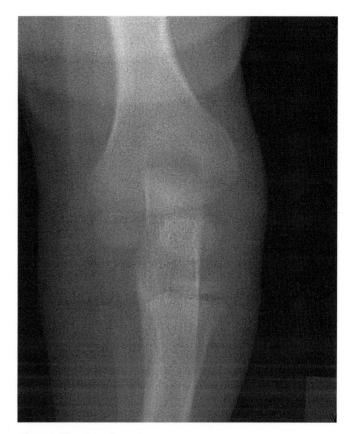

Figure 93   Age 4 weeks.

Figures 93, 94, 95, 96, 97, 98   Craniocaudal projection of elbow joint. Samoyed crossbred dog, entire male, at 4, 8, 13, 17, 25 and 34 weeks of age.

  A   Humerus
     1 Distal epiphysis
        1(a) Medial condylar centre
        1(b) Lateral condylar centre
     2 Epiphysis of medial epicondyle
     3 Distal growth plate
        3(a) Open
        3(b) Closing
        3(c) Remnant

  B   Radius
     4 Proximal epiphysis
     5 Proximal growth plate
        5(a) Open
        5(c) Remnant

  C   Ulna
     6 Proximal epiphysis

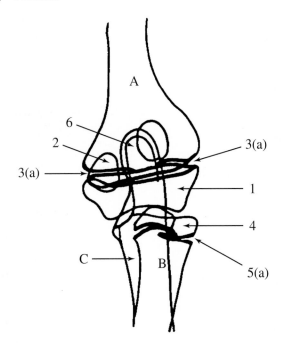

Figure 94

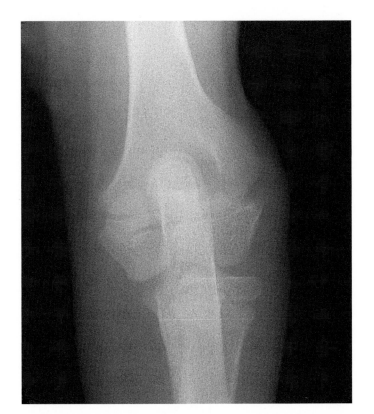

Figure 94   Age 8 weeks.

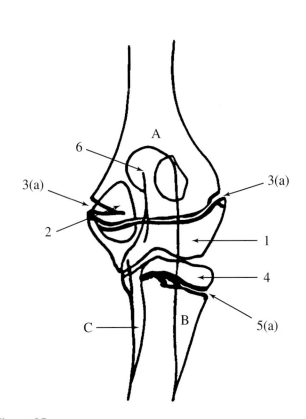

Figure 95

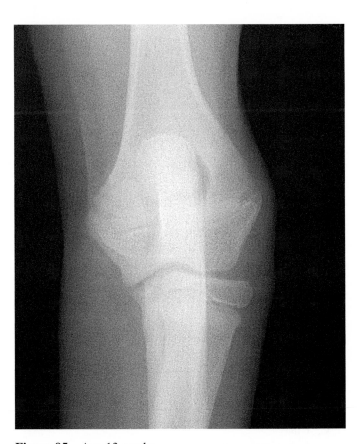

Figure 95   Age 13 weeks.

An Atlas of Interpretative Radiographic Anatomy of the Dog and Cat

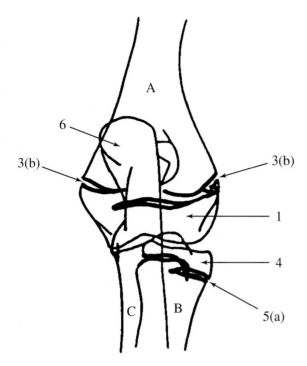

Figure 96

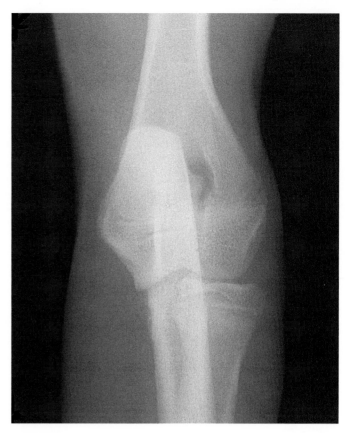

Figure 96   Age 17 weeks.

Figures 93, 94, 95, 96, 97, 98   Craniocaudal projection of elbow joint. Samoyed crossbred dog entire male at 4, 8, 13, 17, 25, and 34 weeks of age.

A   Humerus
   1 Distal epiphysis
      1(a) Medial condylar centre
      1(b) Lateral condylar centre
   2 Epiphysis of medial epicondyle
   3 Distal growth plate
      3(a) Open
      3(b) Closing
      3(c) Remnant

B   Radius
   4 Proximal epiphysis
   5 Proximal growth plate
      5(a) Open
      5(c) Remnant

C   Ulna
   6 Proximal epiphysis

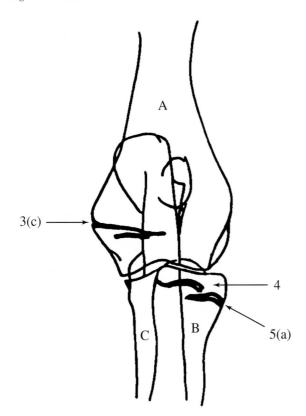

Figure 97

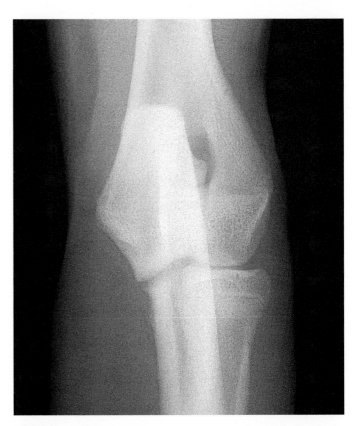

Figure 97 Age 25 weeks.

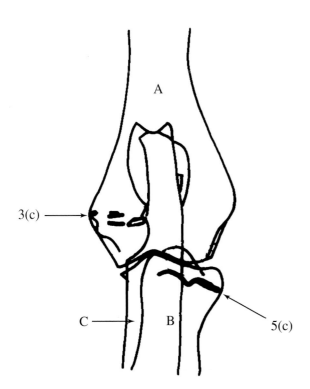

Figure 98

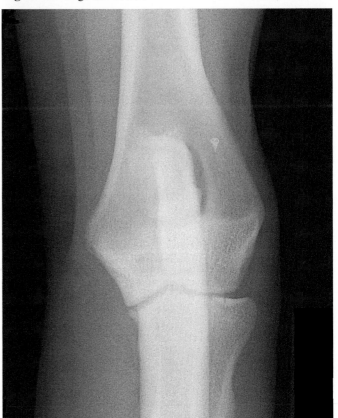

Figure 98 Age 34 weeks.

An Atlas of Interpretative Radiographic Anatomy of the Dog and Cat

Figures 99, 100, 101, 102, 103, 104   Dorsopalmar projection of carpus, metacarpal bones and phalanges. Samoyed crossbred dog, entire male, at 4, 8, 13, 17, 25 and 34 weeks of age.

A Radius
   1 Distal epiphysis
   2 Distal growth plate
     2(a) Open
     2(b) Closing

B Ulna
   3 Distal epiphysis
   4 Distal growth plate
     4(a) Open
     4(c) Remnant

C Carpus

D Metacarpal bone 5 (2, 3 and 4 similar)
   5 Epiphysis.
Note that there is only a distal epiphysis in these metacarpal bones.

   6 Growth plate
     6(a) Open
   7 Proximal sesamoid bone (lateral identified)

E Proximal phalanx of digit 5 (2, 3 and 4 similar)
   8 Epiphysis.
Note that there is only a proximal epiphysis in the proximal phalanges.

   9 Growth plate
     9(a) Open
     9(c) Remnant

F Middle phalanx of digit 5 (2, 3 and 4 similar)
   10 Epiphysis.
Note that there is only a proximal epiphysis in the middle phalanges.

   11 Growth plate
     11(a) Open

G Distal phalanx of digit 5 (2, 3 and 4 similar)

H Metacarpal bone 1
   12 Epiphysis.
Note that there is only a proximal epiphysis in this metacarpal bone.

   13 Growth plate
     13(a) Open

I Proximal phalanx of digit 1
   14 Epiphysis.
Note that there is only a proximal epiphysis.

   15 Growth plate
     15(a) Open

J Distal phalanx of digit 1

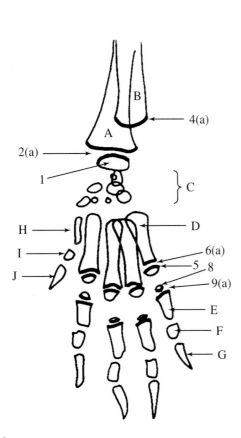

Figure 99

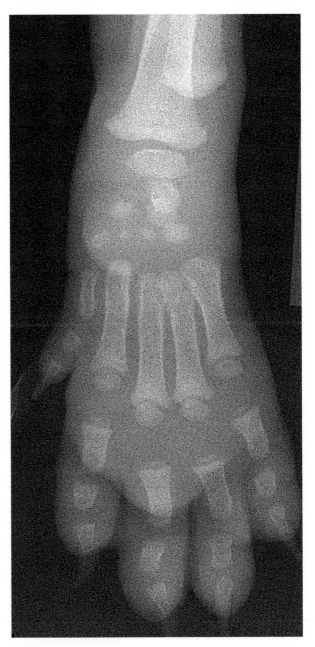

Figure 99   Age 4 weeks.

An Atlas of Interpretative Radiographic Anatomy of the Dog and Cat

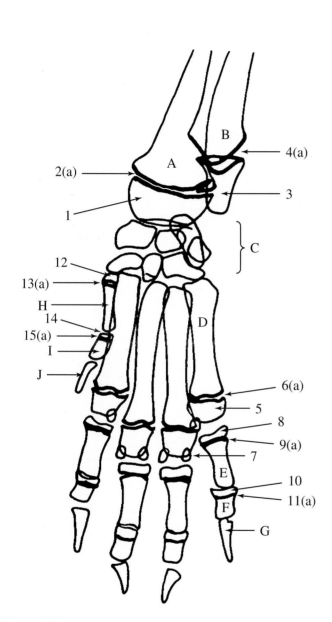

Figure 100

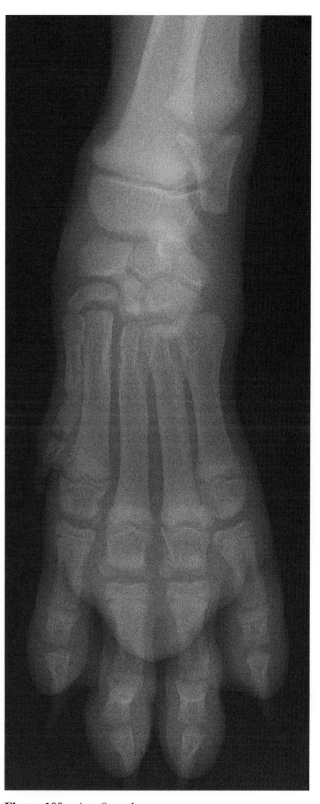

Figure 100 Age 8 weeks.

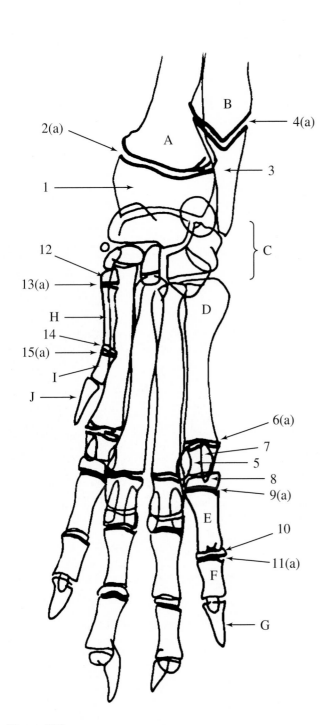

Figure 101

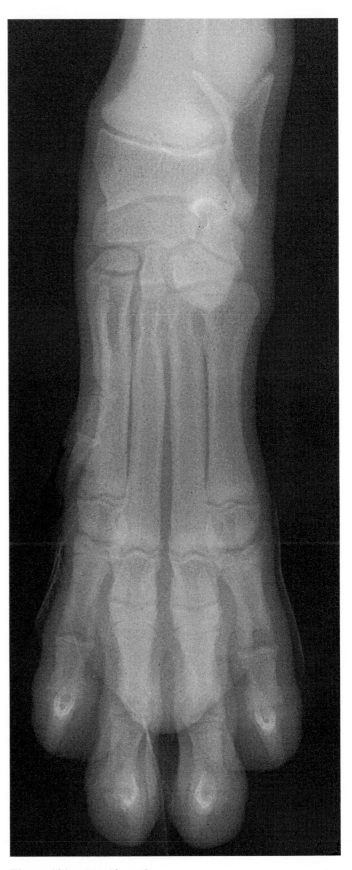

Figure 101 Age 13 weeks.

An Atlas of Interpretative Radiographic Anatomy of the Dog and Cat

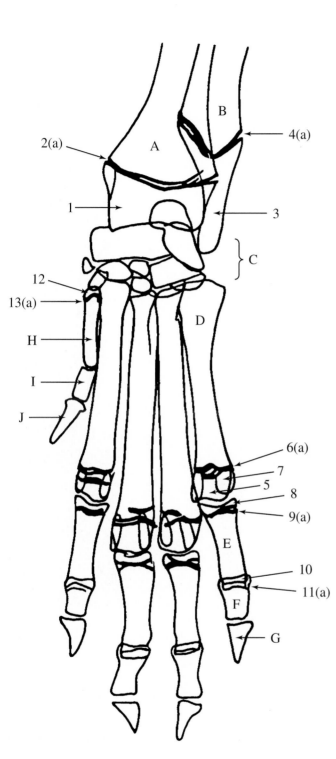

Figure 102

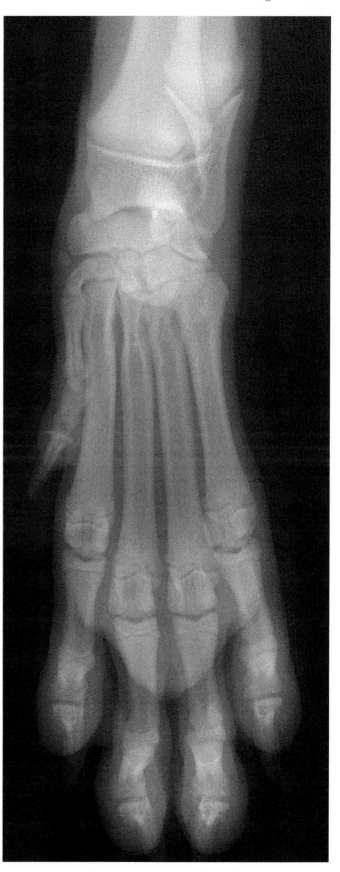

Figure 102   Age 17 weeks.

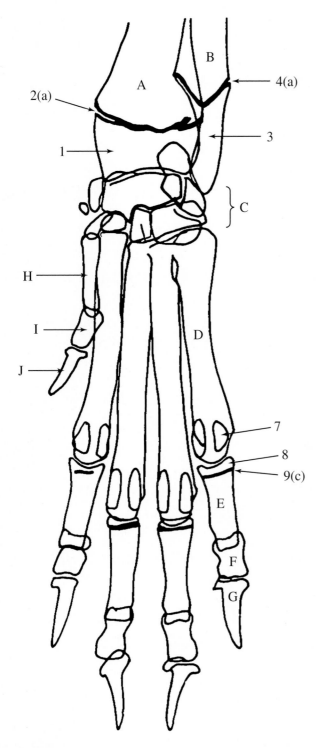

Figure 103

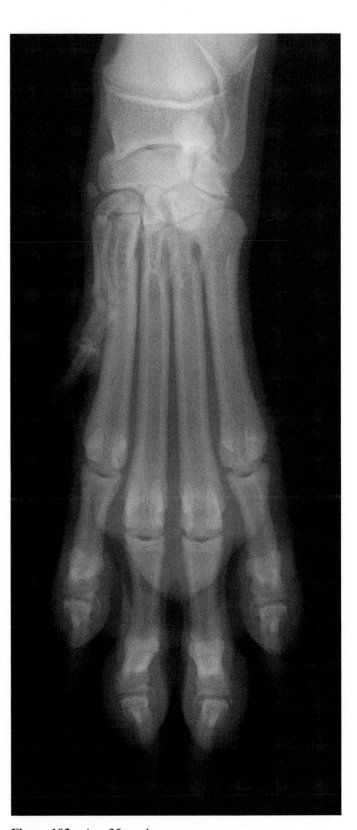

Figure 103 Age 25 weeks.

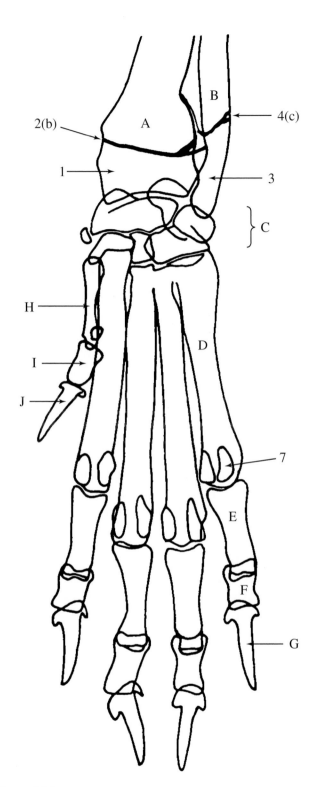

Figure 104

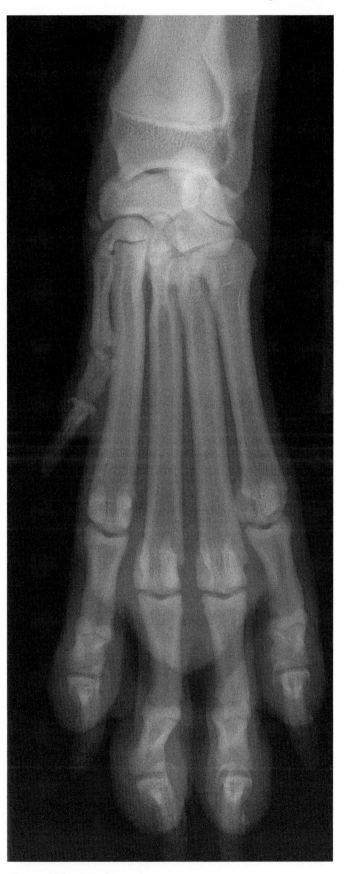

Figure 104 Age 34 weeks.

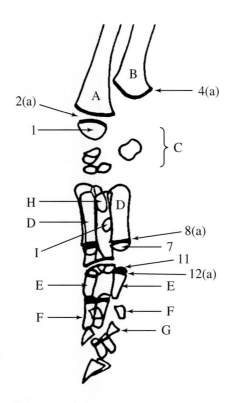

Figure 105

Figures 105, 106, 107, 108, 109, 110   Mediolateral projection of carpus, metacarpal bones and phalanges. Samoyed crossbred dog, entire male, at 4, 8, 13, 17, 25 and 34 weeks of age.

A Radius
   1 Distal epiphysis
   2 Distal growth plate
     2(a) Open
     2(b) Closing

B Ulna
   3 Distal epiphysis
   4 Distal growth plate
     4(a) Open
     4(c) Remnant

C Carpus
   5 Epiphysis of accessory carpal bone
   6 Accessory carpal bone growth plate
     6(a) Open

D Metacarpal bone 2 or 5 (3 and 4 similar but longer)
   7 Epiphysis.
Note that there is only a distal epiphysis in these metacarpal bones.

   8 Growth plate
     8(a) Open
     8(c) Remnant
   9 Proximal sesamoid bone
   10 Dorsal sesamoid bone associated with digits 3 and 4

E Proximal phalanx digits 2 or 5 (3 and 4 similar)
   11 Epiphysis.
Note that there is only a proximal epiphysis in the proximal phalanges.

12 Growth plate
   12(a) Open
   12(c) Remnant

F Middle phalanx digits 2 or 5 (3 and 4 similar)
   13 Epiphysis.
Note that there is only a proximal epiphysis in the middle phalanges.

   14 Growth plate
     14(a) Open

G Distal phalanx digit 2 or 5 (3 and 4 similar)

H Metacarpal bone 1
   15 Epiphysis.
Note that there is only a proximal epiphysis in this metacarpal bone.

   16 Growth plate
     16(a) Open
   17 Proximal sesamoid bone

I Proximal phalanx digit 1
   18 Epiphysis.
Note that there is only a proximal epiphysis.

   19 Growth plate
     19(a) Open

J Distal phalanx digit 1

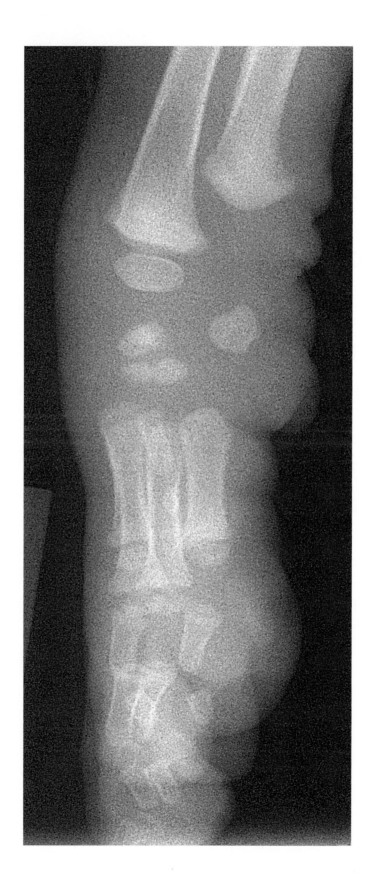

Figure 105   Age 4 weeks.

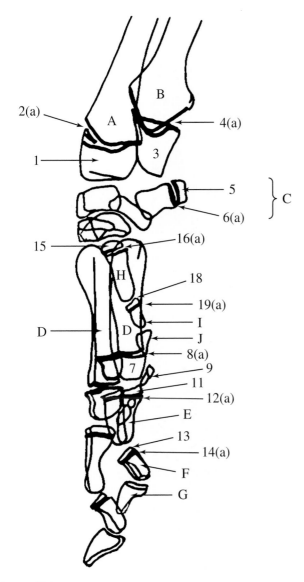

Figure 106

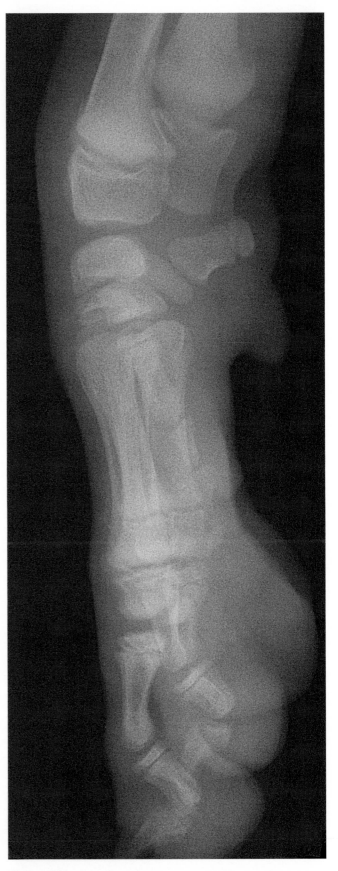

Figure 106 Age 8 weeks.

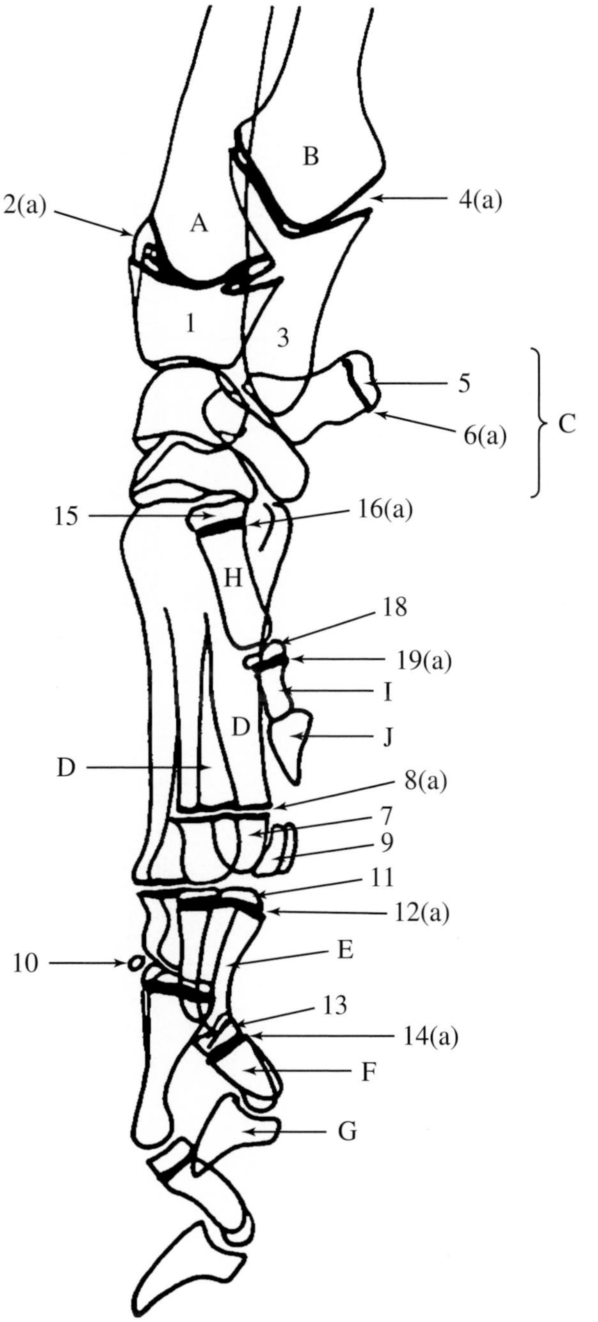

Figure 107

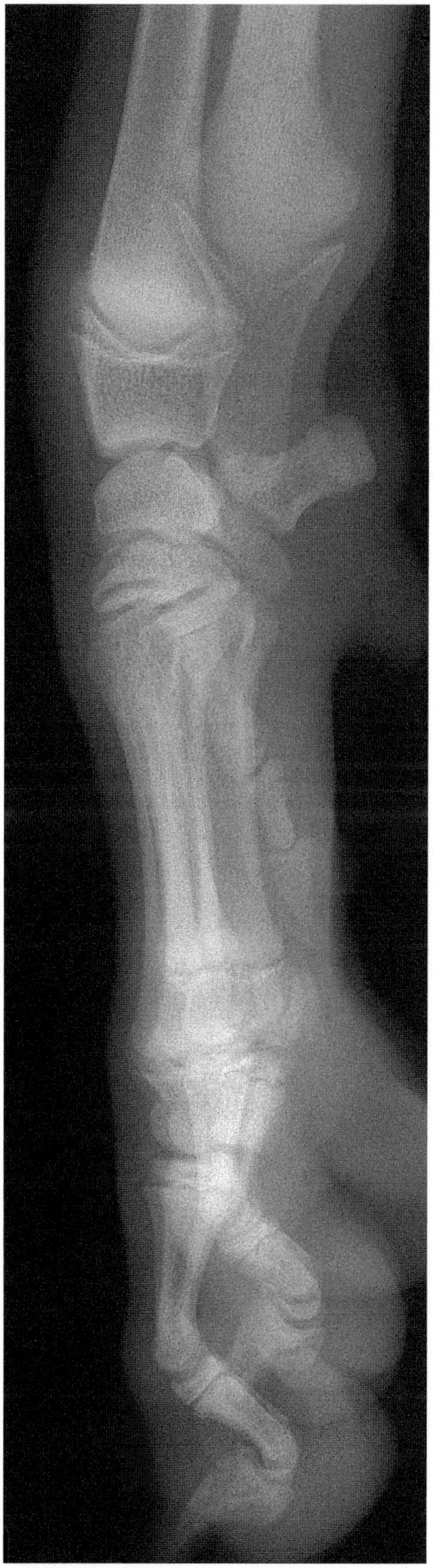

Figure 107 Age 13 weeks.

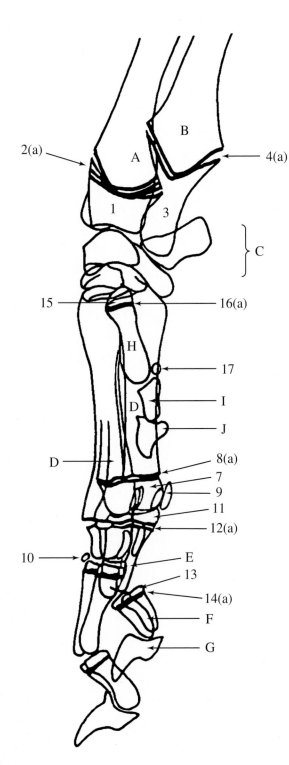

Figure 108

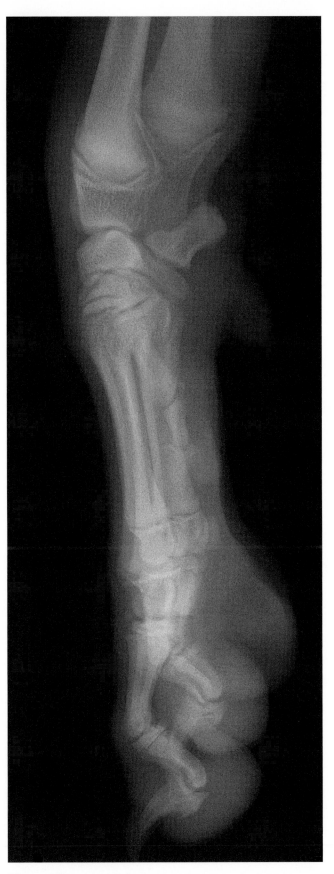

Figure 108   Age 17 weeks.

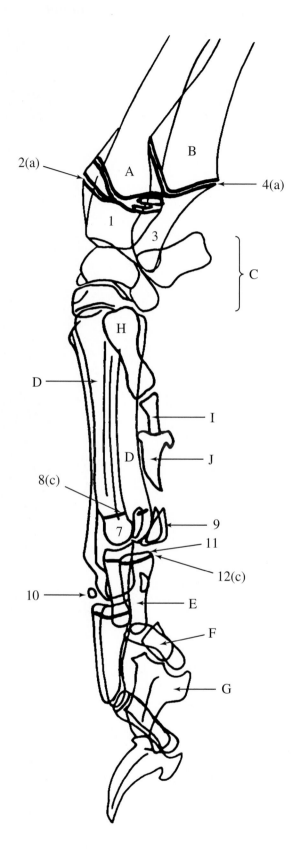

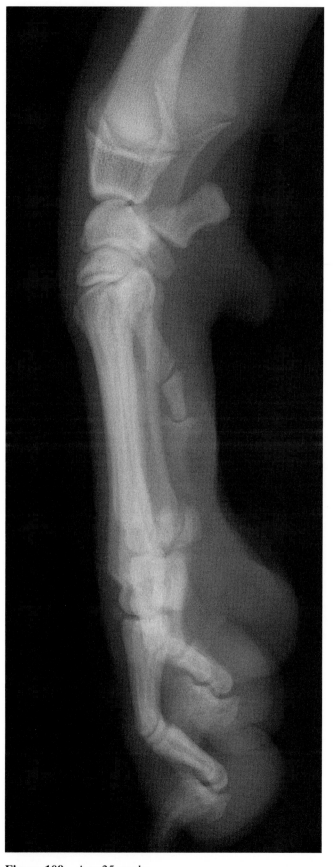

Figure 109

Figure 109 Age 25 weeks.

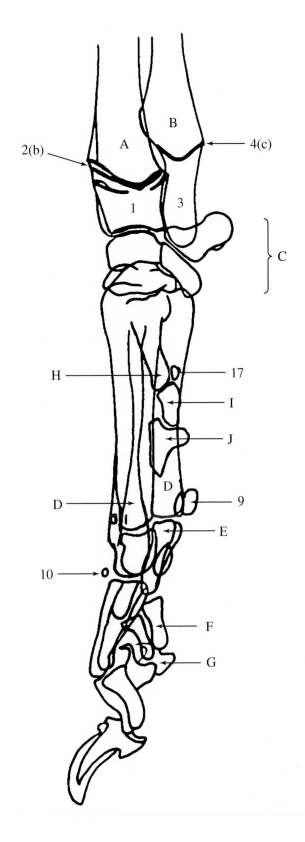

Figure 110

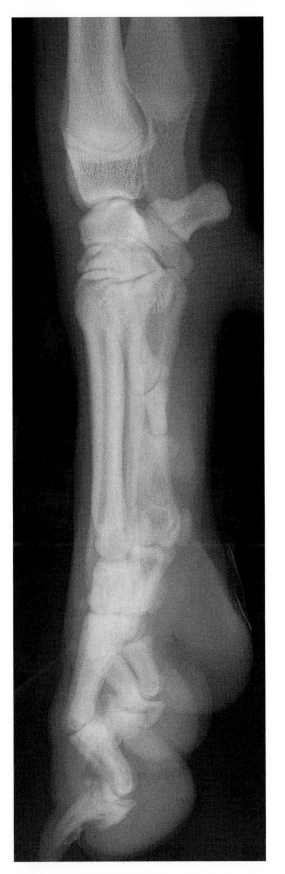

Figure 110   Age 34 weeks.

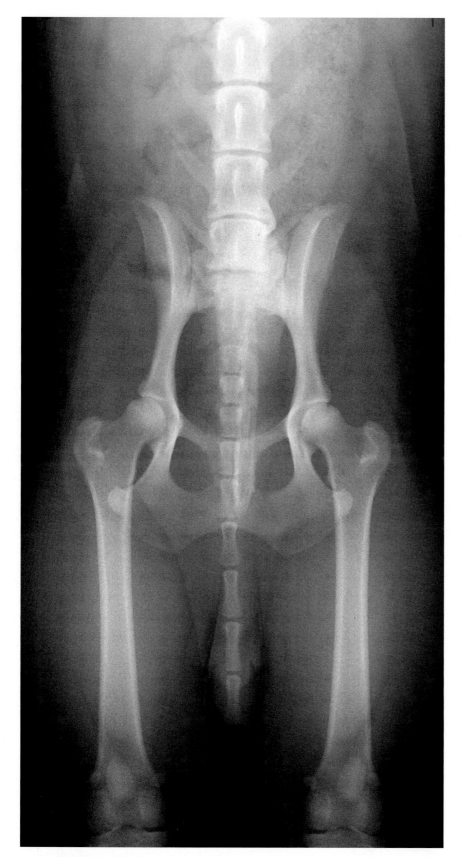

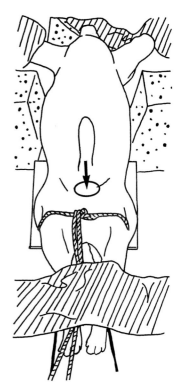

Figure 112 Line drawing of photograph representing radiographic positioning for Figure 111.

Figure 111 Ventrodorsal projection of hip joints and pelvis with full extension of femurs (stifle joints included for hip dysplasia evaluation). Beagle dog 2.5 years old, entire male.

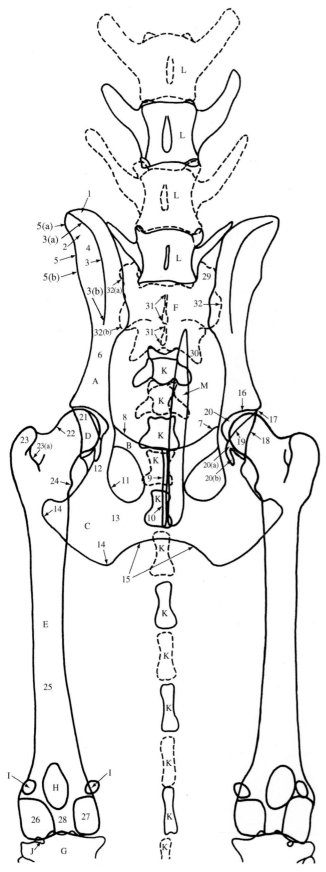

Figure 113   Ventrodorsal projection of hip joints and pelvis with full extension of femurs. To simplify the labelling each structure has been numbered on one side or the other but not on both sides. Also, the vertebral column has not been fully labelled.

A Ilium
1 Crest
2 Gluteal surface
3 Tuber sacrale or dorsal iliac spine
  3(a) Cranial dorsal iliac spine
  3(b) Caudal dorsal iliac spine
4 Wing
5 Tuber coxae or ventral iliac spine
  5(a) Cranial ventral iliac spine
  5(b) Caudal ventral iliac spine
6 Body

B Pubis
7 Position of iliopubic eminence. Eminence is often seen as a distinct process where cranial pubic border joins ilium.
8 Pecten
9 Pubic symphysis. Part of symphysis of pelvis.

C Ischium
10 Ischiatic symphysis. Part of symphysis of pelvis.
11 Obturator foramen
12 Ischiatic spine
13 Ischiatic table
14 Ischiatic tuberosity
15 Ischiatic arch

D Acetabulum
16 Cranial acetabular edge
17 Cranial effective acetabular rim
18 Dorsal acetabular edge
19 Ventral acetabular edge
20 Acetabular fossa
  20(a) Acetabular notch
  20(b) Acetabular fissure

E Femur
21 Head
22 Neck
23 Greater trochanter
  23(a) Trochanteric fossa
24 Lesser trochanter (more distinct in left leg)
25 Body
26 Lateral condyle
27 Medial condyle
28 Intercondyloid fossa

F Sacrum
29 Wing
30 Lateral sacral crest
31 Median sacral crest
32 Articular surface with ilium wing
  32(a) Synovial part of articular surface
  32(b) Cartilaginous part of articular surface

G Tibia

H Patella

I Fabella of m.gastrocnemius (lateral and medial heads)

J Fabella of m.popliteus

K Coccygeal vertebra

L Lumbar vertebra. (Chronic degenerative changes are present on the left side of 6th. and 7th. vertebrae at disc space level. Please see 'normality' in the Introduction.)

M Os penis

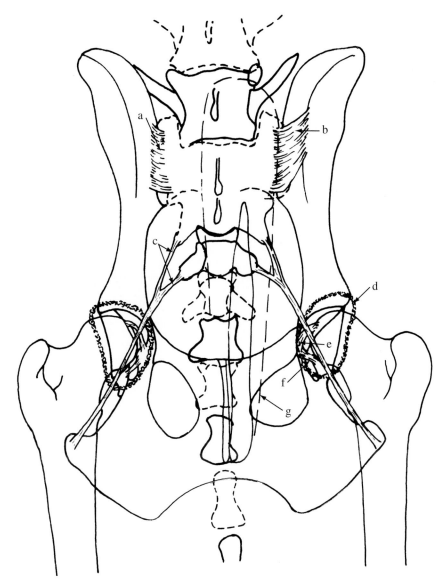

Figure 114 Schematic drawing of ventrodorsal projection of hip joints and pelvis with full extension of femurs to demonstrate extent of joints and ligaments.

Sacroiliac joint

This is a combination of a synovial and cartilaginous joint. The joint capsule is very thin and the two wings are united by a layer of fibrocartilage. Both ventrally and dorsally wide bands of sacroiliac ligaments cover the joint capsule. The dorsal group is more substantial.

a = Dorsal sacroiliac ligament
b = Ventral sacroiliac ligament
c = Sacrotuberous ligament

Hip joint

d = Joint capsule
e = Ligament of the head of the femur. Formerly called the round ligament. It extends from the fovea capitis of the femoral head to the acetabular fossa. The fovea capitus is not clearly seen in this radiograph but is often visible as a flattening on the medial aspect of the femoral head.
f = Transverse acetabular ligament
g = Soft tissue shadow of prepuce. This shadow often causes confusion if it is not identified and traced along its entire length. The increase in radiopacity created by its superimposition over bony structures may lead to misdiagnosis.

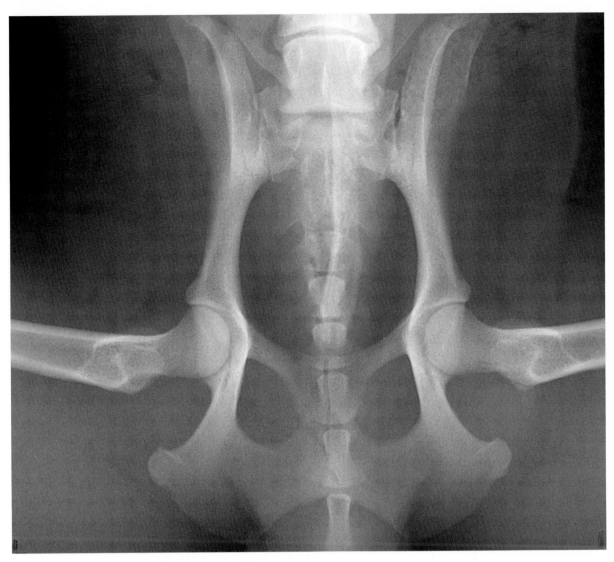

Figure 115   Ventrodorsal projection of hip joints and pelvis with abduction of femurs. The so-called 'frog legged' projection. Beagle dog 2.5 years old, entire male (same dog as in Figure 111).

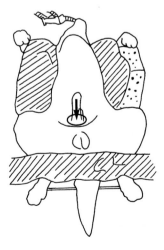

Figure 116   Line drawing of photograph representing radiographic positioning for Figure 115.

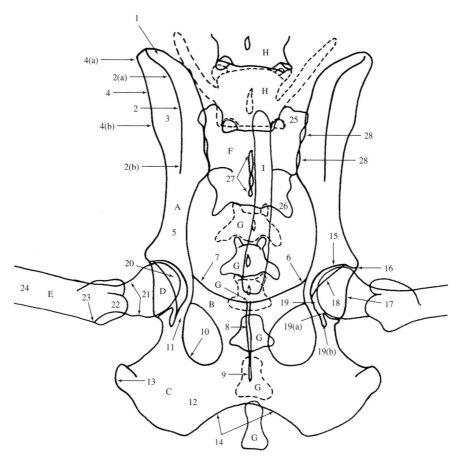

Figure 117 Ventrodorsal projection of hip joints and pelvis with abduction of femurs. The so-called 'frog legged' projection.

A Ilium
  1 Crest
  2 Tuber sacrale or dorsal iliac spine
    2(a) Cranial aspect of dorsal iliac spine
    2(b) Caudal aspect of dorsal iliac spine
  3 Wing
  4 Tuber coxae or ventral iliac spine
    4(a) Cranial ventral iliac spine
    4(b) Caudal ventral iliac spine
  5 Body

B Pubis
  6 Position of iliopubic eminence. (The eminence is more prominent in this projection than in the corresponding fully extended femora projection, Figure 113.)
  7 Pecten
  8 Pubic symphysis. Part of symphysis of pelvis.

C Ischium
  9 Ischiatic symphysis. Part of symphysis of pelvis.
  10 Obturator foramen
  11 Ischiatic spine
  12 Ischiatic table
  13 Ischiatic tuberosity
  14 Ischiatic arch

D Acetabulum
  15 Cranial acetabular edge
  16 Cranial effective acetabular rim
  17 Dorsal acetabular edge
  18 Ventral acetabular edge
  19 Acetabular fossa
    19(a) Acetabular notch
    19(b) Acetabular fissure

E Femur
  20 Head
  21 Neck
  22 Greater trochanter
  23 Lesser trochanter
  24 Body

F Sacrum
  25 Wing
  26 Lateral sacral crest
  27 Median sacral crest
  28 Sacroiliac articulation. Synovial part cranial to cartilaginous part of joint.

G Coccygeal vertebra

H Lumbar vertebra (see comments on fully extended femora projection, Figure 113)

I Os penis

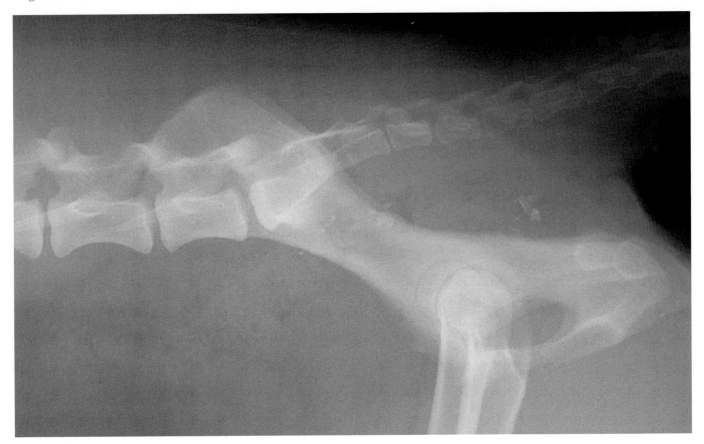

Figure 118 Lateral projection of hip joints and pelvis. Beagle dog 2.5 years old, entire male.

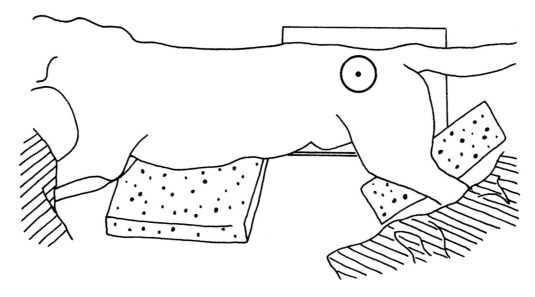

Figure 119 Line drawing of photograph representing radiographic positioning for Figure 118.

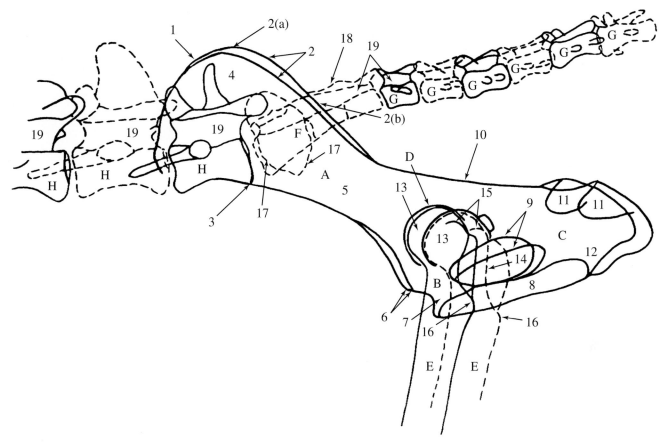

Figure 120   Lateral projection of hip joints and pelvis.

A Ilium
   1 Crest
   2 Tuber sacrale or dorsal iliac spine
     2(a) Cranial aspect of spine
     2(b) Caudal aspect of spine
   3 Caudal ventral iliac spine. (Cranial ventral iliac spine
     is not visible in this film.) Cranial and caudal ventral
     iliac spines form the tuber coxae or ventral iliac spine.
   4 Wing
   5 Body

B Pubis
   6 Iliopubic eminence
   7 Pecten of pubis

C Ischium
   8 Pelvic symphysis
   9 Obturator foramen
  10 Ischiatic spine
  11 Ischiatic tuberosity
  12 Ischiatic table

D Acetabulum

E Femur
  13 Head
  14 Neck
  15 Greater trochanters (shadows are not clearly visible
     but they will extend almost, if not quite, as far
     proximal as do the femoral heads on a truly lateral
     projection)
  16 Lesser trochanter

F Sacrum
  17 Sacroiliac articulation
  18 Sacral lamina (dorsal surface is not clearly
     distinguishable)
  19 Vertebral canal

G Coccygeal vertebra

H Lumbar vertebra

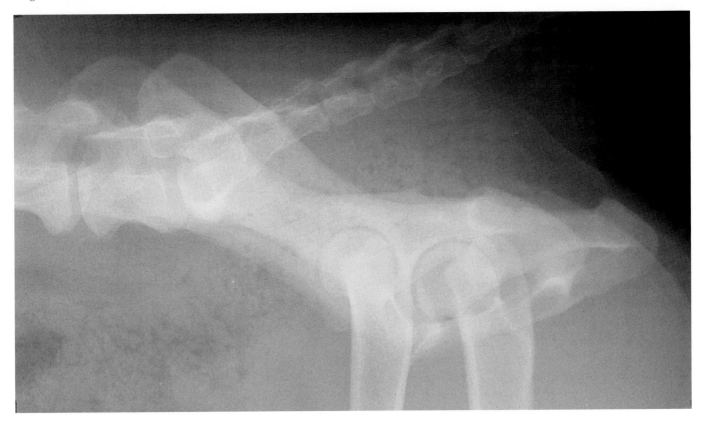

Figure 121   Lateral oblique projection of hip joints and pelvis. Beagle dog 7 years old, entire male.

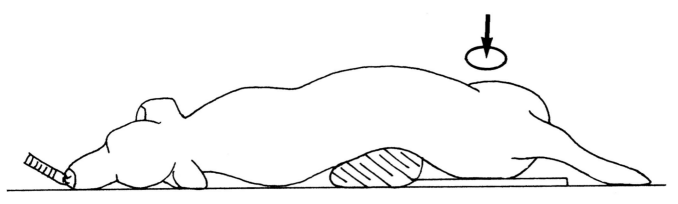

Figure 122   Line drawing of photograph representing radiographic positioning for Figure 121.

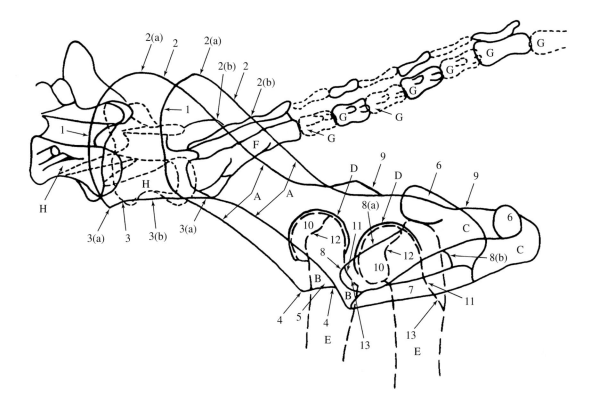

Figure 123   Lateral oblique projection of hip joints and pelvis.

A Ilium
   1 Crest
   2 Tuber sacrale or dorsal iliac spine
      2(a) Cranial dorsal iliac spine
      2(b) Caudal dorsal iliac spine
   3 Tuber coxae or ventral iliac spine
      3(a) Cranial ventral iliac spine
      3(b) Caudal ventral iliac spine

B Pubis
   4 Iliopubic eminence
   5 Pecten

C Ischium
   6 Ischiatic tuberosity
   7 Pelvic symphysis

8 Obturator foramen
      8(a) Obturator foramen recumbent side
      8(b) Obturator foramen non-recumbent side
   9 Ischiatic spine

D Acetabulum

E Femur
   10 Head
   11 Neck
   12 Greater trochanter
   13 Lesser trochanter

F Sacrum

G Coccygeal vertebra

H Lumbar vertebra

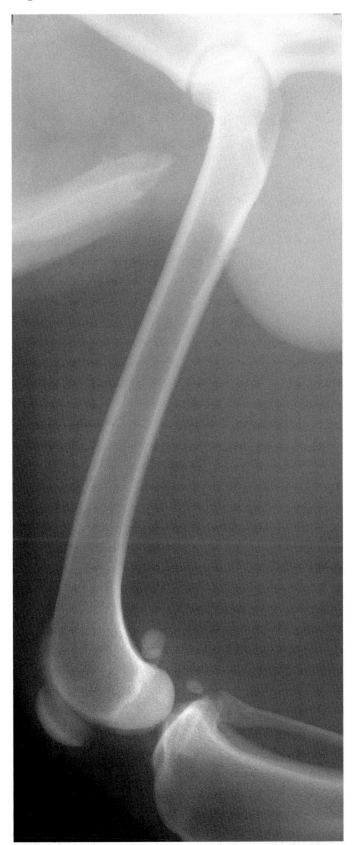

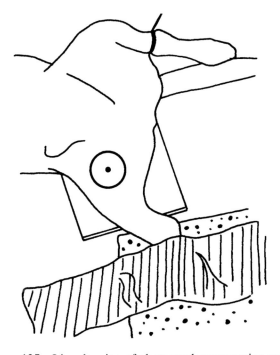

Figure 125 Line drawing of photograph representing radiographic positioning for Figure 124.

Figure 124 Mediolateral projection of femur. Beagle dog 7 years old, entire male.

An Atlas of Interpretative Radiographic Anatomy of the Dog and Cat

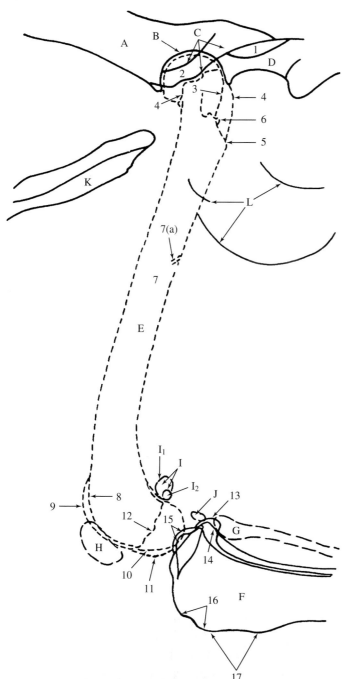

Figure 126 Mediolateral projection of femur.

A Ilium

B Acetabulum

C Pubis

D Ischium
   1 Obturator foramen

E Femur
   2 Head
   3 Neck
   4 Greater trochanter
   5 Lesser trochanter
   6 Trochanteric fossa
   7 Body
     7(a) Nutrient foramen
         (just visible as a
         radiolucent track
         through cortex)
   8 Trochlear groove
   9 Trochlear ridge
  10 Lateral condyle
  11 Medial condyle
  12 Base of intercondyloid
     fossa

F Tibia
  13 Lateral condyle
  14 Medial condyle
  15 Intercondyloid
     eminence. More
     caudal shadow is
     lateral.
  16 Tibial tuberosity
  17 Cranial border or
     'tibial crest' as
     formerly known

G Fibula

H Patella

I Fabellae of
   m.gastrocnemius
  I_1 Lateral fabella
  I_2 Medial fabella

J Fabella of
   m.popliteus

K Os penis

L Scrotal shadow

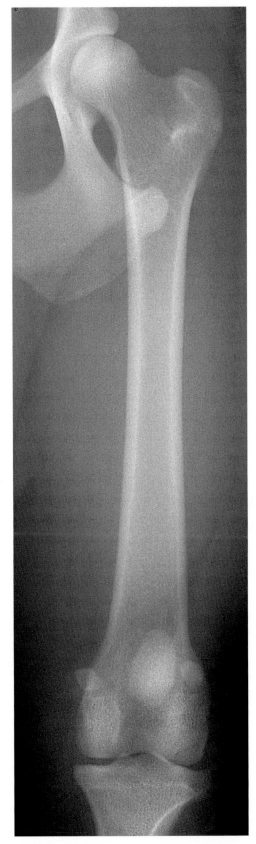

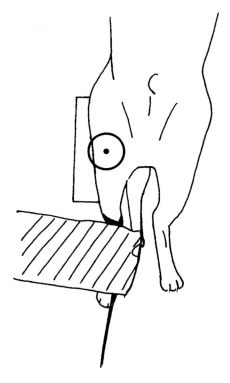

Figure 128   Line drawing of photograph representing radiographic positioning for Figure 127.

Figure 127   Craniocaudal projection of femur. Beagle dog 2.5 years old, entire male.

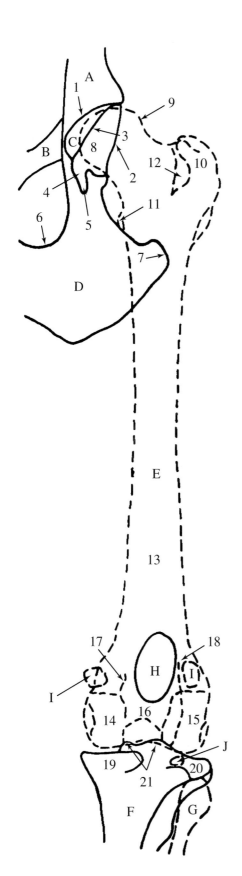

Figure 129   Craniocaudal projection of femur.

A Ilium

B Pubis

C Acetabulum
   Acetabular features:
   1 Cranial acetabular edge
   2 Dorsal acetabular edge
   3 Ventral acetabular edge
   4 Acetabular notch
   5 Acetabular fissure

D Ischium
   6 Obturator foramen
   7 Ischiatic tuberosity

E Femur
   8 Head
   9 Neck
   10 Greater trochanter

11 Lesser trochanter
12 Trochanteric fossa
13 Body
14 Medial condyle
15 Lateral condyle
16 Intercondyloid fossa
17 Medial trochlear ridge
18 Lateral trochlear ridge

F Tibia
   19 Medial condyle
   20 Lateral condyle
   21 Intercondyloid eminence

G Fibula

H Patella

I Fabella of m.gastrocnemius

J Fabella of m.popliteus

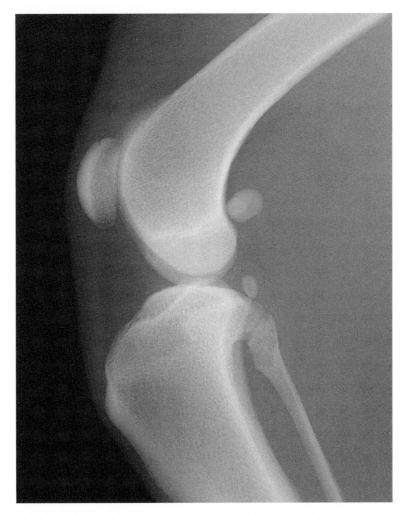

Figure 130   Mediolateral projection of stifle joint. Beagle dog 7 years old, entire male.

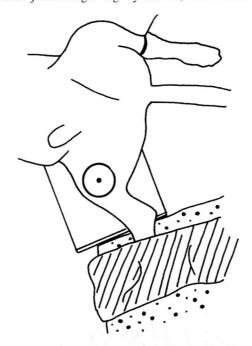

Figure 131   Line drawing of photograph representing radiographic positioning for Figure 130.

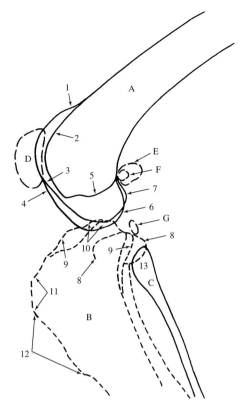

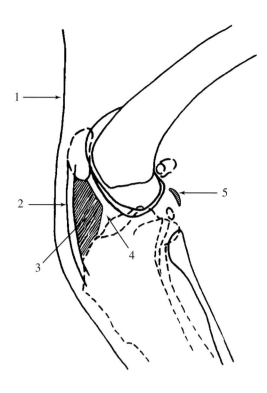

Figure 132 Mediolateral projection of stifle joint.

A Femur
  1 Trochlear ridges.
    Medial is more dorsal
    than lateral
  2 Trochlear groove
  3 Medial trochlear ridge
  4 Lateral trochlear ridge
  5 Base of intercondyloid
    fossa
  6 Lateral condyle (inden-
    tation of extensor fossa
    only just visible)
  7 Medial condyle

B Tibia
  8 Lateral condyle
  9 Medial condyle
  10 Intercondyloid emi-
  nence or intercondyloid
  tubercles. More caudal
  is lateral.
  11 Tibial tuberosity
  12 Cranial border or
    'tibial crest' as
    formerly known

C Fibula
  13 Head

D Patella

E Lateral fabella of
  m.gastrocnemius

F Medial fabella of
  m.gastrocnemius

G Fabella of m.popliteus

Figure 133 Line drawing of mediolateral projection of stifle joint to demonstrate soft tissue shadows seen in radiograph Figure 130.

1 Skin at cranial aspect of limb

2 Patellar ligament

3 Infrapatellar fat pad. Reduction of this grey shadow is normally seen with joint enlargement, most commonly secondary to effusion.

4 Soft tissue opacity from joint capsule, synovial fluid, menisci, ligaments and tendons in this region

5 Fat tissue shadow from adipose tissue within fascial planes in this region. Disturbance of this shadow usually reflects joint enlargement most commonly due to effusion.

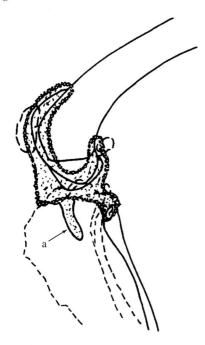

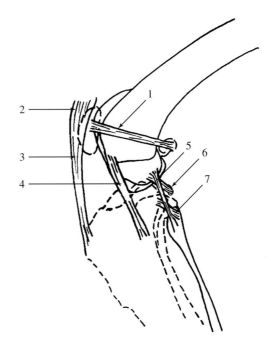

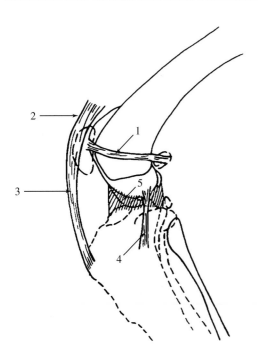

Figure 134 Schematic drawing of mediolateral projection of stifle joint to demonstrate extent of joint capsule.

🐾 = Joint capsule

⣿ = Synovial space

a = Distolateral extension around tendon of the m.extensor digitorum longus where it traverses the extensor groove of the lateral tibial condyle.

Note that the stifle joint cavity extends into the synovial joints made by the patella, lateral and medial fabellae and the fibula as well as the femorotibial joint.

Figure 135 Schematic drawing of mediolateral projection of stifle joint. The positions of ligaments and tendons on the axial and lateral aspects are indicated.

1 = Lateral femoropatellar ligament

2 = Tendon insertion of m.quadriceps femoris into the patella

3 = Patellar ligament

4 = Tendon of m.extensor digitorum longus

5 = Lateral collateral ligament

6 = Tendon of m.popliteus plus sesamoid bone

7 = Ligament of fibular head

Meniscal and cruciate ligaments not shown but will be found in the femorotibial joint between the tendons of m.extensor digitorum longus and m.popliteus.

Figure 136 Schematic drawing of mediolateral projection of stifle joint. The positions of ligaments and tendons on the axial and medial aspects are indicated.

1 = Medial femoropatellar ligament

2 = Tendon insertion of m.quadriceps femoris into the patella

3 = Patellar ligament

4 = Medial collateral ligament

5 = Region of menisci

Meniscal and cruciate ligaments not shown but will be found in the region of menisci.

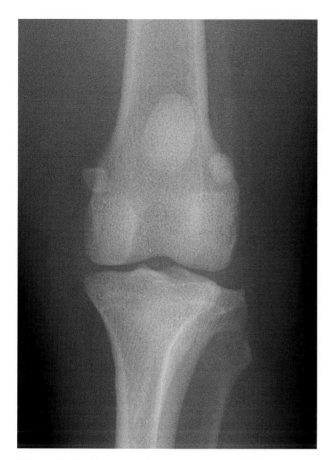

Figure 137 Caudocranial projection of stifle joint. Beagle dog 2.5 years old, entire male.

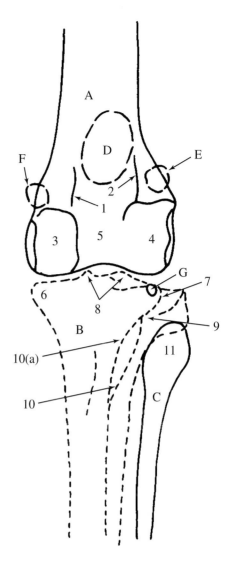

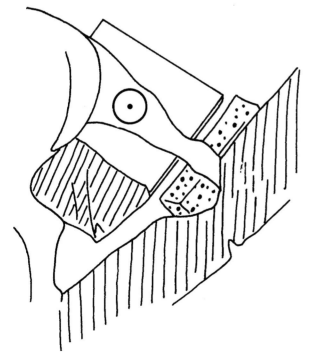

Figure 138 Line drawing of photograph representing radiographic positioning for Figure 137.

Figure 139 Caudocranial projection of stifle joint.

A Femur
  1 Medial trochlear ridge
  2 Lateral trochlear ridge
  3 Medial condyle
  4 Lateral condyle
  5 Intercondyloid fossa

B Tibia
  6 Medial condyle
  7 Lateral condyle
  8 Intercondyloid eminence or medial and lateral inter-condyloid tubercles
  9 Tibial tuberosity
  10 Cranial border or 'tibial crest' as formerly known

10(a) Outline for the extensor muscles, especially m.cranialis tibialis

C Fibula
  11 Head

D Patella

E Lateral fabella of m.gastrocnemius

F Medial fabella of m.gastrocnemius

G Fabella of m.popliteus

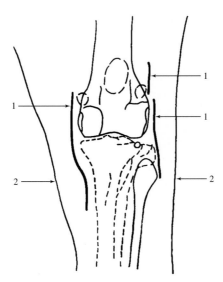

Figure 140   Line drawing of caudocranial projection of stifle joint to demonstrate soft tissue shadows seen in radiograph Figure 137.

1   Fat tissue shadow from adipose tissue within fascial planes. Disturbances of these shadows usually reflect joint enlargement, most commonly due to joint effusions.

2   Skin limits

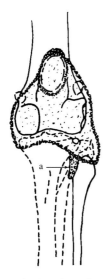

Figure 141   Schematic drawing of caudocranial projection of stifle joint. Extent of the joint capsule on the cranial aspect of the joint has been indicated.

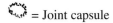 = Joint capsule

= Synovial space. Note that patella is not in synovial space.

a   = Distal extension surrounding tendon of m.extensor digitorum longus. Only present on cranial aspect.

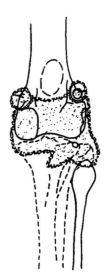

Figure 142   Schematic drawing of caudocranial projection of stifle joint. Extent of the joint capsule on the caudal aspect of the joint has been indicated.

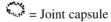 = Joint capsule

= Synovial space. Note that fabellae are not in the synovial space but the joint cavity extends into the joints between fabellae and femur.

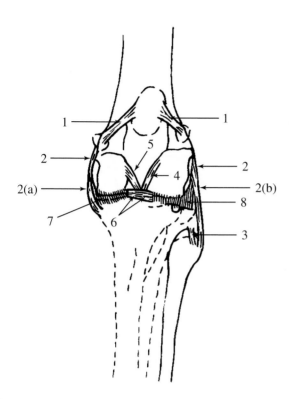

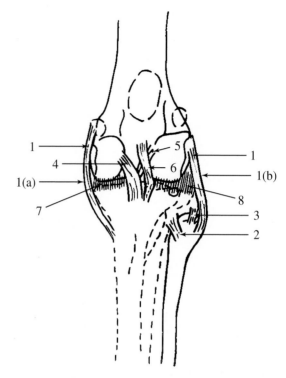

Figure 143 Schematic drawing of caudocranial projection of stifle joint. Positions of ligaments of the medial, lateral and cranial aspects are indicated. Positions of the menisci are also shown.

1 = Femoropatellar ligaments

2 = Collateral ligaments
  2(a) = Medial
  2(b) = Lateral

3 = Cranial fibular ligament

4 = Cranial cruciate ligament

5 = Caudal cruciate ligament

6 = Transverse or intermeniscal ligament

7 = Medial meniscus

8 = Lateral meniscus

Meniscal ligaments attaching menisci to tibia and femur not shown. Patellar ligament excluded to avoid confusion.

Figure 144 Schematic drawing of caudocranial projection of stifle joint. Positions of ligaments of the medial, lateral and caudal aspects are indicated. Positions of the menisci are also shown.

1 = Collateral ligaments
  1(a) = Medial
  1(b) = Lateral

2 = Caudal fibular ligament

3 = Cranial fibular ligament

4 = Caudal cruciate ligament. Extends from axial surface of medial femoral condyle to tibial popliteal notch. It is longer and heavier than cranial.

5 = Cranial cruciate ligament. Extends from caudal part of axial surface of lateral femoral condyle to cranial intercondyloid area of tibia.

6 = Meniscofemoral ligament

7 = Medial meniscus

8 = Lateral meniscus

Meniscal ligaments attaching menisci to tibia and intermeniscal ligament not shown. Patellar ligament excluded to avoid confusion.

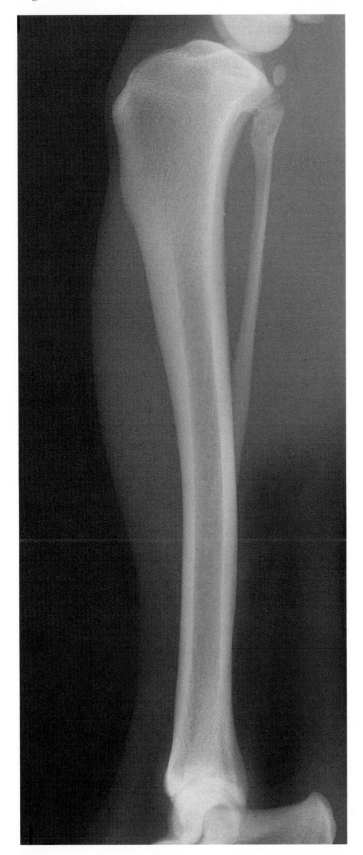

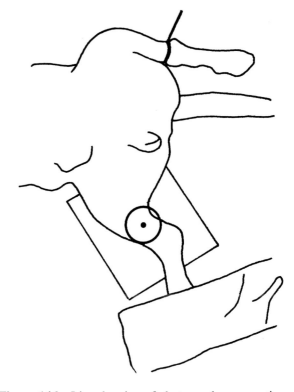

Figure 146 Line drawing of photograph representing radiographic positioning for Figure 145.

Figure 145 Mediolateral projection of tibia and fibula. Beagle dog 7 years old, entire male.

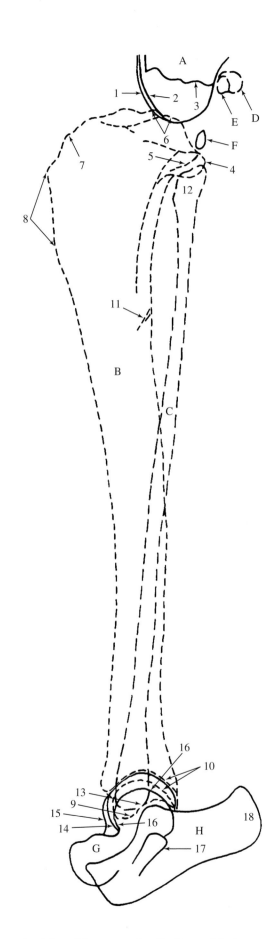

Figure 147   Mediolateral projection of tibia and fibula.

A Femur
  1 Lateral condyle
  2 Medial condyle
  3 Base of intercondyloid
    fossa

B Tibia
  4 Lateral condyle
  5 Medial condyle
  6 Intercondyloid eminence or
    intercondyloid tubercles.
    The more caudal shadow is
    the lateral tubercle

  7 Tibial tuberosity

  8 Cranial border or 'tibial
    crest' as formerly known

  9 Medial malleolus

  10 Distal articular border

  11 Nutrient foramen (only just
    visible but can mimic a

fracture if the tibia is
slightly rotated on
exposure)

C Fibula
  12 Head
  13 Lateral malleolus

D Lateral fabella of
   m.gastrocnemius

E Medial fabella of
   m.gastrocnemius

F Fabella of m.popliteus

G Tibial tarsal bone or talus
  14 Lateral trochlear ridge
  15 Medial trochlear ridge
  16 Trochlear groove

H Fibular tarsal bone or
   calcaneus
  17 Sustentaculum tali
  18 Calcaneal tuber

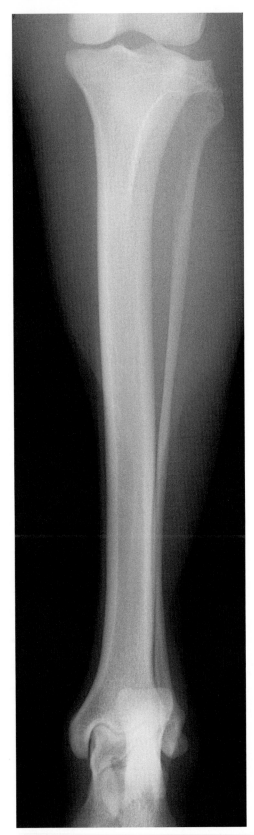

Figure 148 Caudocranial projection of tibia and fibula. Beagle dog 2.5 years old, entire male.

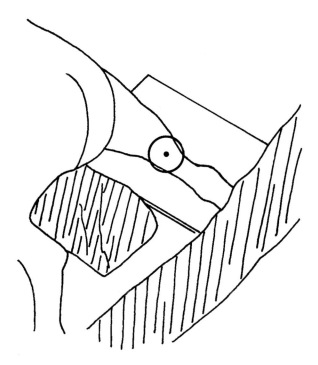

Figure 149 Line drawing of photograph representing radiographic positioning for Figure 148.

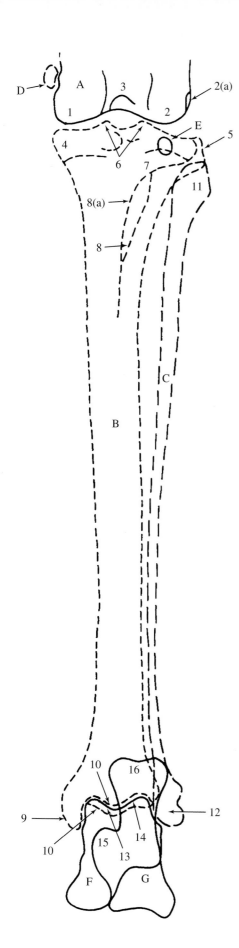

Figure 150 Caudocranial projection of tibia and fibula.

A Femur
  1 Medial condyle
  2 Lateral condyle
    2(a) Extensor fossa.
      Origin of m.flexor
      digitorum longus.
  3 Intercondyloid fossa

B Tibia
  4 Medial condyle
  5 Lateral condyle
  6 Intercondyloid eminence
    or intercondyloid
    tubercles
  7 Tibial tuberosity
  8 Cranial border or 'tibial
    crest' as formerly known
    8(a) Outline of concavity
      in the tibia which
      houses extensor
      muscles
  9 Medial malleolus
 10 Distal articular border

C Fibula
 11 Head
 12 Lateral malleolus

D Medial fabella of m.gastro-
  cnemius. (Note the unusual
  position of this fabella in
  relationship to the medial
  femoral condyle. This is an
  anatomical variant which is
  not to be misdiagnosed as a
  rupture of the m.gastro-
  cnemius.)

E Fabella of m.popliteus

F Tibial tarsal bone or talus
 13 Medial trochlear ridge
 14 Lateral trochlear ridge

G Fibular tarsal bone or
  calcaneus
 15 Sustentaculum tali
 16 Calcaneal tuber

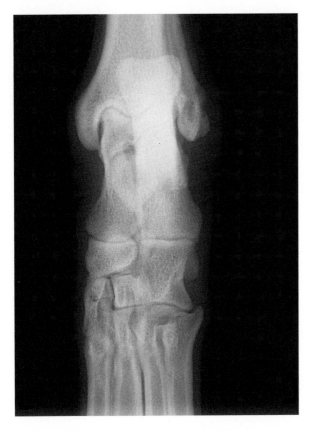

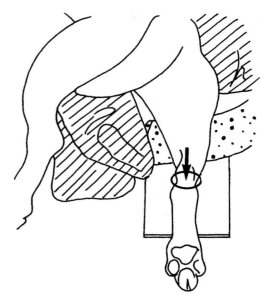

Figure 152   Line drawing of photograph representing radiographic positioning for Figure 151.

Figure 151   Plantarodorsal projection of tarsus. Beagle dog 2.5 years old, entire male.

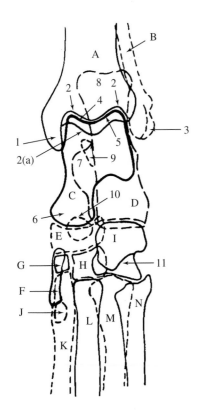

Figure 153   Plantarodorsal projection of tarsus.

A Tibia
  1 Medial malleolus
  2 Distal articular border. (Medial and lateral grooves.)
    2(a) Distal articular border. (Cranial aspect.)

B Fibula
  3 Lateral malleolus. (Note the relatively proximal position of the lateral malleolus compared to the medial malleolus. In many dogs the malleoli are at an equal distal level.)

C Tibial tarsal bone or talus
  4 Medial trochlear ridge
  5 Lateral trochlear ridge
  6 Head

D Fibular tarsal bone or calcaneus
  7 Sustentaculum tali
  8 Calcaneal tuber

  9 Tarsal sinus. (Radiolucent shadow which is the space between talus and calcaneus extends more distally than can be seen in this projection.)

E Central tarsal bone
  10 Plantar process

F Tarsal bone 1

G Tarsal bone 2

H Tarsal bone 3

I Tarsal bone 4
  11 Shadow formed by large tuberosity on the plantar surface

J Metatarsal bone 1

K Metatarsal bone 2

L Metatarsal bone 3

M Metatarsal bone 4

N Metatarsal bone 5

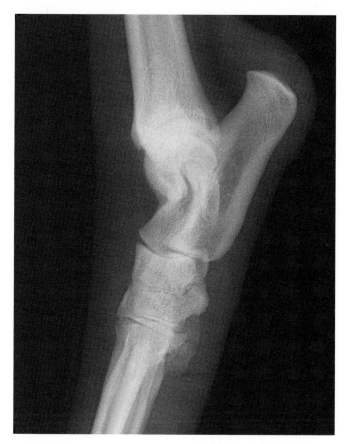

Figure 154 Extended mediolateral projection of tarsus. Beagle dog 2.5 years old, entire male.

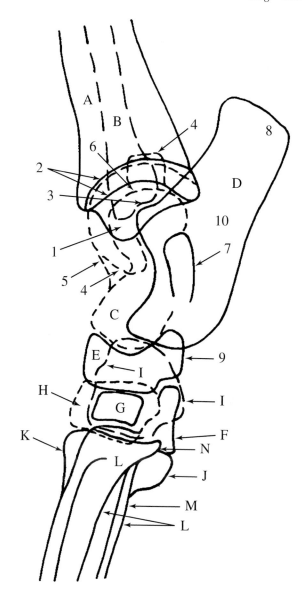

Figure 156 Extended mediolateral projection of tarsus.

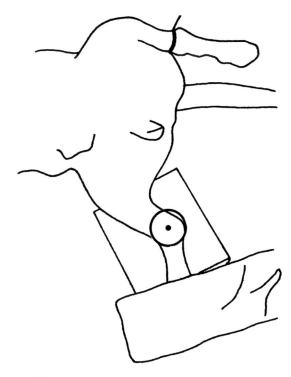

Figure 155 Line drawing of photograph representing radiographic positioning for Figure 154.

A Tibia
  1 Medial malleolus
  2 Distal articular border

B Fibula
  3 Lateral malleolus

C Tibial tarsal bone or talus
  4 Lateral trochlear ridge
  5 Medial trochlear ridge
  6 Trochlear groove

D Fibular tarsal bone or calcaneus
  7 Sustentaculum tali
  8 Calcaneal tuber

E Central tarsal bone
  9 Plantar process

F Tarsal bone 1

G Tarsal bone 2

H Tarsal bone 3

I Tarsal bone 4

J Metatarsal bone 1

K Metatarsal bone 3

L Combined shadows of metatarsal bones 2, 4 and 5

M Metatarsal bone 2

N Metatarsal bone 5

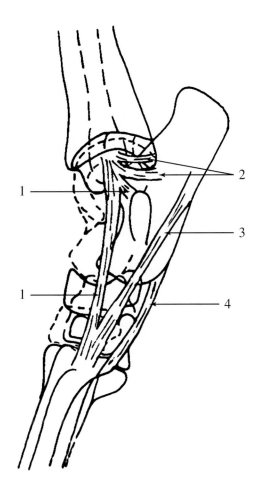

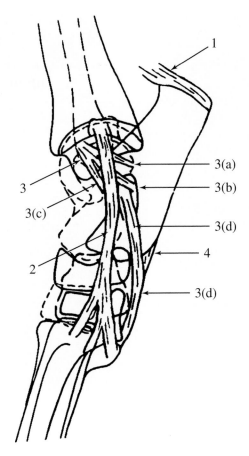

Figure 157 Schematic drawing of extended medio-lateral projection of tarsus. Positions of ligaments of the lateral aspect are indicated.

1 = Lateral collateral ligament. Long part.

2 = Lateral collateral ligament. Short part.

3 = Lateral collateral ligament. Calcaneometatarsal part.

4 = Plantar ligament

Figure 158 Schematic drawing of extended mediolateral projection of tarsus. Positions of ligaments of the medial aspect are indicated. Position of the Achilles' tendon is also shown.

1 = Achilles' tendon or calcanean tendon. Components are mainly superficial digital flexor and m.gastrocnemius. Also present are the m.biceps femoris, m.semitendinosus and m.gracilis.

2 = Medial collateral ligament. Long part.

3 = Medial collateral ligament. Short part.
   3(a) To tibial tarsal bone
   3(b) To sustentaculum tali
   3(c) To long part of medial collateral ligament
   3(d) From sustentaculum tali to base of metatarsal bones 2, 3 and 4

4 = Origin of long plantar ligament

Dorsal tarsal ligaments not shown. Intertarsal ligaments, proximal extensor retinaculum and distal extensor retinaculum not shown.

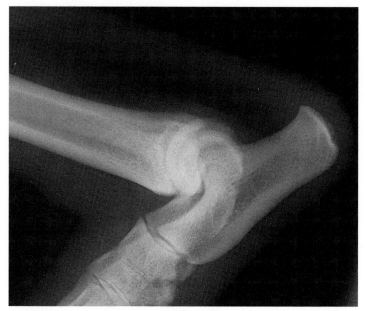

Figure 159 Flexed mediolateral projection of tarsus. Beagle dog 2.5 years old, entire male.

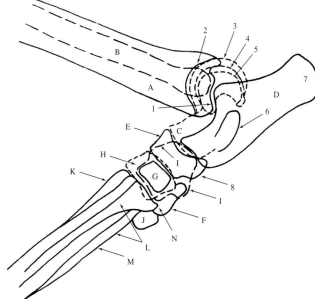

Figure 161 Flexed mediolateral projection of tarsus.

A Tibia 　1 Medial malleolus 　2 Distal articular border	E Central tarsal bone 　8 Plantar process
	F Tarsal bone 1
B Fibula Lateral malleolus cannot be identified as a separate structure	G Tarsal bone 2
	H Tarsal bone 3
	I Tarsal bone 4
C Tibial tarsal bone or talus 　3 Lateral trochlear ridge 　4 Medial trochlear ridge 　5 Trochlear groove	J Metatarsal bone 1
	K Metatarsal bone 3
	L Combined shadows of metatarsal bones 2, 4 and 5
D Fibular tarsal bone or calcaneus 　6 Sustentaculum tali 　7 Calcaneal tuber	M Metatarsal bone 2
	N Metatarsal bone 5

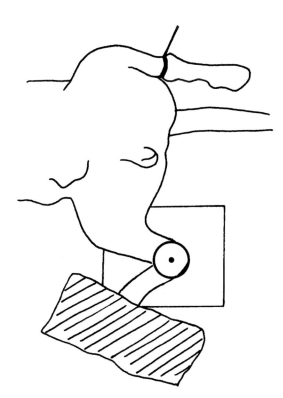

Figure 160 Line drawing of photograph representing radiographic positioning for Figure 159.

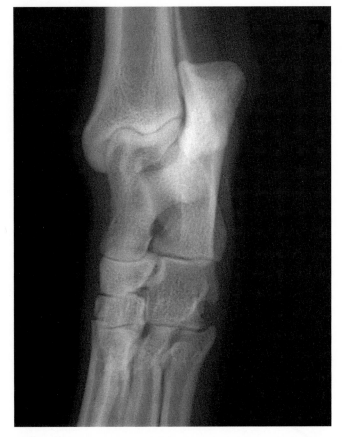

Figure 162 Plantaromedial-dorsolateral oblique projection of tarsus. Beagle dog 2.5 years old, entire male.

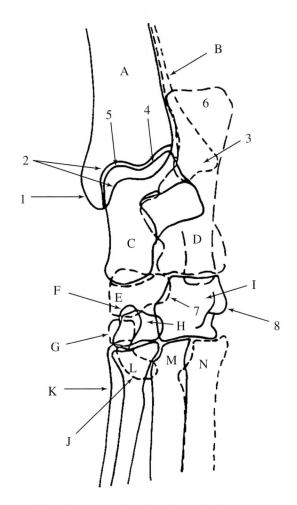

Figure 164 Plantaromedial–dorsolateral oblique projection of tarsus.

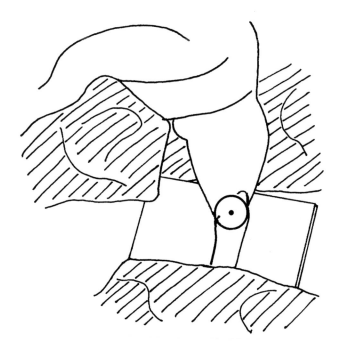

Figure 163 Line drawing of photograph representing radiographic positioning for Figure 162.

A Tibia
  1 Medial malleolus
  2 Distal articular border

B Fibula
  3 Lateral malleolus

C Tibial tarsal bone or talus
  4 Lateral trochlear ridge
  5 Medial trochlear ridge

D Fibular tarsal bone or calcaneus
  6 Calcaneal tuber

E Central tarsal bone
  7 Plantar process

F Tarsal bone 1

G Tarsal bone 2

H Tarsal bone 3

I Tarsal bone 4
  8 Tuberosity on plantar aspect

J Metatarsal bone 1

K Metatarsal bone 2

L Metatarsal bone 3

M Metatarsal bone 4

N Metatarsal bone 5

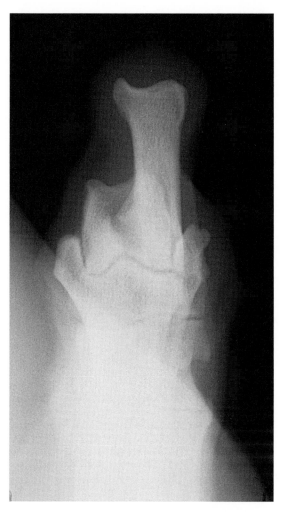

Figure 165 Dorsoplantar projection of calcaneus and talus (flexed). Beagle dog 2.5 years old, entire male.

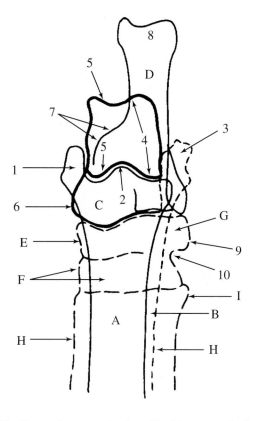

Figure 167 Dorsoplantar projection of calcaneus and talus (flexed).

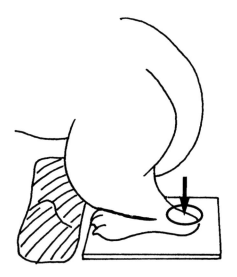

Figure 166 Line drawing of photograph representing radiographic positioning for Figure 165.

A Tibia
  1 Medial malleolus
  2 Distal articular border
B Fibula
  3 Lateral malleolus
C Tibial tarsal bone or talus
  4 Lateral trochlear ridge
  5 Medial trochlear ridge
  6 Medial surface of head
D Fibular tarsal bone or
  calcaneus

  7 Sustentaculum tali
  8 Calcaneal tuber
E Central tarsal bone
F Proximal tarsal bones 1, 2
  and 3
G Tarsal bone 4
  9 Tuberosity on plantar
    surface
  10 Groove for tendon of
    m.fibularis longus
H Metatarsal bones

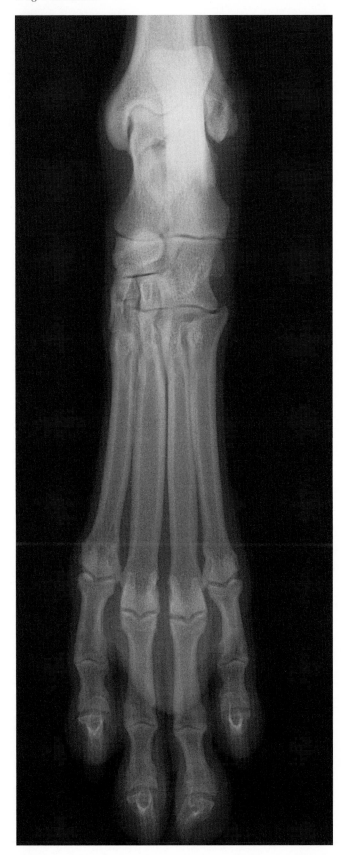

Figure 168 Plantarodorsal projection of metatarsus and phalanges. Beagle dog 2.5 years old, entire male.

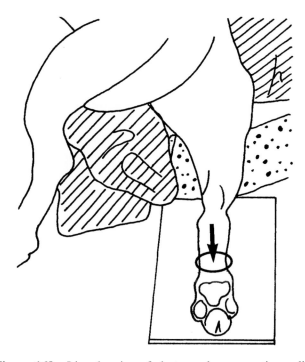

Figure 169 Line drawing of photograph representing radiographic positioning for Figure 168.

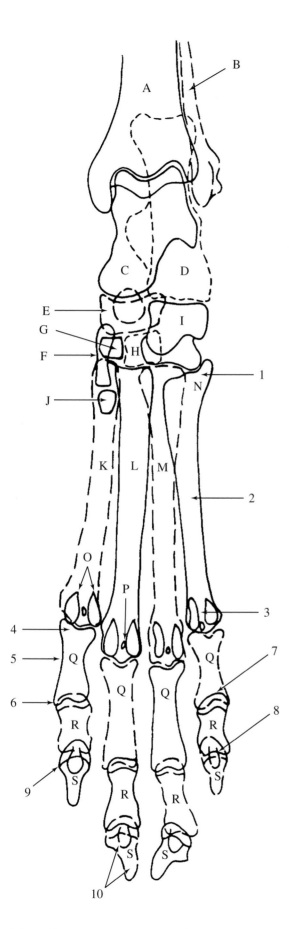

Figure 170 Plantarodorsal projection of metatarsus and phalanges.

A Tibia

B Fibula

C Tibial tarsal bone or talus

D Fibular tarsal bone or calcaneus

E Central tarsal bone (Note bony shadow of plantar process which appears as a radiopaque body)

F Tarsal bone 1

G Tarsal bone 2

H Tarsal bone 3

I Tarsal bone 4

J Metatarsal bone 1
   1 Base
   2 Body
   3 Head

K Metatarsal bone 2

L Metatarsal bone 3

M Metatarsal bone 4

N Metatarsal bone 5

O Proximal sesamoid bones. Present on plantar aspect.

P Dorsal sesamoid bones (Just visible)

Q Proximal phalanges or 1st. phalanges
   4 Base
   5 Body
   6 Head
   The metatarsal pad is seen as a distinct soft tissue shadow superimposed on the proximal phalanges

R Middle phalanges or 2nd. phalanges

   Divided into base, body and head as proximal phalanges
   7 Proximal articular border
   8 Distal articular border

S Distal phalanges or 3rd. phalanges
   9 Ungual crest
   10 Ungual process

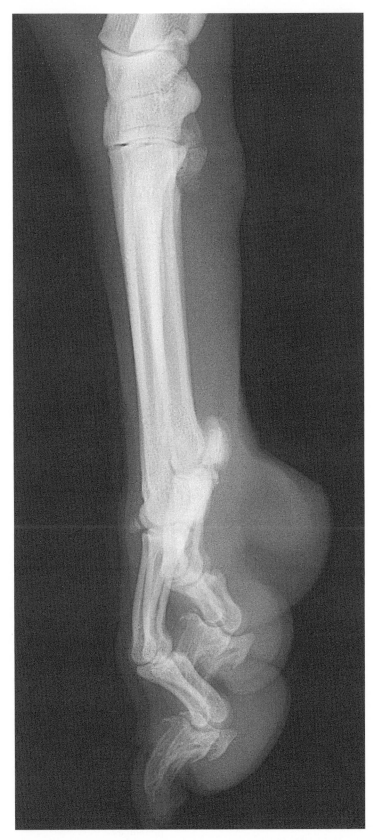

Figure 171 Mediolateral projection of metatarsus and phalanges. Beagle dog 7 years old, entire male.

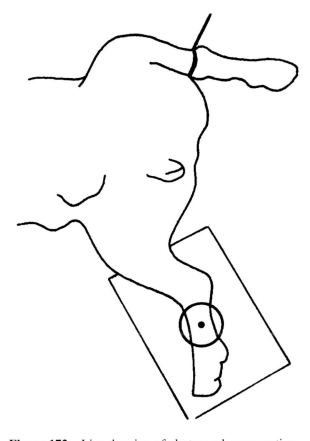

Figure 172 Line drawing of photograph representing radiographic positioning for Figure 171.

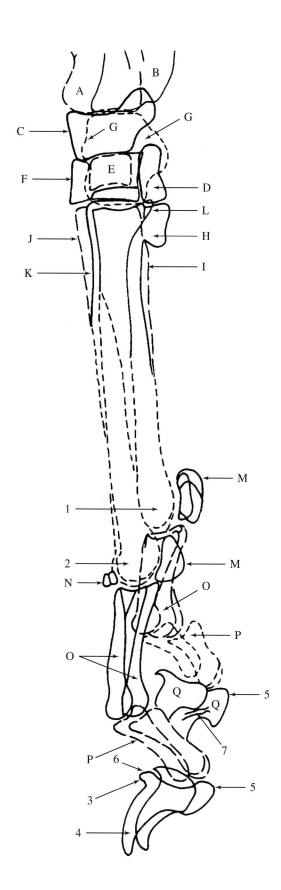

Figure 173 Mediolateral projection of metatarsus and phalanges.

A Tibial tarsal bone or talus

B Fibular tarsal bone or calcaneus

C Central tarsal bone

D Tarsal bone 1

E Tarsal bone 2

F Tarsal bone 3

G Tarsal bone 4

H Metatarsal bone 1

I Metatarsal bone 2

J Metatarsal bone 3

K Metatarsal bone 4

L Metatarsal bone 5

 1 Superimposed heads of metatarsal bones 2 and 5

 2 Superimposed heads of metatarsal bones 3 and 4

M Proximal sesamoid bones. Two in number at plantar aspect of each proximal interphalangeal joint.

N Dorsal sesamoid bones. One in number at dorsal aspect of each proximal interphalangeal joint.

O Proximal phalanges or 1st. phalanges

P Middle phalanges or 2nd. phalanges

Q Distal phalanges or 3rd. phalanges

 3 Ungual crest

 4 Ungual process

 5 Flexor tuberosity

 6 Extensor tuberosity

 7 Nutrient canal

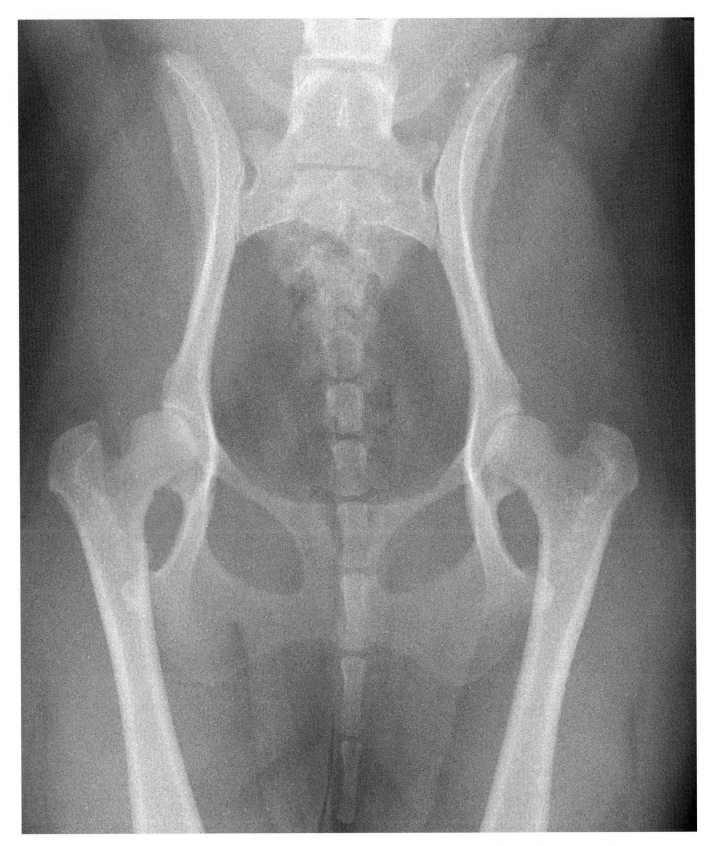

Figure 174   Ventrodorsal projection of pelvis and hip joints. Toy breed of dog. Yorkshire Terrier dog 2 years old, entire female.

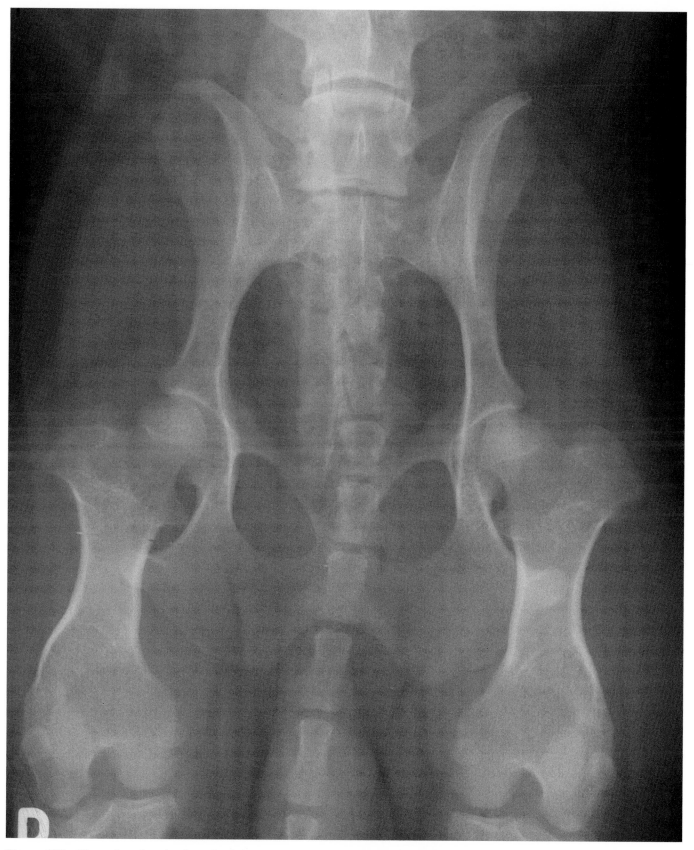

Figure 175 Ventrodorsal projection of pelvis and hip joints. Chondrodystrophic breed of dog. Standard Dachshund dog 7 years old, entire male.

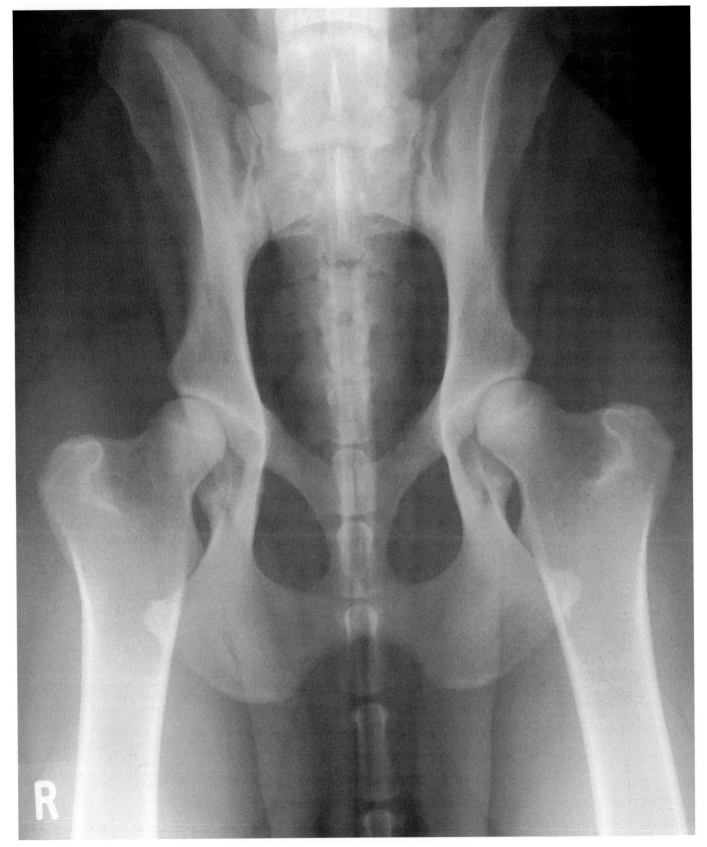

Figure 176   Ventrodorsal projection of pelvis and hip joints. Giant breed of dog. English Bull Mastiff dog 21 months old, entire male.

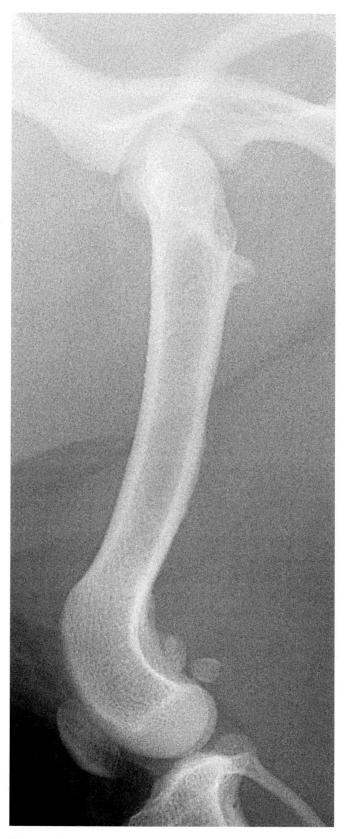

Figure 177   Mediolateral projection of femur. Chondrodystrophic breed of dog. Miniature Dachshund dog 6 years old, neutered female.

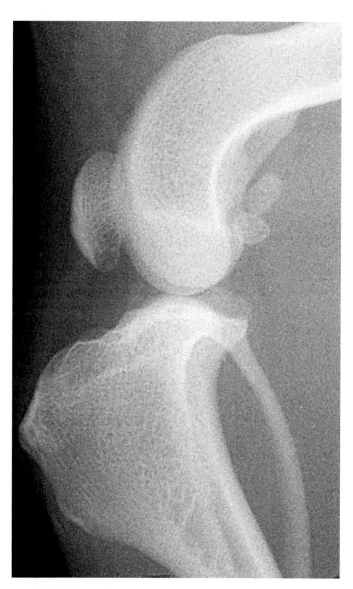

Figure 178   Mediolateral projection of stifle joint. Chondrodystrophic breed of dog. Miniature Dachshund dog 6 years old, neutered female.

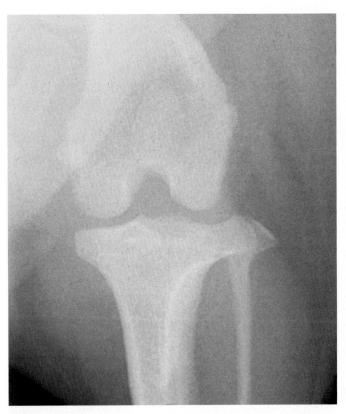

Figure 179   Caudocranial projection of stifle joint.
Chondrodystrophic breed of dog. Miniature Dachshund dog
6 years old, neutered female.

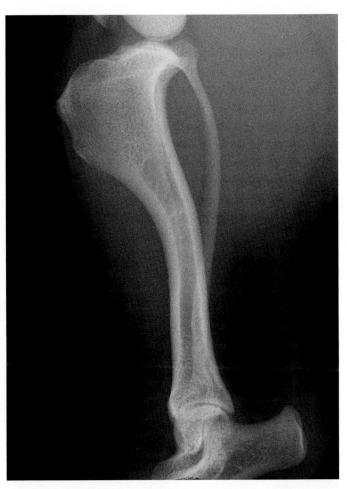

Figure 180   Mediolateral projection of tibia and fibula. Chondrodystrophic breed of dog. Miniature Dachshund dog
6 years old, neutered female.

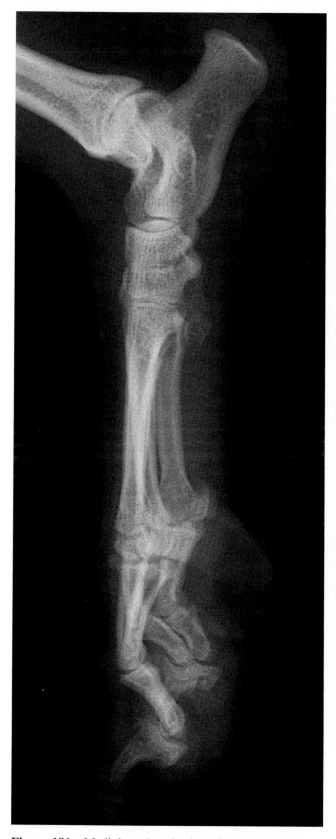

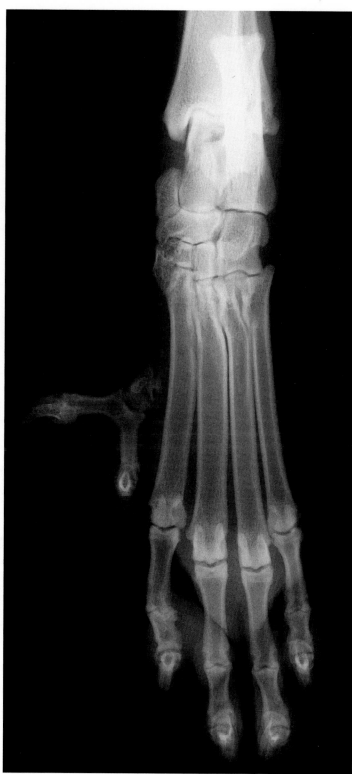

Figure 181   Mediolateral projection of tarsus and phalanges. Chondrodystrophic breed of dog. Miniature
Dachshund dog 6 years old, neutered female.

Figure 182   Plantarodorsal projection of tarsus and phalanges.
Giant breed of dog. Pyrenean Mountain dog 4 years old, entire
female. The radiograph demonstrates the unusual bony appendage of
the central tarsal bone that can be found in a number of giant breeds
of dog. More obvious for the Pyrenean Mountain dog is the congenital development of the 1st. digit which is a breed point for showing.

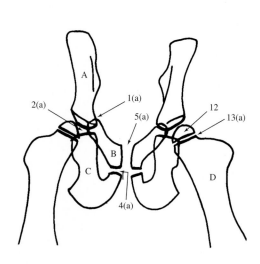

Figure 183

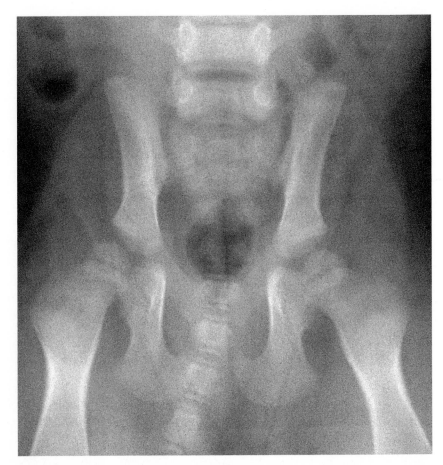

Figure 183 Age 4 weeks.

Figures 183, 184, 185, 186, 187, 188, 189, 190 Ventrodorsal projection of pelvis and craniocaudal projection of proximal femur. Samoyed Crossbred dog, entire male, at 4, 8, 13, 17, 21, 25, 34 and 47 weeks of age.

A Ilium

B Pubis

C Ischium
   1   Iliopubic growth plate
      1(a) Open
   2   Ilioischial growth plate
      2(a) Open
      2(b) Closing
   3   Acetabular bone
   4   Ischiopubic growth plate
      4(a) Open
      4(c) Remnant
   5   Symphysis of pelvis
      5(a) Open
   6   Ischiatic tuberosity
   7   Ischiatic tuberosity growth plate
      7(a) Open
      7(b) Closing

   8   Ischial arch centre
   9   Ischial arch growth plate
      9(a) Open
      9(b) Closing
  10 Median ischial arch centre
  11 Median ischial arch growth plate
     11(a) Open

D Femur
  12 Head
  13 Proximal growth plate
     13(a) Open
     13(b) Closing
  14 Greater trochanter
  15 Greater trochanter growth plate
     15(a) Open
     15(b) Closing
  16 Lesser trochanter

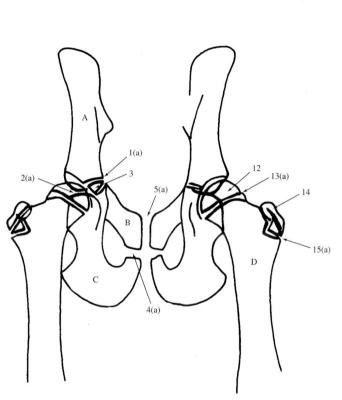

Figure 184

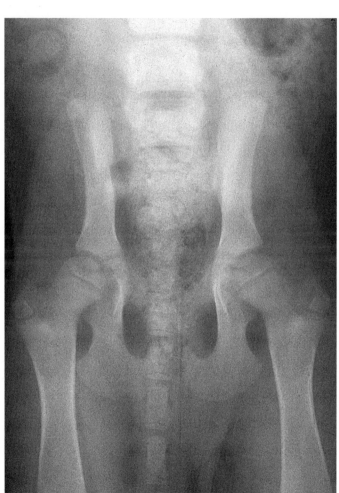

Figure 184 Age 8 weeks.

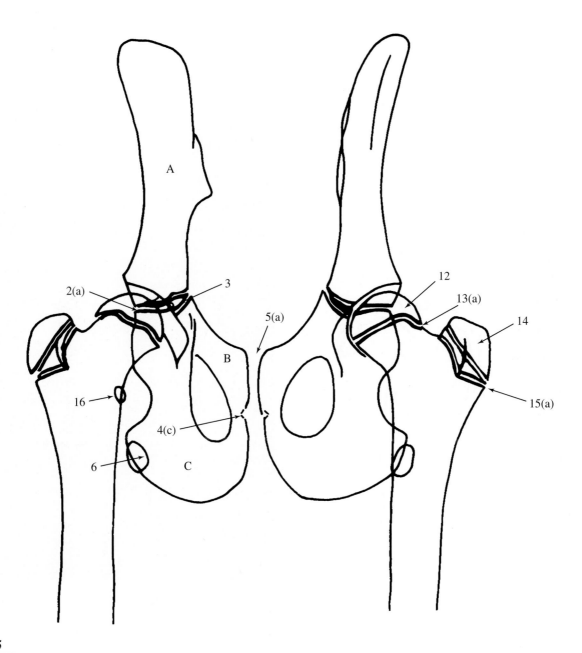

Figure 185

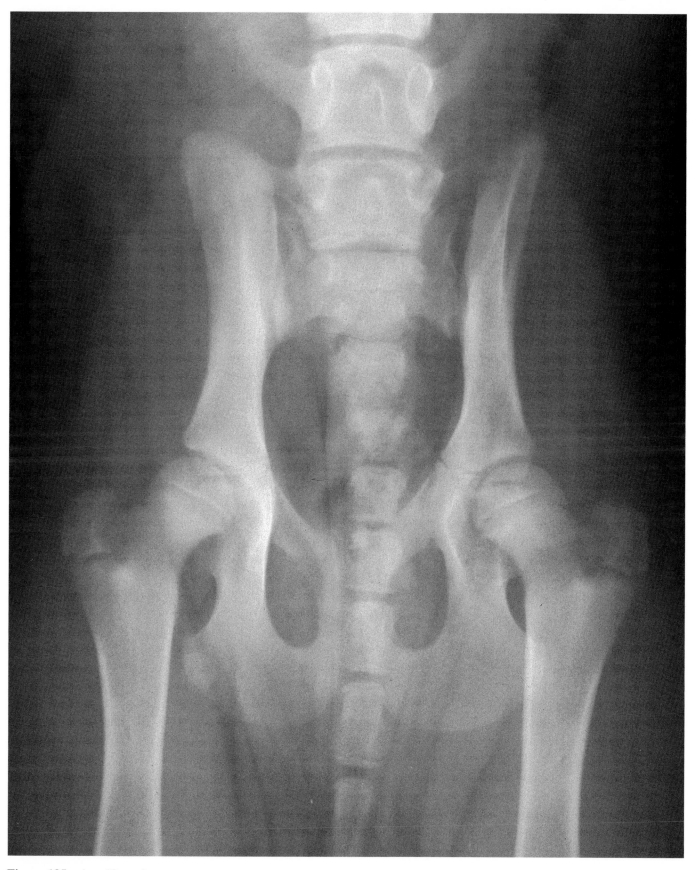

Figure 185   Age 13 weeks.

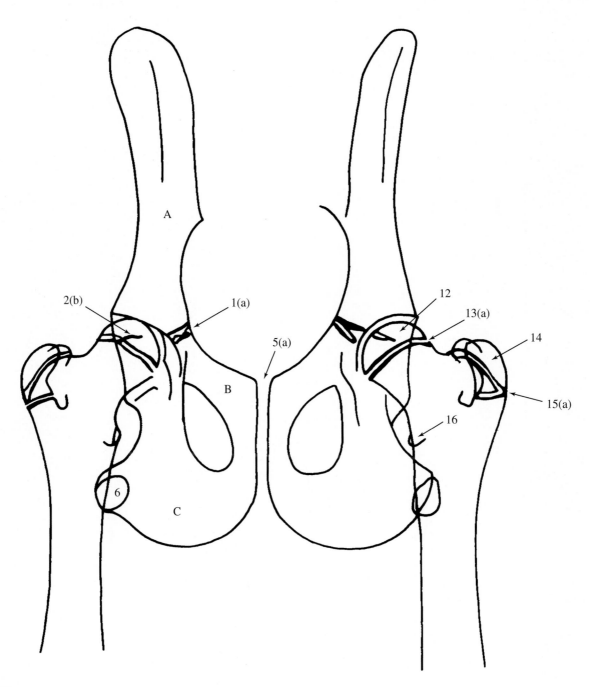

Figure 186

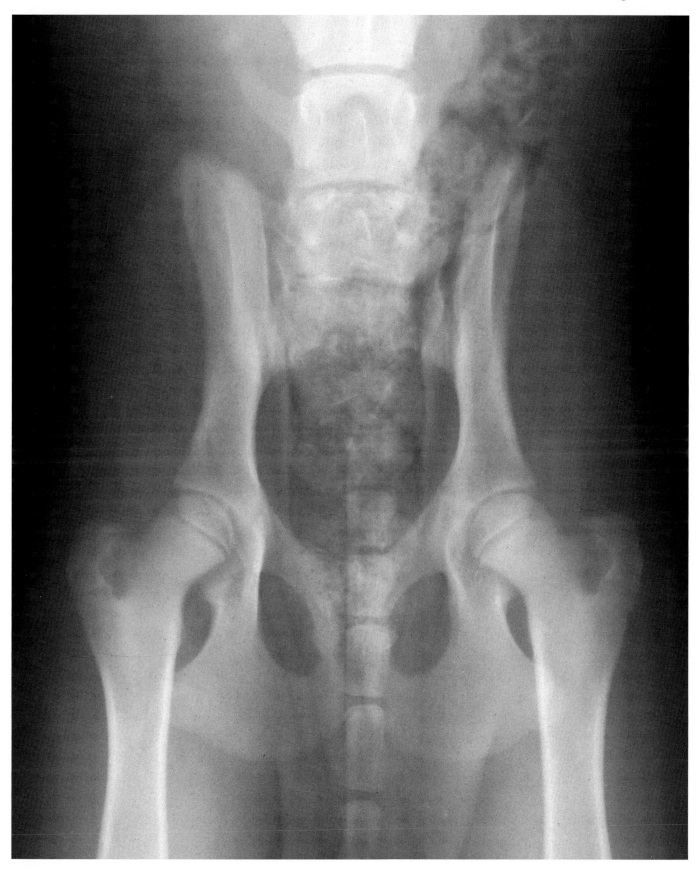

Figure 186 Age 17 weeks.

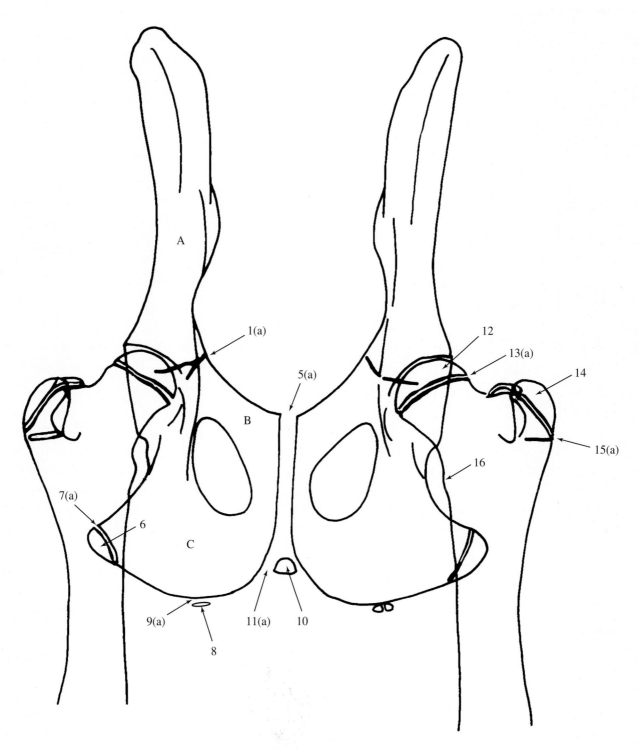

Figure 187

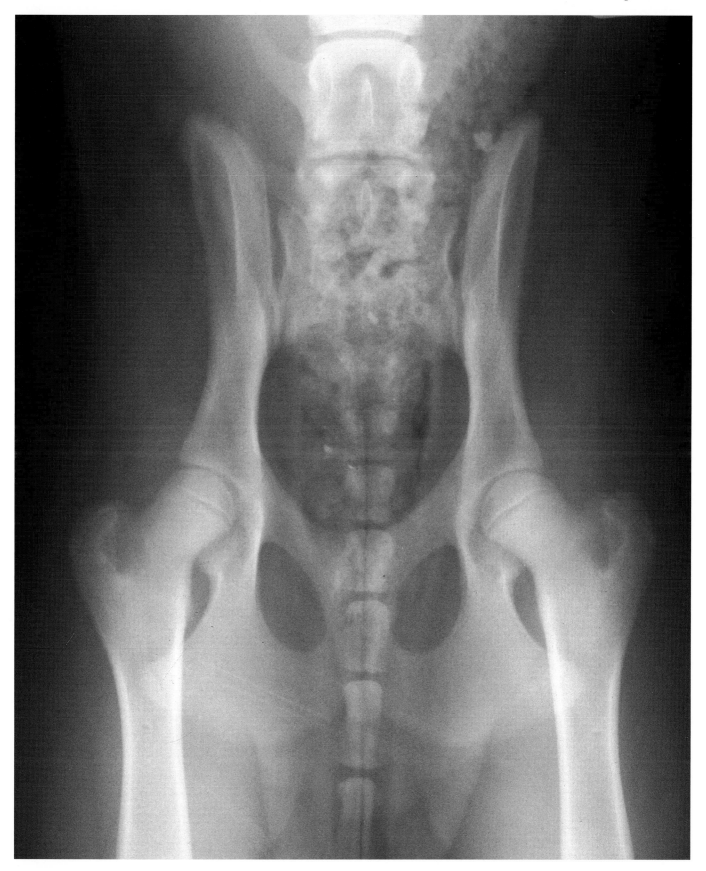

Figure 187   Age 21 weeks.

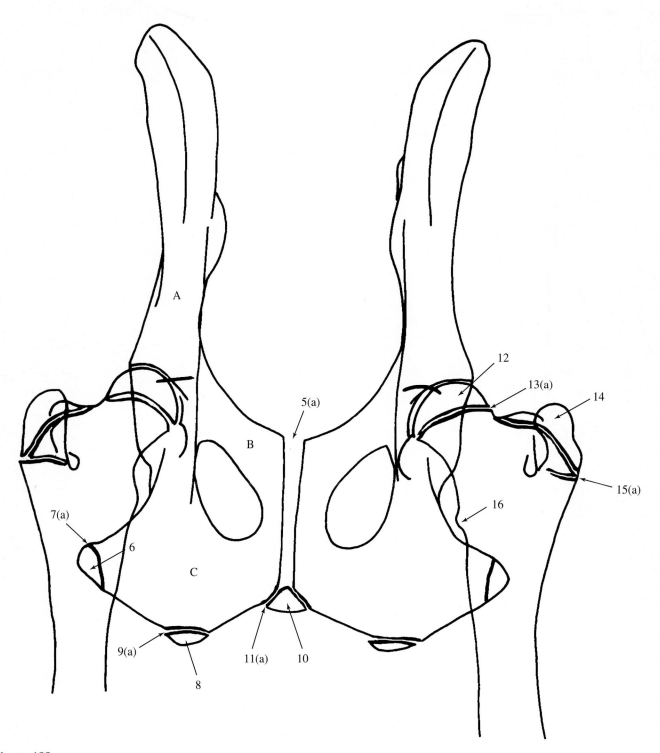

Figure 188

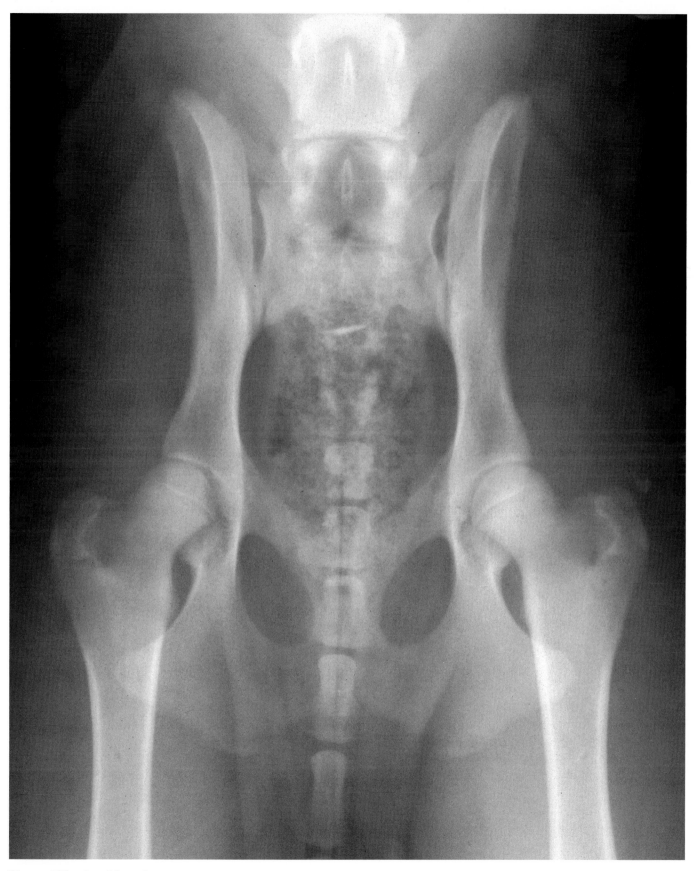

Figure 188 Age 25 weeks.

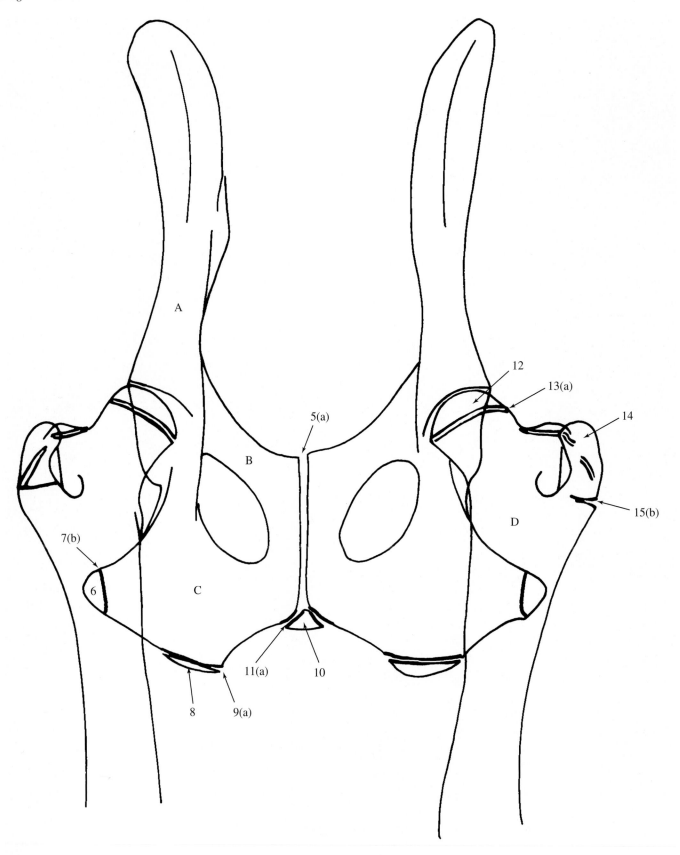

Figure 189

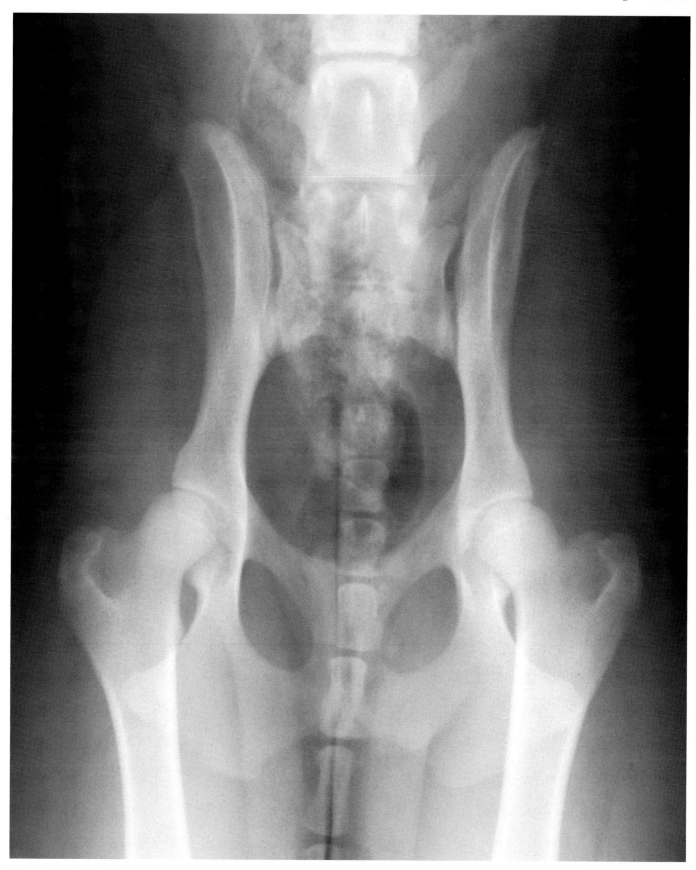

Figure 189 Age 34 weeks.

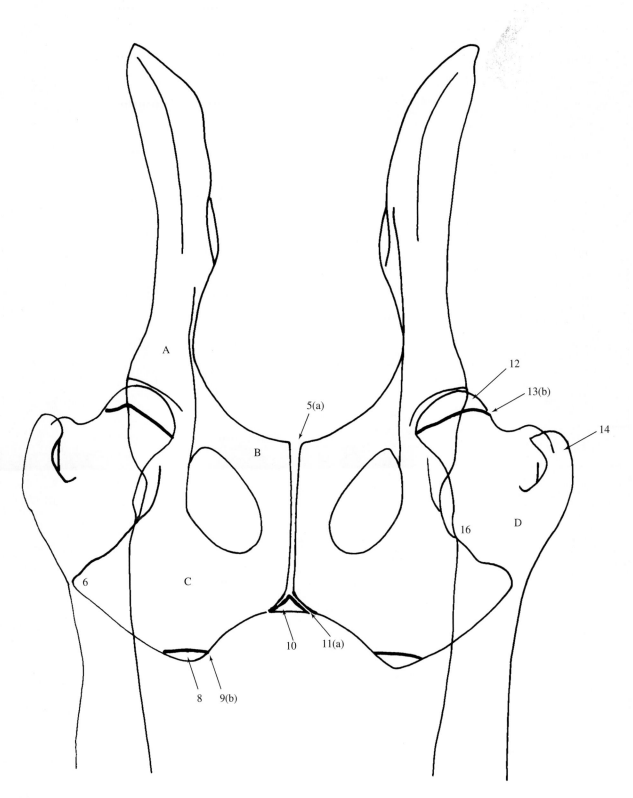

Figure 190

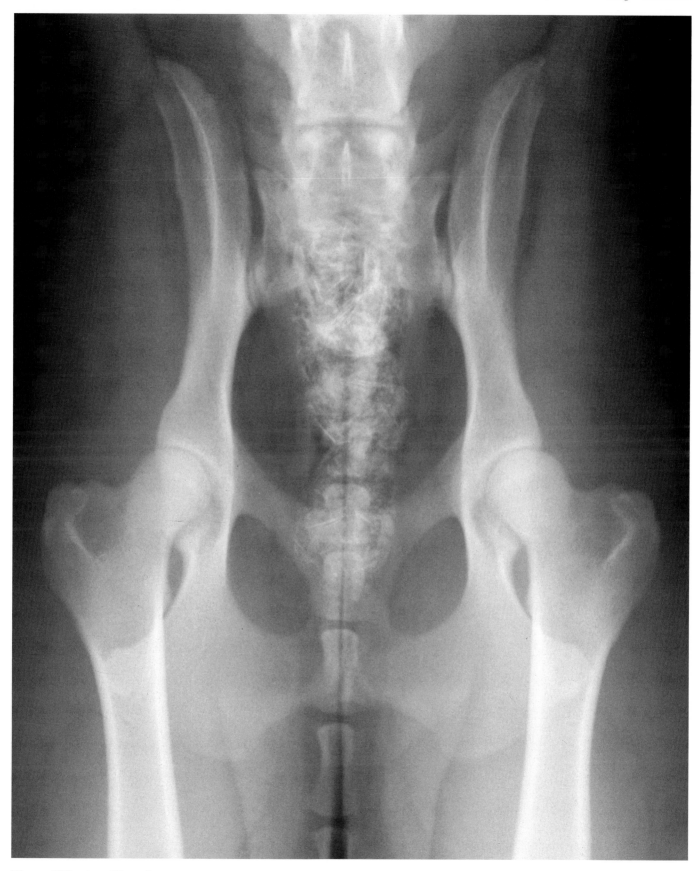

Figure 190 Age 47 weeks.

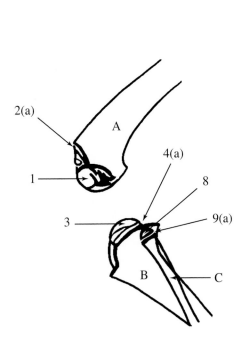

Figure 191

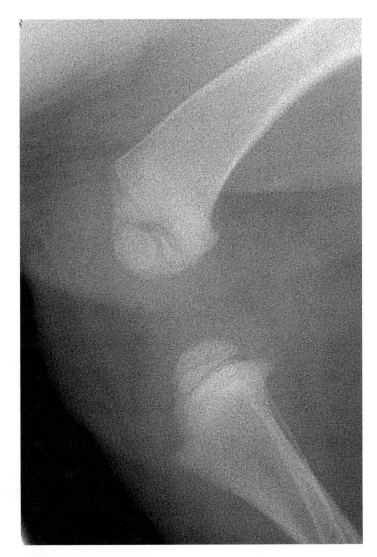

Figure 191   Age 4 weeks.

Figures 191, 192, 193, 194, 195, 196, 197, 198   Mediolateral projection of stifle joint. Samoyed crossbred dog, entire male, at 4, 8, 13, 17, 21, 25, 34 and 43 weeks of age.

A Femur
  1 Distal epiphysis
  2 Distal growth plate
    2(a) Open
    2(b) Closing
    2(c) Remnant

B Tibia
  3 Proximal epiphysis
  4 Proximal growth plate
    4(a) Open
    4(c) Remnant
  5 Tibial tuberosity
  6 Tibial tuberosity growth plate to diaphysis
    6(a) Open
    6(b) Closing

  7 Tibial tuberosity growth plate to proximal epiphysis
    7(a) Open
    7(b) Closing
    7(c) Remnant

C Fibula
  8 Proximal epiphysis
  9 Proximal growth plate
    9(a) Open
    9(c) Remnant

D Patella

E Fabellae of m.gastrocnemius

F Fabella of m.popliteus

An Atlas of Interpretative Radiographic Anatomy of the Dog and Cat

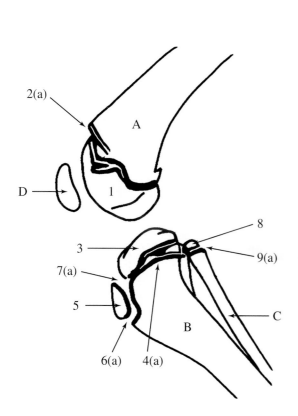

Figure 192

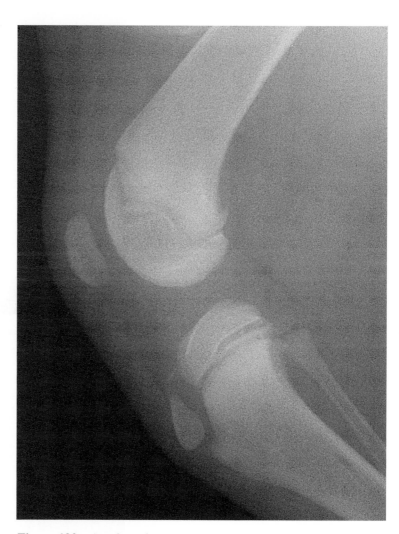

Figure 192 Age 8 weeks.

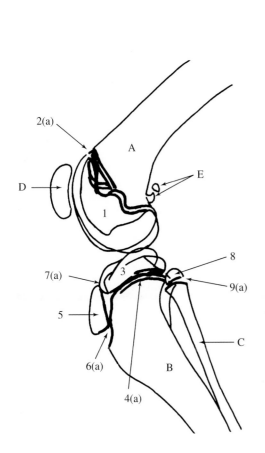

Figure 193

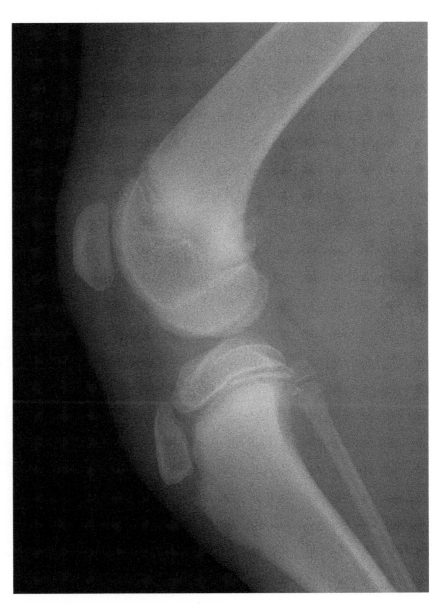

Figure 193   Age 13 weeks.

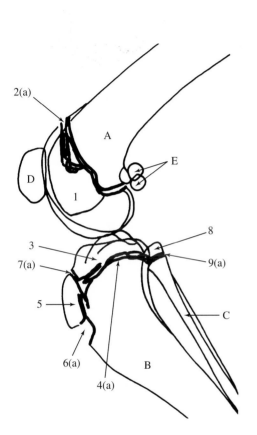

Figure 194

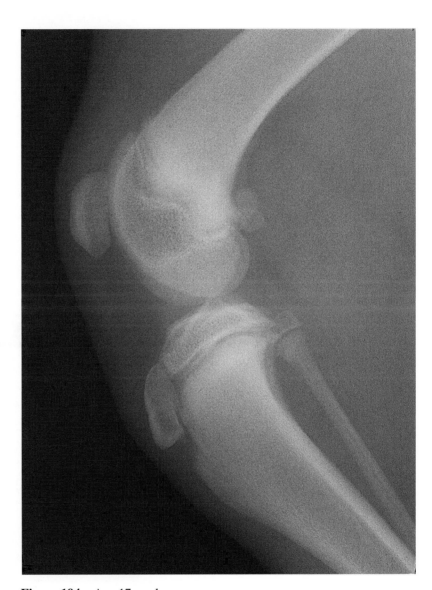

Figure 194   Age 17 weeks.

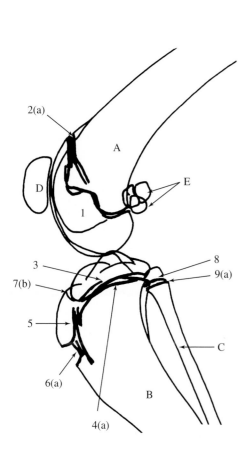

Figure 195

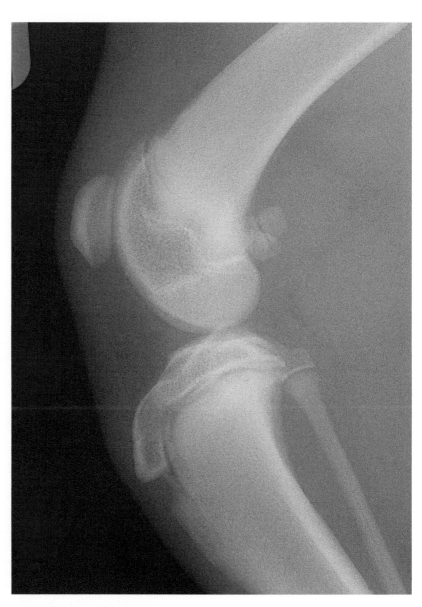

Figure 195   Age 21 weeks.

An Atlas of Interpretative Radiographic Anatomy of the Dog and Cat

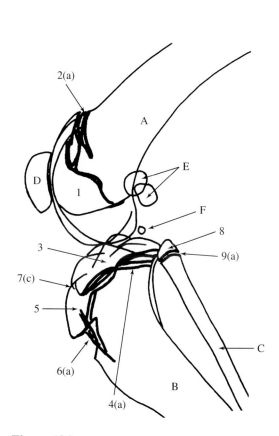

Figure 196

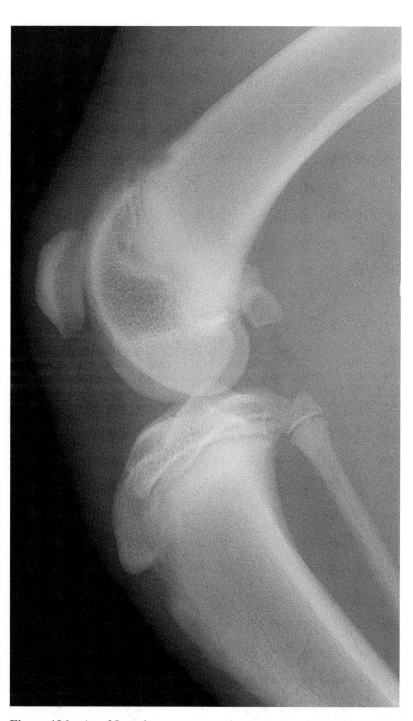

Figure 196   Age 25 weeks.

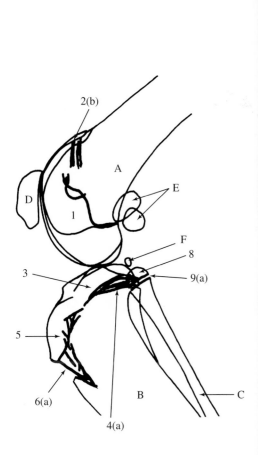

Figure 197

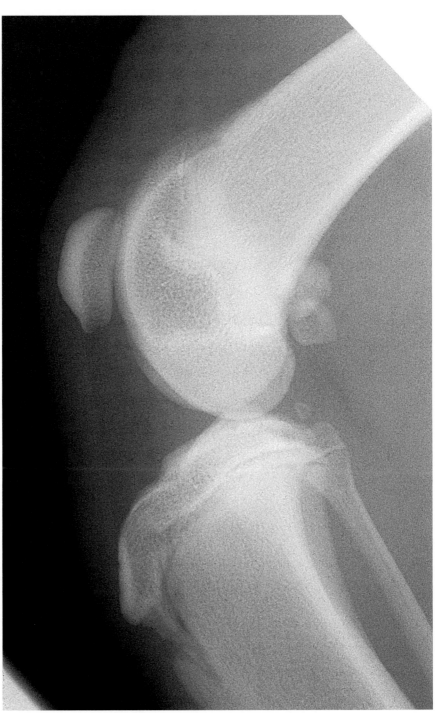

Figure 197 Age 34 weeks.

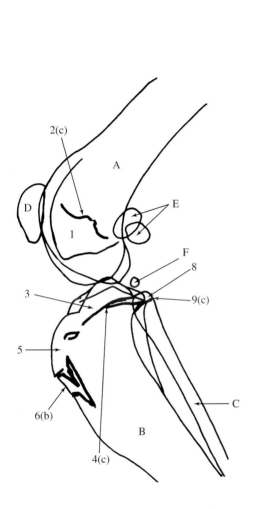

Figure 198

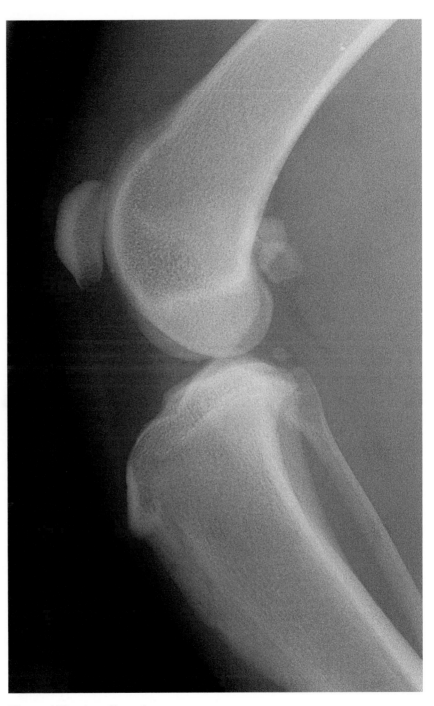

Figure 198   Age 43 weeks.

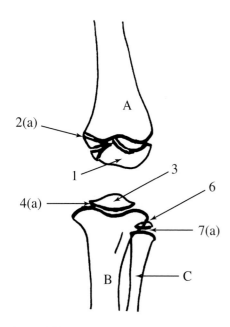

Figure 199

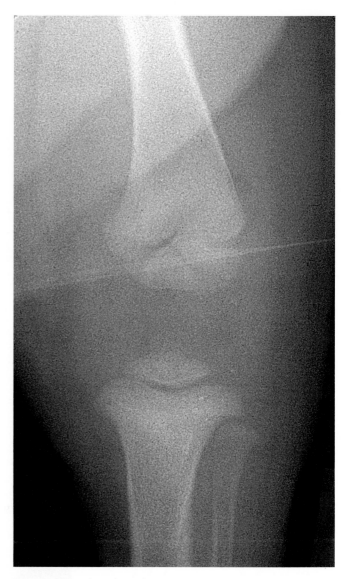

Figure 199   Age 4 weeks.

Figures 199, 200, 201, 202, 203, 204, 205, 206   Craniocaudal projection of stifle joint. Samoyed Crossbred dog, entire male, at 4, 8, 13, 17, 21, 25, 34 and 43 weeks of age.

A Femur
  1 Distal epiphysis
  2 Distal growth plate
    2(a) Open
    2(b) Closing
    2(c) Remnant

B Tibia
  3 Proximal epiphysis
  4 Proximal growth plate
    4(a) Open
    4(c) Remnant
  5 Tibial tuberosity

C Fibula
  6 Proximal epiphysis
  7 Proximal growth plate
    7(a) Open
    7(c) Remnant

D Patella

E Fabella of m.gastrocnemius

Fabella of m.popliteal is not visible on any of these films.

An Atlas of Interpretative Radiographic Anatomy of the Dog and Cat

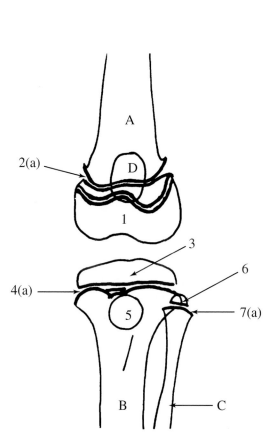

Figure 200

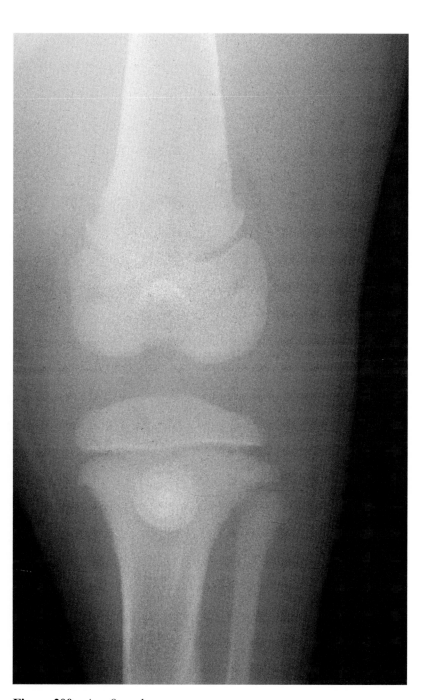

Figure 200 Age 8 weeks.

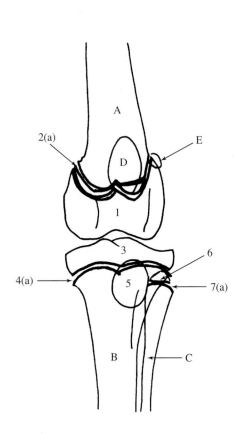

Figure 201

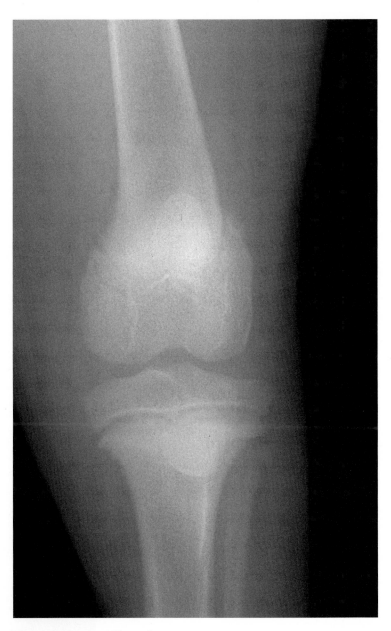

Figure 201   Age 13 weeks.

An Atlas of Interpretative Radiographic Anatomy of the Dog and Cat

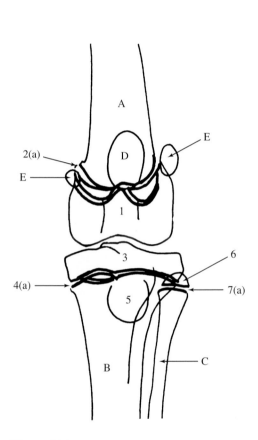

Figure 202

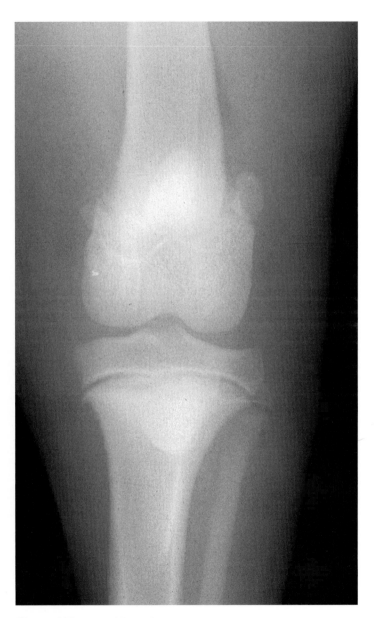

Figure 202   Age 17 weeks.

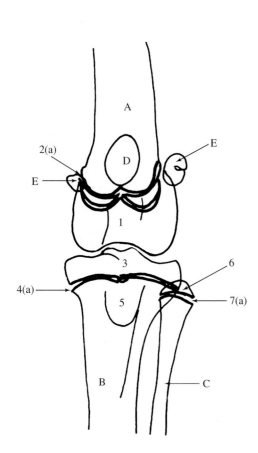

Figure 203

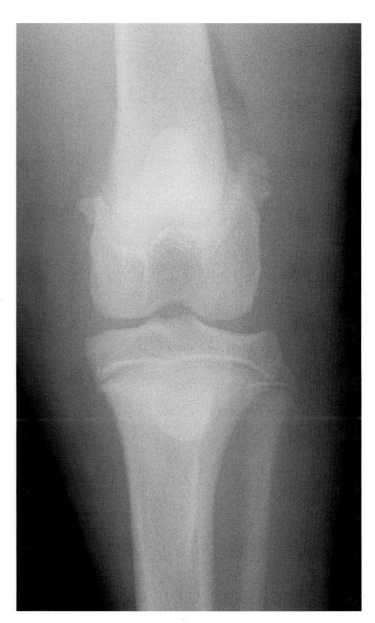

Figure 203   Age 21 weeks.

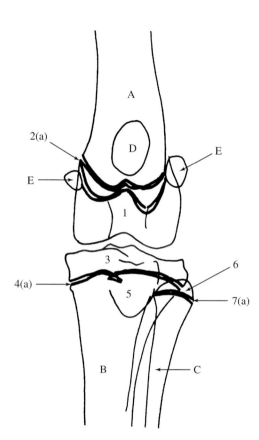

Figure 204

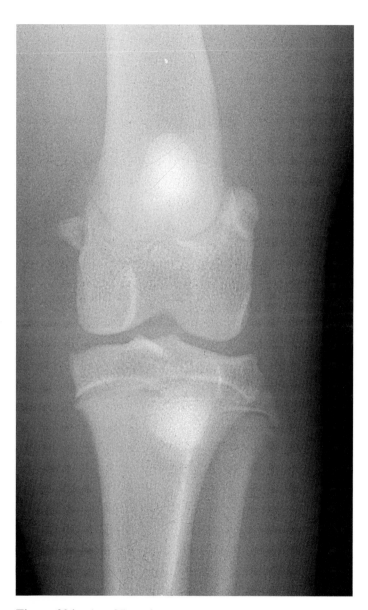

Figure 204   Age 25 weeks.

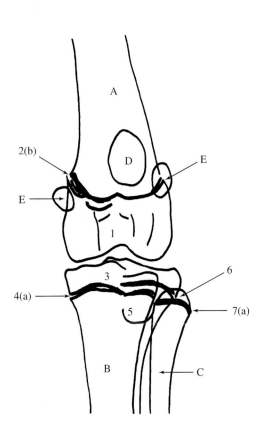

Figure 205

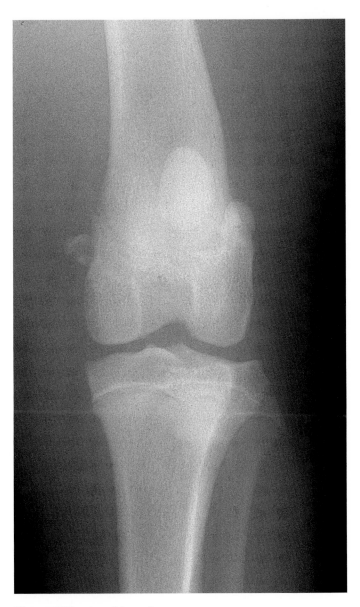

Figure 205   Age 34 weeks.

An Atlas of Interpretative Radiographic Anatomy of the Dog and Cat

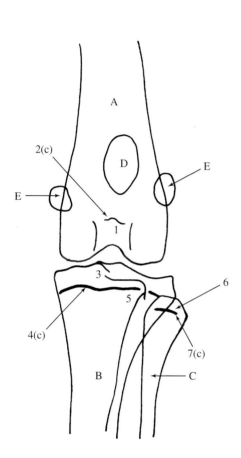

Figure 206

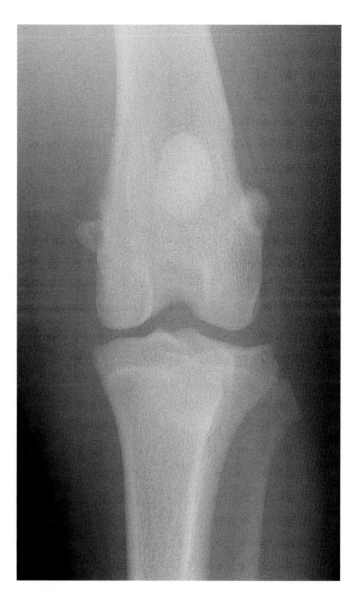

Figure 206 Age 43 weeks.

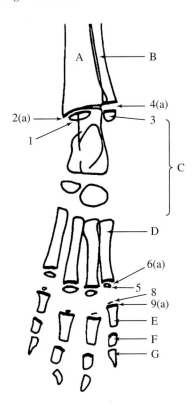

Figure 207

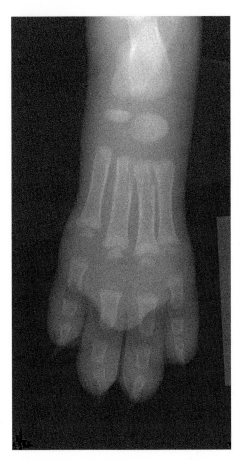

Figure 207 Age 4 weeks.

Figures 207, 208, 209, 210, 211, 212 Dorsoplantar projection of tarsus, metatarsal bones and phalanges. Samoyed Crossbred dog, entire male, at 4, 8, 13, 21, 25 and 34 weeks of age.

A Tibia
  1 Distal epiphysis.
     Initially with separate ossification centre for medial malleolus.
  2 Distal growth plate
     2(a) Open
     2(b) Closing
     2(c) Remnant

B Fibula
  3 Distal epiphysis
  4 Distal growth plate
     4(a) Open
     4(b) Closing

C Tarsus.
  Only tibial tarsal bone, body of fibular tarsal bone, central tarsal bone and tarsal bone 4 are seen at 4 weeks of age.

D Metatarsal bone 5 (2, 3 and 4 are similar)
  5 Epiphysis.
     Note that there is only a distal epiphysis in these metatarsal bones.

  6 Growth plate
     6(a) Open
     6(b) Closing
  7 Proximal sesamoid bones

E Proximal phalanx of digit 5 (2, 3 and 4 are similar)
  8 Epiphysis.
     Note that there is only a proximal epiphysis in the proximal phalanges.
  9 Growth plate
     9(a) Open
     9(b) Closing

F Middle phalanx of digit 5 (2, 3 and 4 are similar)
  10 Epiphysis.
      Note that there is only a proximal epiphysis in the middle phalanges.
  11 Growth plate
      11(a) Open

G Distal phalanx of digit 5 (2, 3 and 4 are similar)

H Metatarsal bone 1

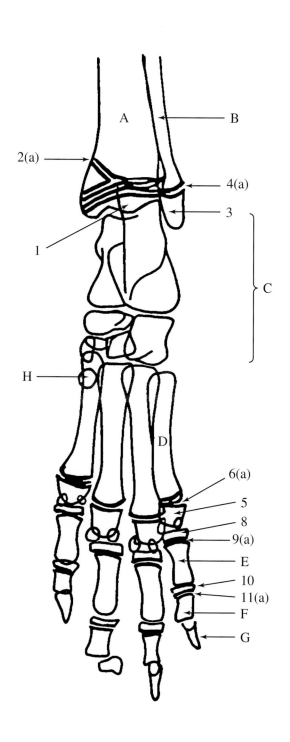

Figure 208

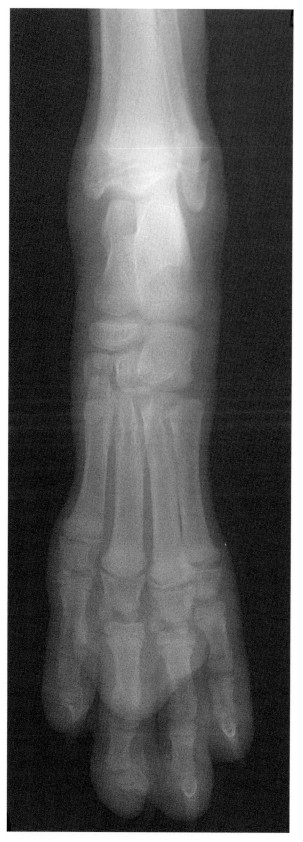

Figure 208   Age 8 weeks.

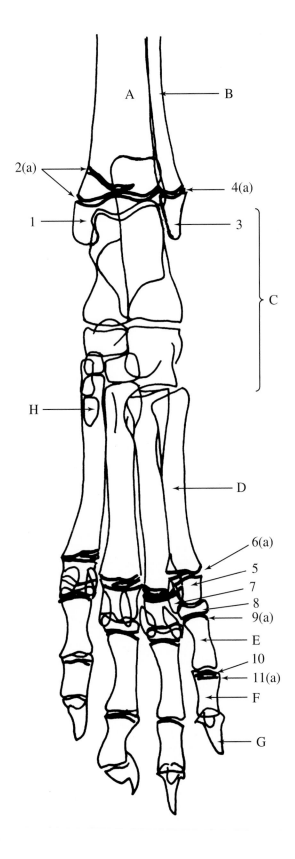

Figure 209

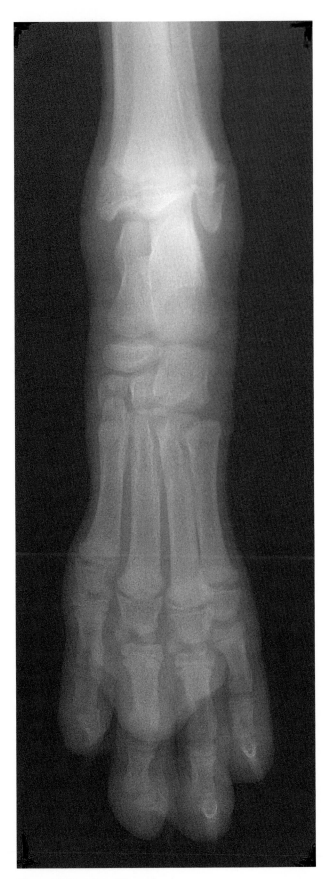

Figure 209   Age 13 weeks.

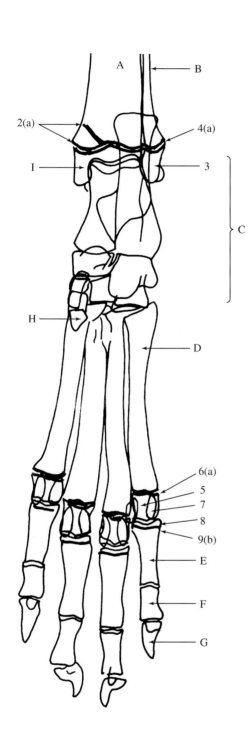

Figure 210

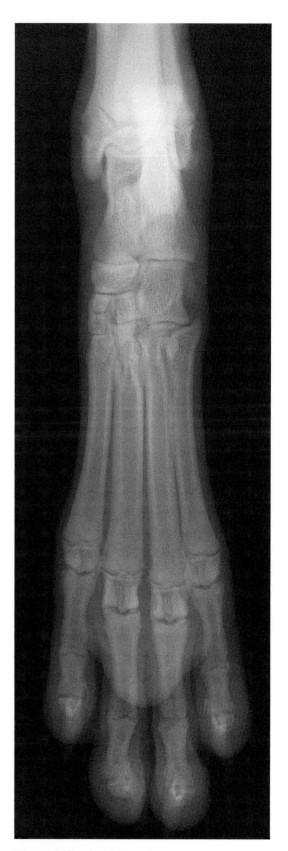

Figure 210   Age 21 weeks.

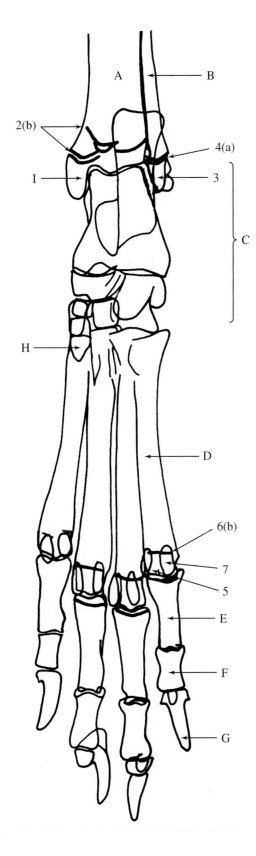

Figure 211

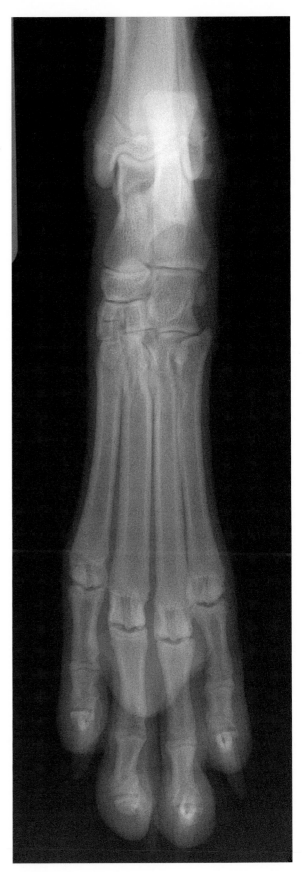

Figure 211   Age 25 weeks.

An Atlas of Interpretative Radiographic Anatomy of the Dog and Cat

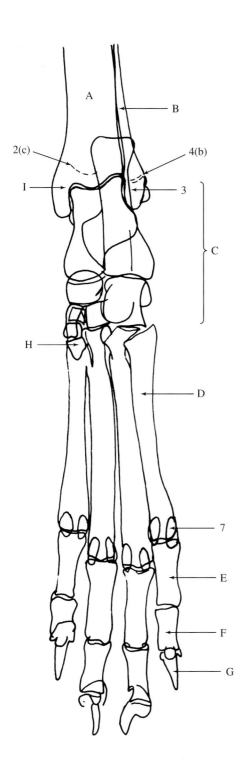

A

B

2(c)

4(b)

I

3

C

H

D

7

E

F

G

Figure 212

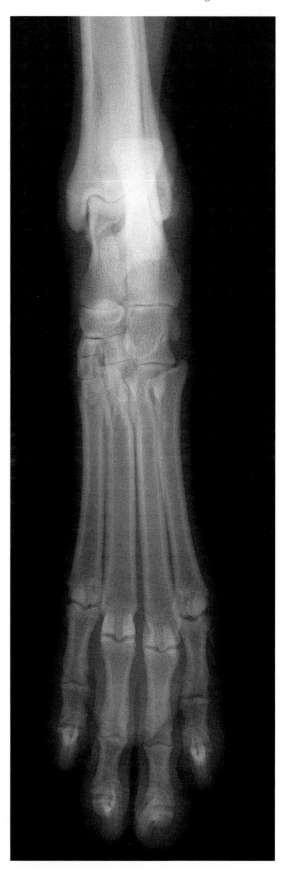

Figure 212 Age 34 weeks.

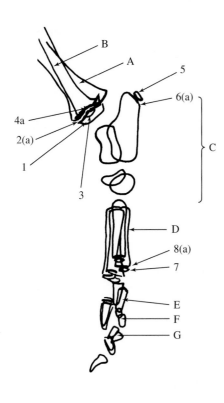

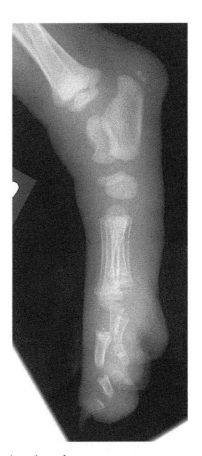

Figure 213

Figure 213   Age 4 weeks.

Figures 213, 214, 215, 216, 217, 218   Mediolateral projection of tarsus, metatarsal bones and phalanges. Samoyed Crossbred dog, entire male, at 4, 8, 13, 21, 25 and 34 weeks of age.

A Tibia
  1 Distal epiphysis
  2 Distal growth plate
    2(a) Open
    2(b) Closing
    2(c) Remnant

B Fibula
  3 Distal epiphysis
  4 Distal growth plate
    4(a) Open
    4(b) Closing

C Tarsus.
  Only tibial tarsal bone, body of fibular tarsal bone, central tarsal bone and tarsal bone 4 are seen at 4 weeks of age.
  5 Epiphysis of fibular tarsal bone
  6 Fibular tarsal bone growth plate
    6(a) Open
    6(b) Closing
    6(c) Remnant

D Metatarsal bone 2 or 5 (3 and 4 are similar)
  7 Epiphysis.
    Note that there is only a distal epiphysis in these metatarsal bones.

8 Growth plate
  8(a) Open
  8(b) Closing
9 Proximal sesamoids

E Proximal phalanx 2 or 5 (3 and 4 are similar)
  10 Epiphysis.
    Note that there is only a proximal epiphysis in the proximal phalanges.
  11 Growth plate
    11(a) Open
    11(b) Closing

F Middle phalanx 2 or 5
  12 Epiphysis.
    Note that there is only a proximal epiphysis in the middle phalanges.
  13 Growth plate
    13(a) Open
    13(b) Closing

G Distal phalanx 2 or 5

H Metatarsal bone 1

I Dorsal sesamoid bone

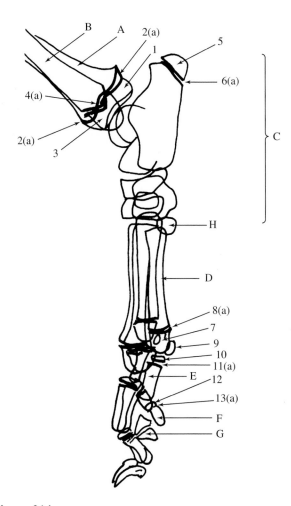

Figure 214

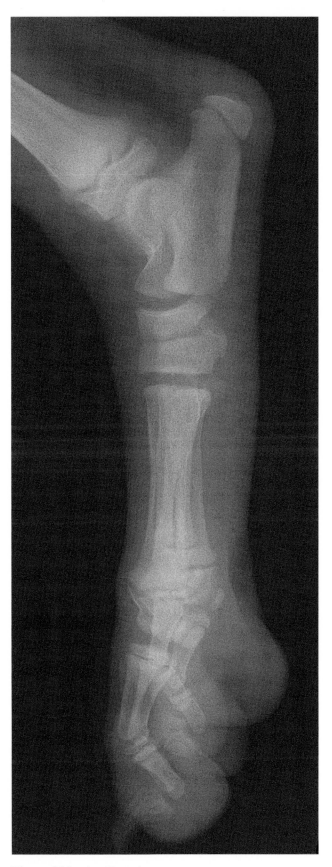

Figure 214   Age 8 weeks.

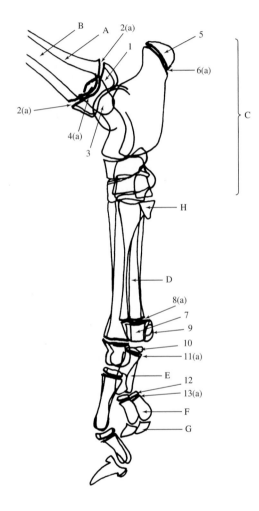

Figure 215

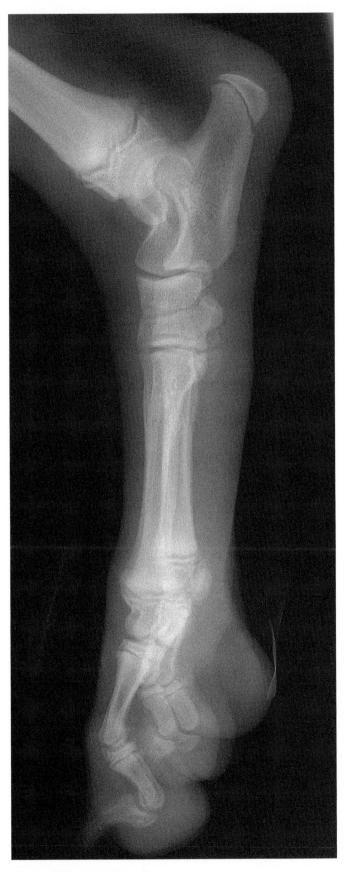

Figure 215 Age 13 weeks.

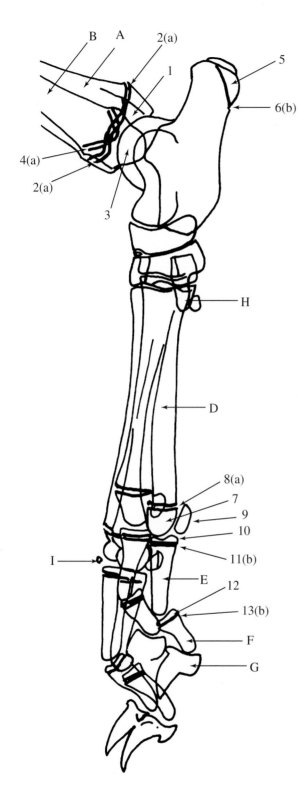

Figure 216

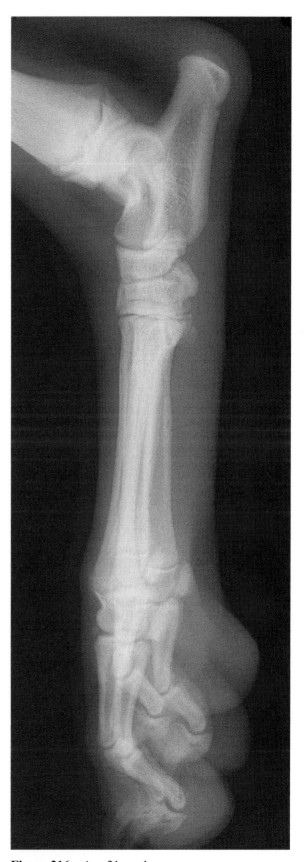

Figure 216   Age 21 weeks.

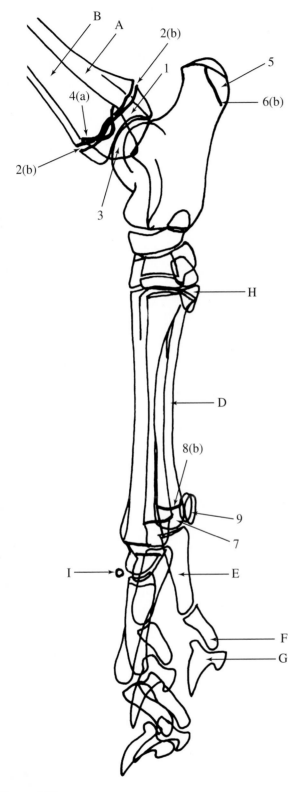

Figure 217

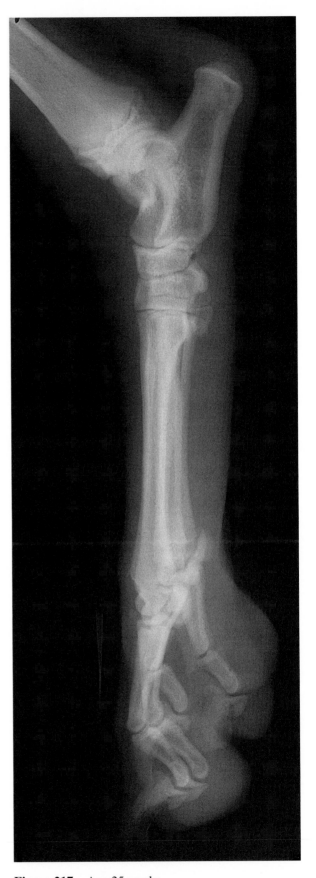

Figure 217 Age 25 weeks.

An Atlas of Interpretative Radiographic Anatomy of the Dog and Cat

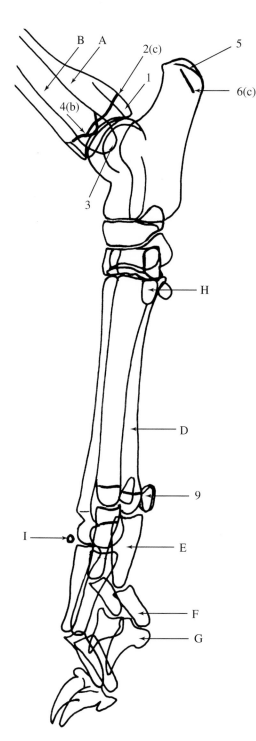

Figure 218

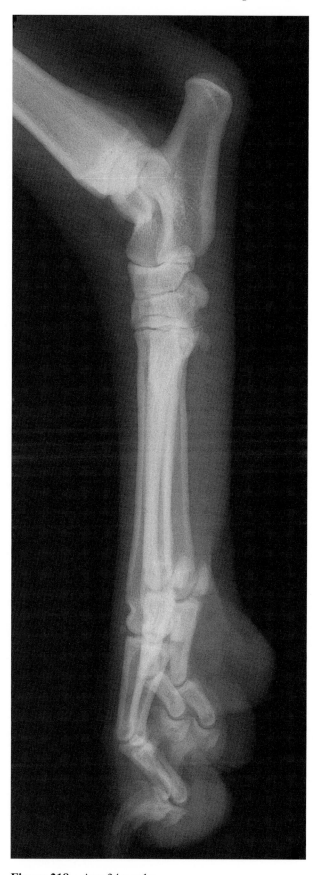

Figure 218 Age 34 weeks.

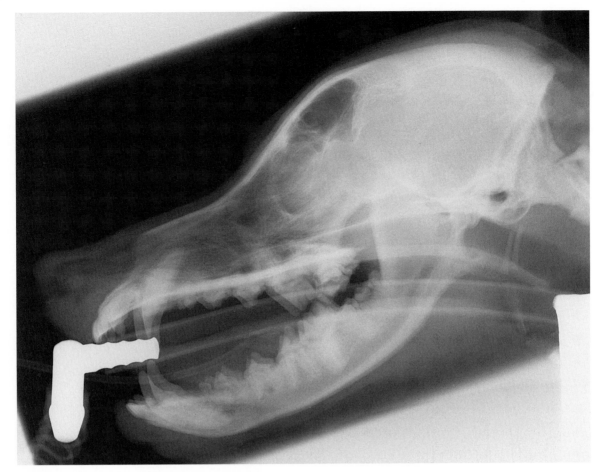

Figure 219   Lateral projection of skull. Beagle dog 2.5 years old, entire male.

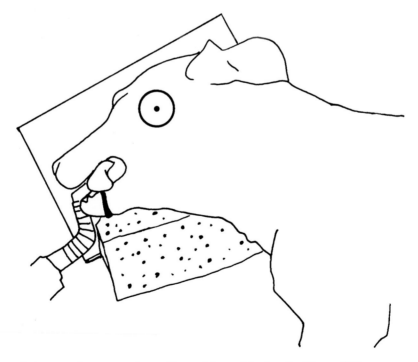

Figure 220   Line drawing of photograph representing radiographic positioning for Figure 219.

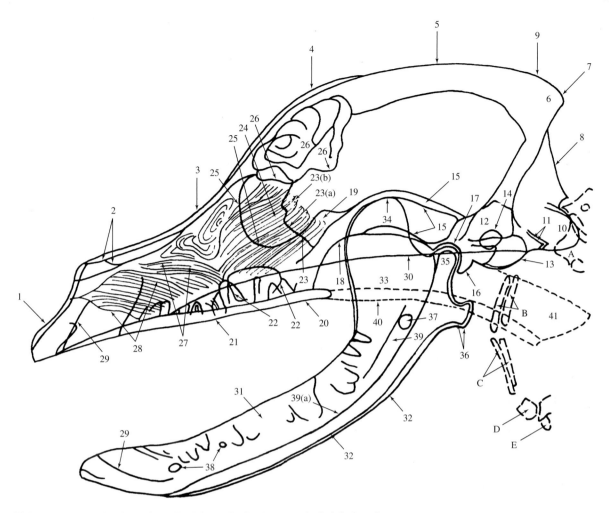

Figure 221 Lateral projection of skull with teeth shadows excluded for clarity.

A Atlas

B Stylohyoid bones

C Epihyoid bones

D Ceratohyoid bones

E Basihyoid bone
  1 Incisive bone
  2 Nasal bone
  3 Maxilla or maxillary bone
  4 Frontal bone
  5 Parietal bone
  6 Occipital bone
  7 External occipital protuberance
  8 External occipital crest
  9 Interparietal process of occipital bone
  10 Occipital bone
  11 Paracondylar process of occipital bone or jugular process
  12 Petrous temporal bone or temporal bone; petrosal part.

13 Tympanic bulla of temporal bone or temporal bone; tympanic part.
14 External acoustic meatus of temporal bone
15 Zygomatic process of temporal bone or temporal bone; squamous part.
16 Retroarticular process of temporal bone
17 Mandibular fossa of temporal bone
18 Masseteric border of zygomatic bone
19 Frontal process of zygomatic bone
20 Palatine bone
21 Vomer
22 Maxillary sinus of maxilla
23 Cribriform plate of ethmoid bone
   23(a) Rostral limit
   23(b) Caudal limit

24 Ethmoturbinates of ethmoid bone
25 Orbital margin
26 Frontal sinuses. Total of six; three on each side.
27 Dorsal nasal concha of ethmoid bone
28 Ventral nasal concha of maxilla
29 Lamina dura
30 Basisphenoid bone
31 Mandible
32 Mandibular body
33 Mandibular ramus
34 Coronoid process of mandible
35 Condyloid or articular process of mandible
36 Angular processes of mandible
37 Mandibular foramen
38 Mental foramen
39 Mandibular canal
   39(a) Ventral border
40 Soft palate
41 Nasopharynx

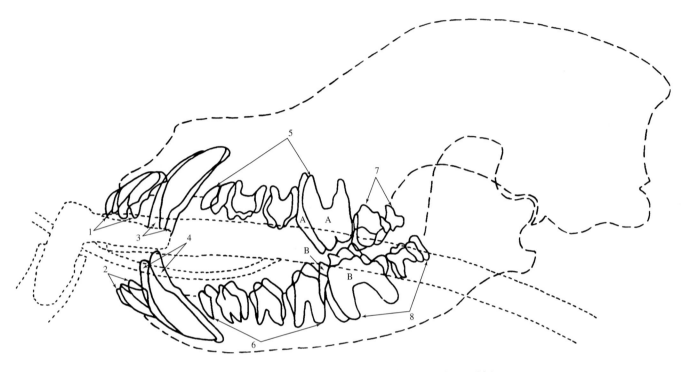

Figure 222 Lateral projection of skull to demonstrate details of teeth excluded in Figure 221.

1 Upper incisors. Total of six.
2 Lower incisors. Total of six.
3 Upper canines. Total of two.
4 Lower canines. Total of two.
5 Upper premolars. Total of eight.
6 Lower premolars. Total of eight.
7 Upper molars. Total of four.
8 Lower molars. Total of six.

A Upper carnassial; 4th. premolar

B Lower carnassial; 1st. molar

Line drawing only illustrates gross details of teeth as seen in radiograph, Figure 219. More detailed drawings are given in the section on dentition.

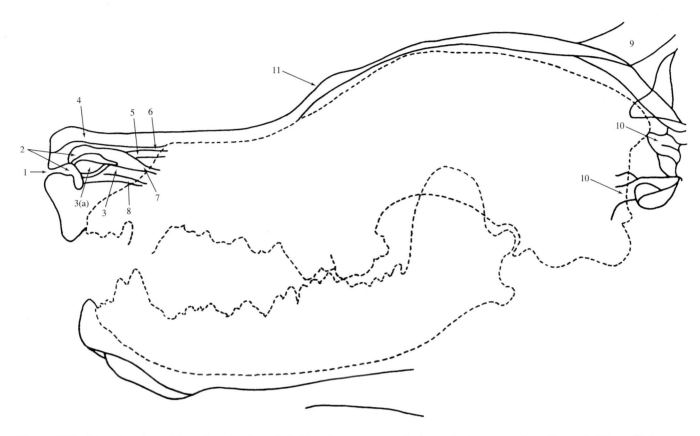

Figure 223   Line drawing of lateral projection of skull to demonstrate soft tissue shadows seen in radiograph, Figure 219.

External nose
1 Nostril
2 Nasal vestibule
3 Alar nasal fold
   3(a) Bulbous terminal enlargement
4 Dorsolateral nasal cartilage
5 Straight nasal fold
6 Dorsal nasal meatus
7 Middle nasal meatus
8 Ventral nasal meatus

External ear
9 Pinna
10 Ear canals
The superimposed shadows, 9 and 10, of the external ear can be confused as bony abnormalities.

11 Skin fold level with dorsal aspect of orbits

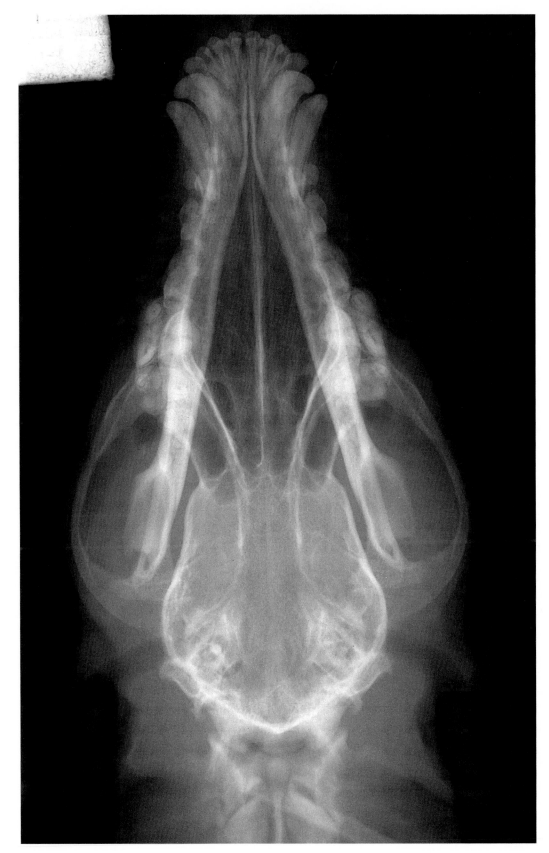

Figure 224 Ventrodorsal projection of skull. Beagle dog 2.5 years old, entire male (same dog as in dorsoventral projection of skull, Figure 230).

An Atlas of Interpretative Radiographic Anatomy of the Dog and Cat

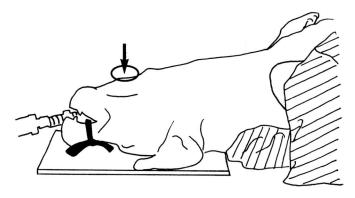

Figure 225 Line drawing of photograph representing radiographic positioning for Figure 224.

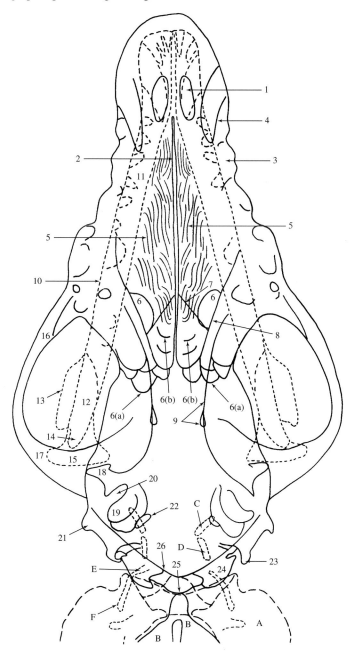

Figure 226 Ventrodorsal projection of skull with teeth shadows excluded for clarity.

A Atlas
B Axis
  Hyoid apparatus. The bony shadows are indistinct but all are visible except for the basihyoid.
C Stylohyoid bone
D Epihyoid bone
E Ceratohyoid bone
F Thyrohyoid bone
  1 Palatine fissure
  2 Vomer
  3 Maxillary teeth obscuring maxilla shadow
  4 Lamina dura
  5 Ventral nasal conchae and ethmoturbinates
  6 Frontal sinuses
    6(a) Frontal sinuses (lateral)
    6(b) Frontal sinuses (medial)
  7 Cribriform plate of ethmoid enclosing ethmoidal fossa
  8 Medial wall of orbit
  9 Border of choanae formed by palatine bone and pterygoid bone. (Hamulus seen as the more opaque shadow at caudal extremity.)
  10 Mandible
  11 Mandibular body
  12 Mandibular ramus

13 Coronoid process of mandible
14 Angular process of mandible
15 Condyloid or articular process of mandible
16 Temporal process of zygomatic bone
17 Zygomatic process of temporal bone 16 and 17 form the zygomatic arch
18 Retroarticular process of temporal bone
19 Tympanic bulla of temporal bone; tympanic part
20 External acoustic meatus of temporal bone; tympanic part
21 Mastoid process of temporal bone; tympanic part
22 Jugular foramen of temporal bone; tympanic part
23 Paracondylar process of occipital bone or jugular process
24 Occipital condyle
25 External occipital protuberance
26 Nuchal crest of occipital bone

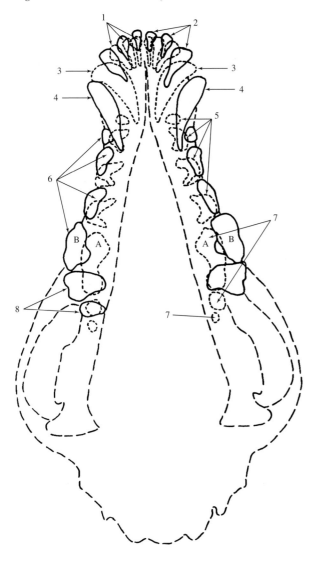

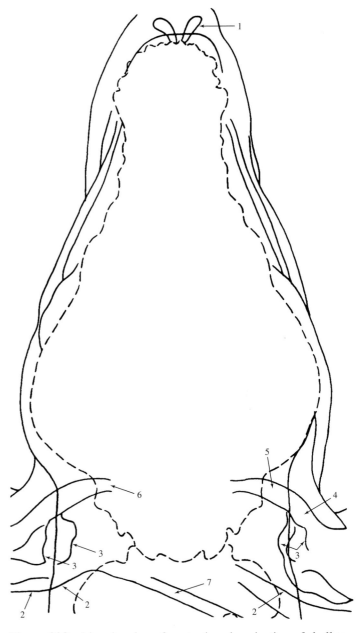

Figure 227 Line drawing to demonstrate teeth shadows excluded in Figure 226. Ventrodorsal projection of skull.

1 Lower incisor teeth. Total of six
2 Upper incisor teeth. Total of six.
3 Lower canine teeth. Total of two.
4 Upper canine teeth. Total of two.
5 Lower premolar teeth. Total of eight.
6 Upper premolar teeth. Total of eight.
7 Lower molar teeth. Total of six.
8 Upper molar teeth. Total of four. (In this dog 2nd. molar on left side is missing.)

A Lower carnassial; 1st. molar
B Upper carnassial; 4th. premolar

The drawing only illustrates gross details of teeth as seen in radiograph. More detailed drawings are given in the section on dentition.

Figure 228 Line drawing of ventrodorsal projection of skull to demonstrate soft tissue shadows seen in radiograph, Figure 224

1 Nostril
2 Caudal limit of pinna
3 Internal folds of pinna
4 Vertical ear canal
5 Horizontal ear canal
6 External acoustic meatus
7 Neck skin fold

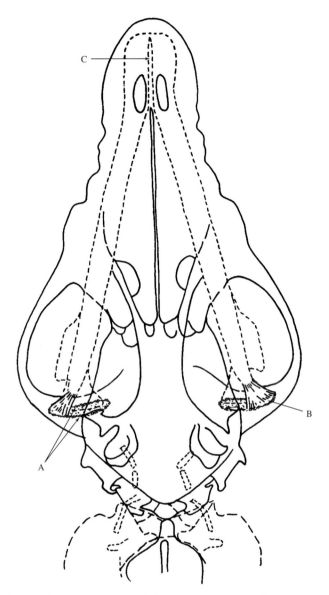

Figure 229 Schematic drawing of ventrodorsal projection of skull to demonstrate the temporomandibular joints and mandibular symphysis.

A = Capsule of temporomandibular joint

B = Lateral ligament

Between the cartilage covered bony articulations is found an articular disc.

C = Symphysis of mandible. (Fibrocartilage is seen as a radiolucent region in the radiograph.)

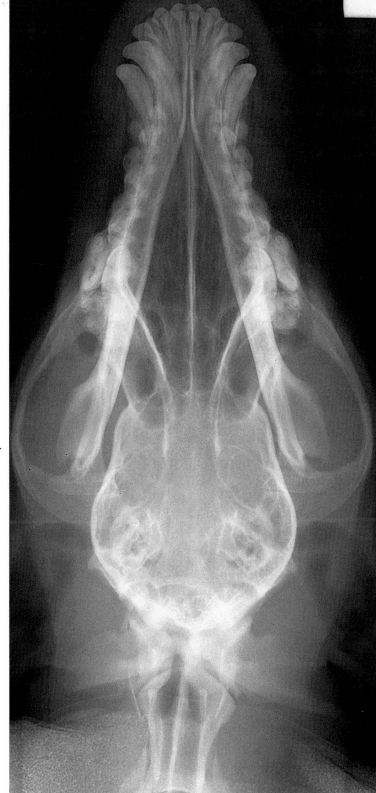

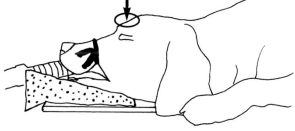

Figure 231 Line drawing of photograph representing radiographic positioning for Figure 230.

Figure 230 Dorsoventral projection of skull. Beagle dog 2.5 years old, entire male (same dog as in ventrodorsal projection of skull, Figure 224).

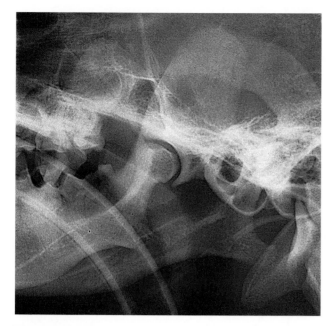

Figure 232   Rostrocaudal oblique (45 degree nose tilt) projection of temporomandibular joints. Doberman dog 7 years old, entire male.

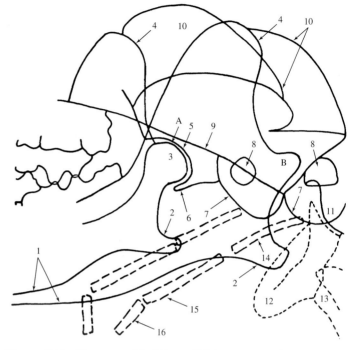

Figure 234   Rostrocaudal oblique (45 degree nose tilt) projection of temporomandibular joints.

A Temporomandibular joint of recumbent side

B Position of temporo-mandibular joint of non-recumbent side obscured by petrous temporal bones

1 Mandibular body
2 Angular process of mandible
3 Condyloid or articular process of mandible
4 Coronoid process of mandible
5 Mandibular fossa of temporal bone

6 Retroarticular process of temporal bone
7 Tympanic bulla of temporal bone
8 External acoustic meatus of temporal bone
9 Basisphenoid bone
10 Temporal process of zygomatic bone
11 Condyle of occipital bone
12 Atlas
13 Axis
14 Stylohoid bone
15 Epihyoid bone
16 Ceratohyoid bone

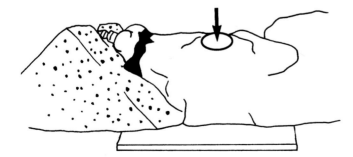

Figure 233   Line drawing of photograph representing radiographic positioning for Figure 232.

An Atlas of Interpretative Radiographic Anatomy of the Dog and Cat

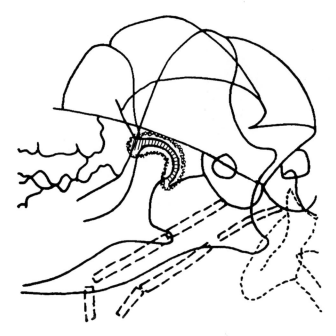

Figure 235   Schematic drawing of rostrocaudal oblique (45 degree nose tilt) projection of temporomandibular joints to demonstrate joint capsule and disc.

= Joint capsule

///// = Articular disc. Divides joint into ventral and dorsal compartments.

Laterally the joint capsule is strengthened to form a fibrous lateral ligament.

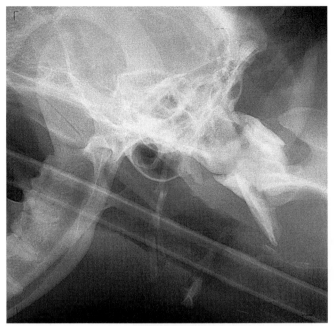

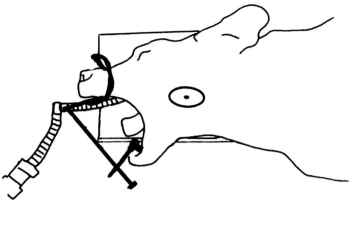

Figure 236   Relaxed lateral (open mouth) projection of tympanic bullae. Beagle dog 2.5 years old, entire male.

Figure 237   Line drawing of photograph representing radiographic postioning for Figure 236.

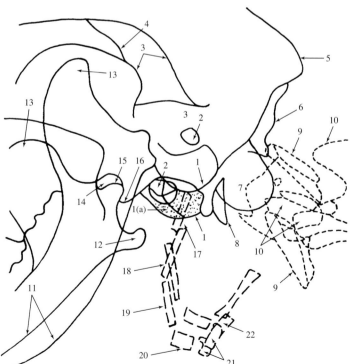

Figure 238   Relaxed lateral (open mouth) projection of tympanic bullae.

1 Tympanic bulla of
   temporal bone
   1(a) Recumbent side
         (shaded in drawing)
2 External acoustic meatus
   of temporal bone
3 Zygomatic process of
   temporal bone
4 Temporozygomatic suture
5 External protuberance of
   occipital bone
6 External occipital crest
7 Occipital condyle
8 Paracondylar process of
   occipital bone or jugular
   process
9 Atlas
10 Axis
11 Mandible
12 Angular process of
   mandible
13 Coronoid process of
   mandible

14 Condyloid or articular
   process of mandible
15 Mandibular fossa of
   temporal bone

Note that 14 and 15 are
superimposed, hence the
temporomandibular joint is
not demonstrated.

16 Retroarticular process of
   temporal bone

Hyoid apparatus

17 Tympanohyoid cartilage
   (seen as a radiolucent
   region between
   tympanic bulla
   and stylohyoid
   bone)
18 Stylohyoid bone
19 Epihyoid bone
20 Ceratohyoid bone
21 Basihyoid bone
22 Thyrohyoid bone

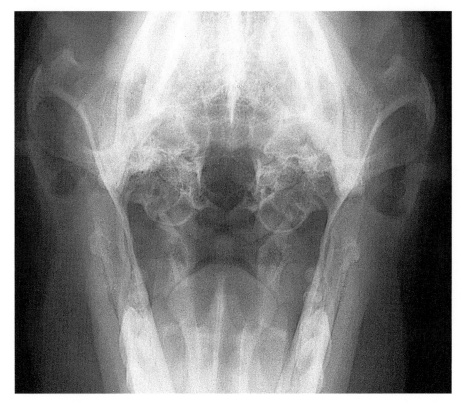

Figure 239   Rostroventral-caudodorsal oblique (open mouth) projection of tympanic bullae. Beagle dog 2.5 years old, entire male.

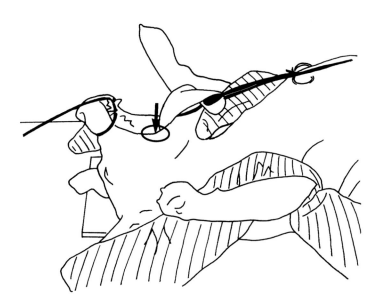

Figure 240   Line drawing of photograph representing radiographic positioning for Figure 239.

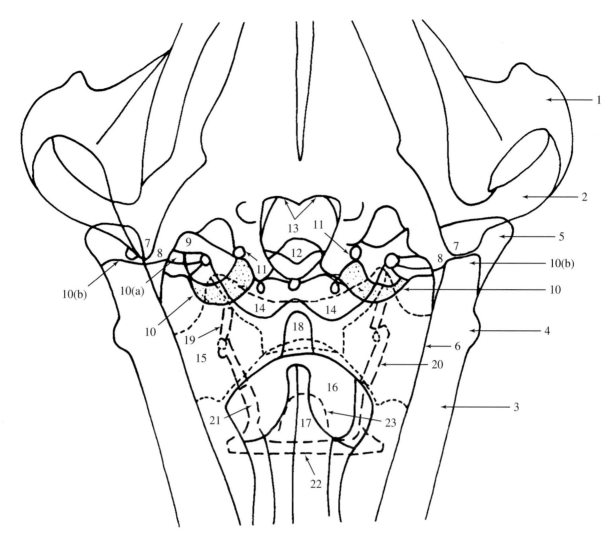

Figure 241   Rostroventral–caudodorsal oblique (open mouth) projection of tympanic bullae.

1   Temporal process of zygomatic bone
2   Zygomatic process of temporal bone
3   Mandibular body
4   Angular process of mandible
5   Condyloid or articular process of mandible
6   Vertical ramus of mandible
7   Retroarticular process of temporal bone
8   Temporomandibular articulation
9   Petrous temporal bone (seen as a radiopaque shadow)
10 Tympanic bulla of temporal bone (shaded in drawing)
   10(a) External acoustic meatus (characteristic 'lip' at bor-
           der of meatus which becomes larger with age)
   10(b) Shadow formed by horizontal ear canal

11 Canal of auditory tube
12 Foramen magnum
13 Caudal edge of palatine bones or hard palate
14 Condyle of occipital bone
15 Atlas
16 Axis
17 Spinous process of axis
18 Dens or odontoid peg of axis
19 Stylohyoid bone
20 Epihyoid bone
21 Ceratohyoid bone
22 Basihyoid bone
23 Epiglottis

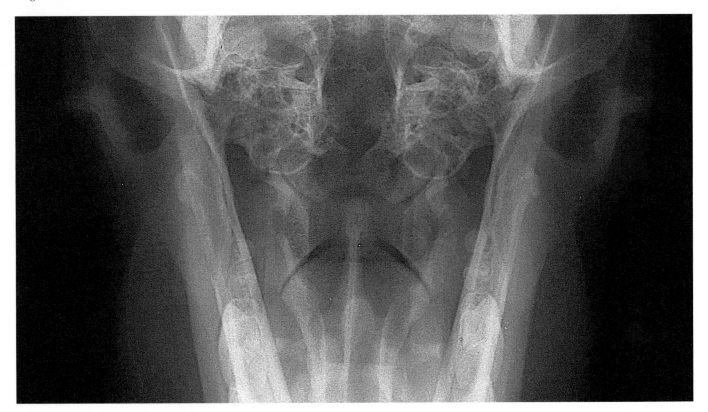

Figure 242   Rostroventral-caudodorsal oblique (open mouth) projection of dens or odontoid peg. Beagle dog 2.5 years old, entire male.

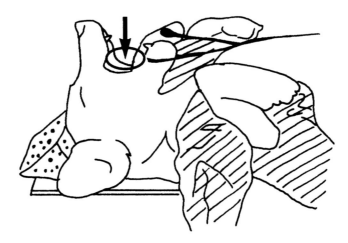

Figure 243   Line drawing of photograph representing radiographic positioning for Figure 242.

An Atlas of Interpretative Radiographic Anatomy of the Dog and Cat

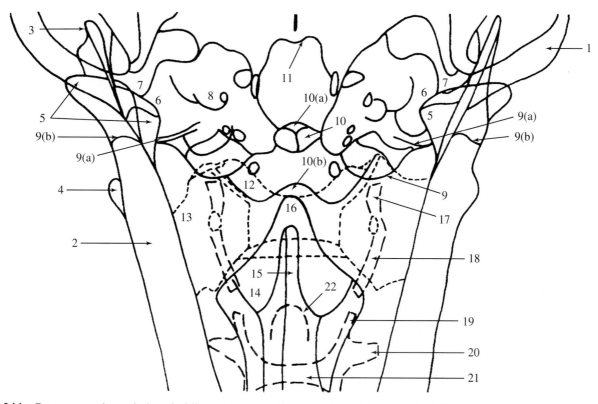

Figure 244 Rostroventral–caudodorsal oblique (open mouth) projection of dens or odontoid peg.

1 Zygomatic process of temporal bone
2 Mandibular ramus
3 Coronoid process of mandible
4 Angular process of mandible
5 Condyloid or articular process of mandible
6 Temporomandibular articulation
7 Upper molar
8 Petrous temporal bone
9 Tympanic bulla of temporal bone
   9(a) External acoustic meatus (Characteristic 'lip' at border of meatus)
   9(b) Shadow formed by horizontal ear canal
10 Foramen magnum
   10(a) Dorsal part
   10(b) Ventral part

11 Caudal border of palatine bones or hard palate
12 Condyle of occipital bone
13 Atlas
14 Axis
15 Spinous process of axis
16 Dens or odontoid peg of axis
17 Stylohoid bone
18 Epihyoid bone
19 Ceratohyoid bone
20 Thyrohoid bone
21 Basihyoid bone
22 Epiglottis

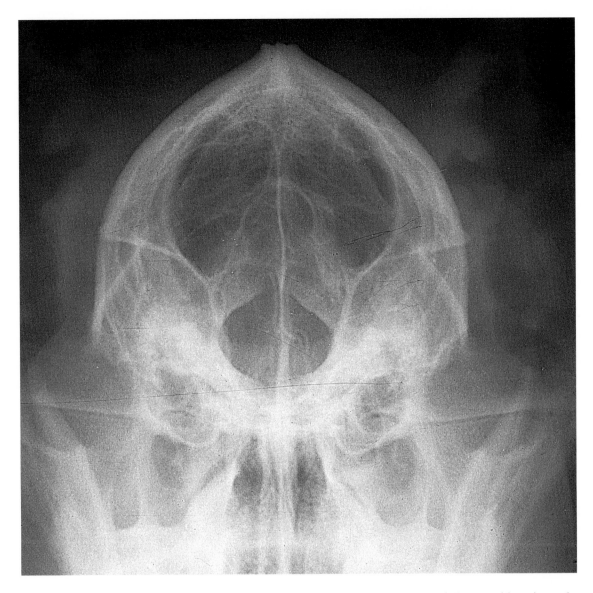

Figure 245   Caudodorsal-rostroventral oblique projection of foramen magnum. Beagle dog 2.5 years old, entire male.

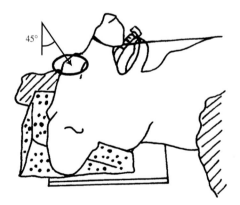

Figure 246   Line drawing of photograph representing radiographic positioning for Figure 245.

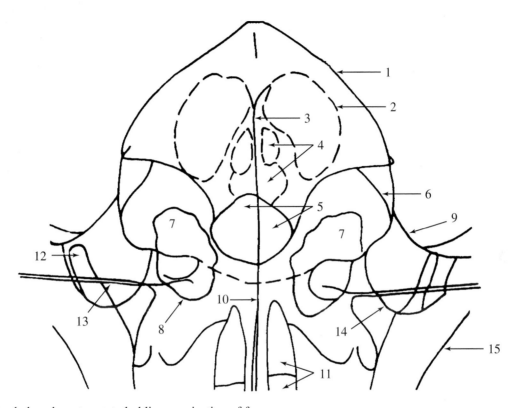

Figure 247 Caudodorsal–rostroventral oblique projection of foramen magnum.

1 Parietal bone
2 Lateral frontal sinus
3 Septum of frontal sinuses
4 Medial and rostral frontal sinuses
5 Foramen magnum
6 Zygomatic process of frontal bone
7 Petrous temporal bone
8 Tympanic bulla of temporal bone

9 Zygomatic process of temporal bone
10 Osseous nasal septum
11 Ethmoturbinates
12 Coronoid process of mandible
13 Condyloid or articular process of mandible
14 Margin of orbit
15 Maxilla or maxillary bone

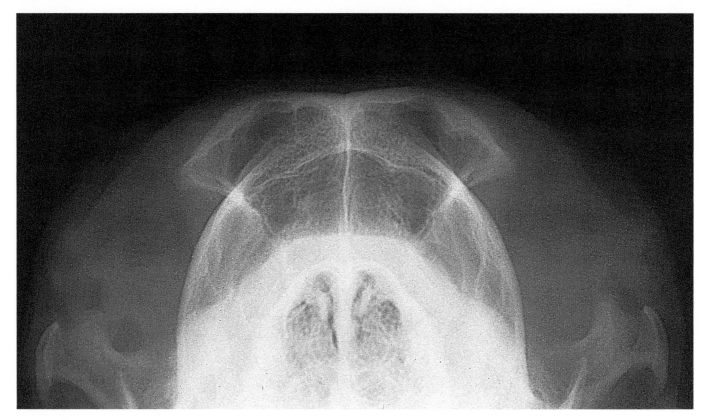

Figure 248   Rostrocaudal projection of frontal sinuses. Beagle dog 2.5 years old, entire male.

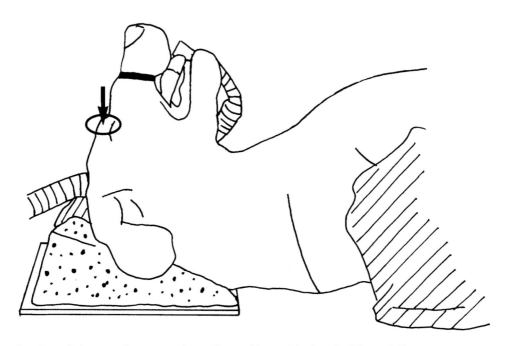

Figure 249   Line drawing of photograph representing radiographic positioning for Figure 248.

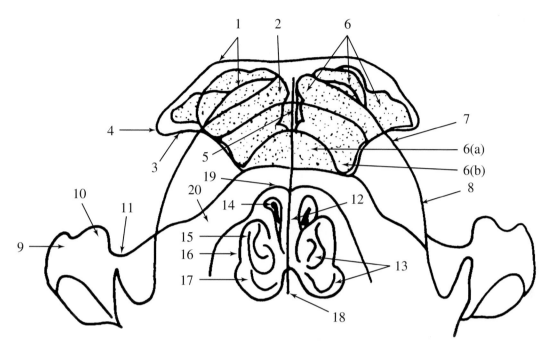

Figure 250 Rostrocaudal projection of frontal sinuses.

1 Frontal bone. The inner and outer tables are separated by the lateral frontal sinus.
2 Medial surface of frontal bone. The septum between the frontal sinuses.
3 Lateral surface of frontal bone; orbital part.
4 Zygomatic process of frontal bone
5 Septum between frontal sinuses. Formed by nasal parts of the frontal bones and septal processes of the nasal bones.
6 Frontal sinuses (shaded in drawing). Usually three separate compartments on each side. Compartments are distinct sinuses with their own openings between ethmoturbinates into nasal cavities.
   6(a) Rostral frontal sinus and its associated ethmo-turbinates. Frontal sinuses extend more rostrally at medial aspect of this region than at lateral aspect.
   6(b) Frontal sinus containing ethmoturbinates
7 Parietal bone
8 Squamous part of temporal bone

9 Zygomatic process of temporal bone
10 Frontal process of zygomatic bone
11 Infraorbital margin of zygomatic bone
12 Osseous nasal septum. Perpendicular plate of the ethmoid. The cartilaginous nasal septum is also part of ethmoid bone and is formed by a rostral prolongation of osseous nasal septum. Articulation is with the vomer ventrally and septal processes of frontal and nasal bones dorsally. Note that the cartilaginous nasal septum is radiolucent.
13 Ethmoturbinates and turbinates of ventral nasal concha
14 Dorsal nasal meatus
15 Middle nasal meatus
16 Conchal crest of maxilla
17 Ventral nasal meatus
18 Vomer
19 Nasal bone
20 Maxilla or maxillary bone

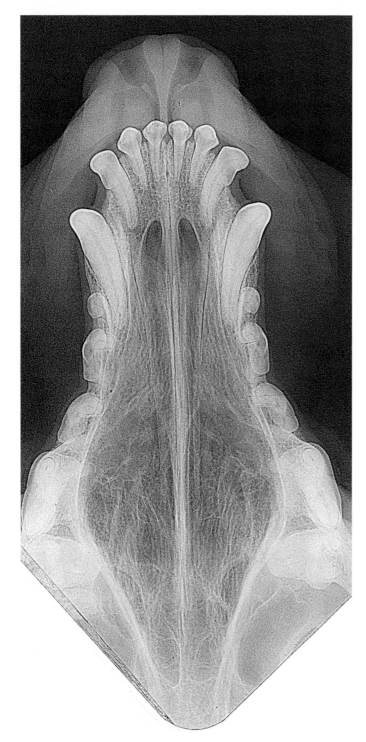

Figure 251 Dorsoventral intraoral projection of nasal chambers. Beagle dog 2.5 years old, entire male.

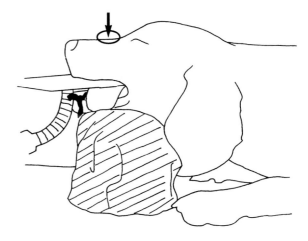

Figure 252 Line drawing of photograph representing radiographic positioning for Figure 251.

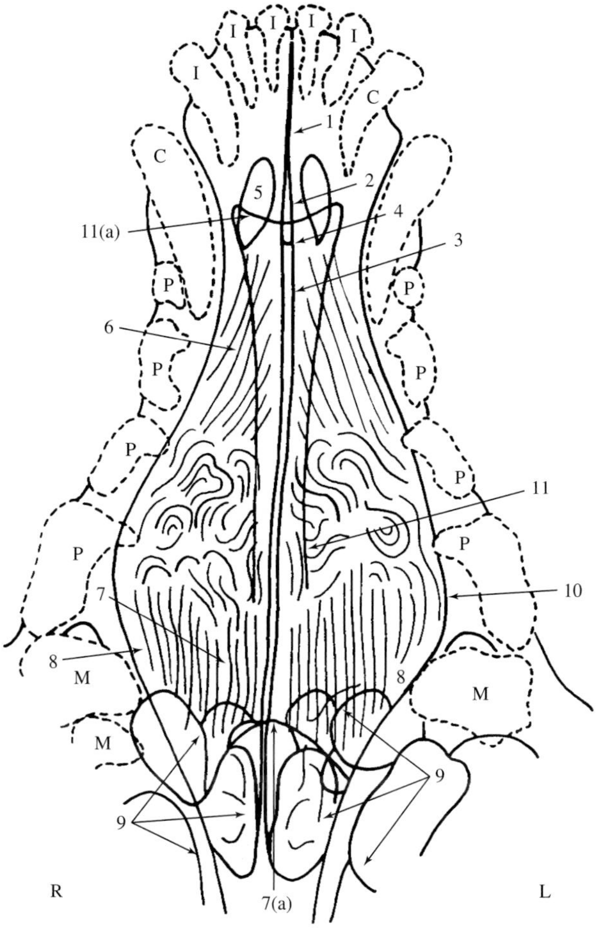

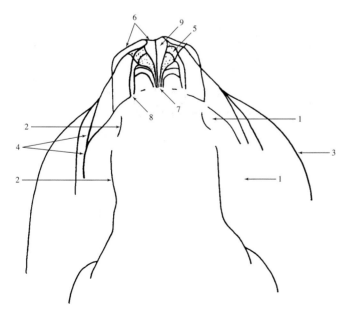

Figure 253 Dorsoventral intraoral projection of nasal chambers.

1 Interincisive suture showing incisive canal
2 Incisive bone palatine process
3 Vomer
4 Suture between incisive bone and vomer
5 Palatine fissure
6 Nasal conchae. (Only ventral turbinates seen in this projection.)
7 Ethmoturbinates. Rostral extent at 2nd. and 3rd. premolar level, with bulk of ethmoturbinates ending at 3rd. and 4th. level. Rostral limit of ethmoidal fossa at 1st. molar level, also the position of the cribriform plate (7(a)).
8 Maxillary sinus or recess of maxilla
9 Frontal sinuses
10 Shadow of external surface of facial bones.
11 Nasal bone
    11(a) Rostral limit

A radiolucent shadow is created within the nasal chambers by the lateral limits of the nasal and vomer bones.

I Upper incisor. Total of six.

C Upper canine. Total of two.

P Upper premolar. Total of eight.

M Upper molar. Total of four. (In this dog left 2nd. molar is missing.)

Note that the term 'upper' can be replaced by 'superior'.

Figure 254 Line drawing of dorsoventral intraoral projection of nasal chambers to demonstrate soft tissue shadows seen in radiograph, Figure 251.

1 Vestibule of mouth
2 Gum
3 Cheek
4 Lip
5 Nostril (shaded in drawing)
6 Nasal plane
7 Ventral nasal meatus
8 Middle and dorsal nasal meatus
9 Cartilaginous nasal septum

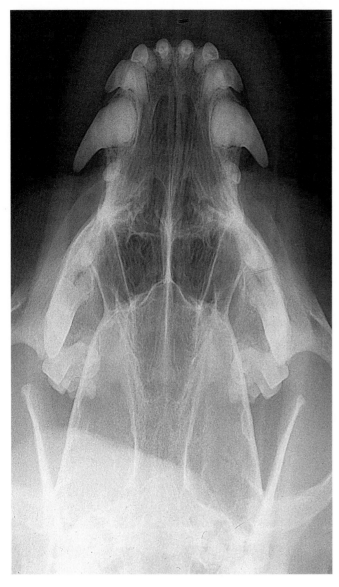

Figure 255 Ventrodorsal oblique (open mouth) projection of nasal chambers. Samoyed dog 6 years old, entire female.

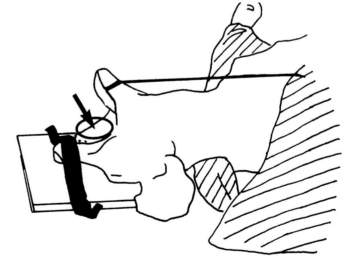

Figure 256 Line drawing of photograph representing radiographic positioning for Figure 255.

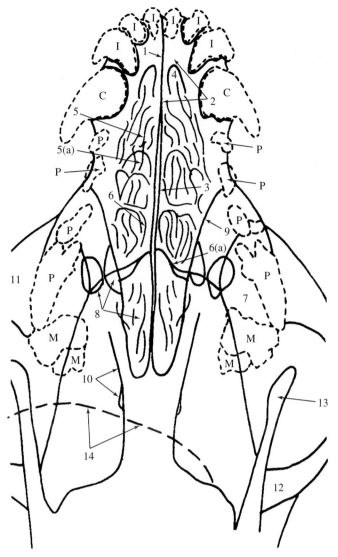

Figure 257   Ventrodorsal oblique (open mouth) projection of nasal chambers.

1 Interincisive suture showing incisive canal
2 Incisive bone palatine process
3 Vomer
4 Palatine fissure
5 Nasal conchae. Nasal and maxillary turbinate
    bones.

The radiolucent shadow created within the nasal chambers
by the lateral limits of the nasal and vomer bones is only
just visible on the right side (5(a)).

6 Ethmoturbinates
    6(a) Rostral limit of ethmoid fossa. This is also the
           position of the cribriform plate.
7 Maxillary sinus or recess of maxilla
8 Frontal sinuses
9 Medial wall of orbit

10 Border of choanae formed by palatine bone and
     pterygoid bone (Hamulus seen as the opaquer shadow
     at the caudal extremity)
11 Temporal process of zygomatic bone
12 Zygomatic process of temporal bone
The zygomatic arch is formed by 11 and 12.

13 Coronoid process of mandible
14 Soft tissue shadow of the tongue

I Upper incisor. Total of six.

C Upper canine. Total of two.

P Upper premolar. Total of eight.

M Upper molar. Total of four.

Note that the term 'upper' can be replaced by 'superior'.

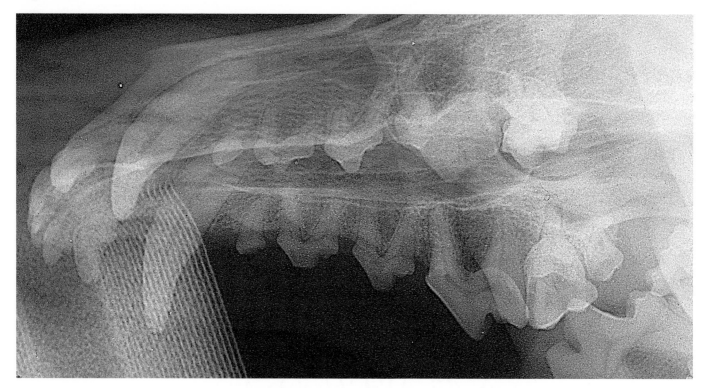

Figure 258 Ventrodorsal oblique (open mouth) projection of maxilla right lateral recumbency. Beagle dog 2.5 years old, entire male.

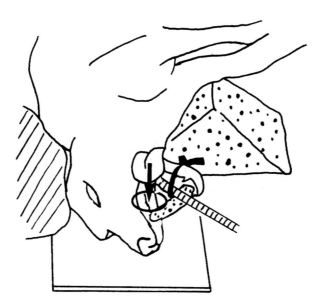

Figure 259 Line drawing of photograph representing radiographic positioning for Figure 258.

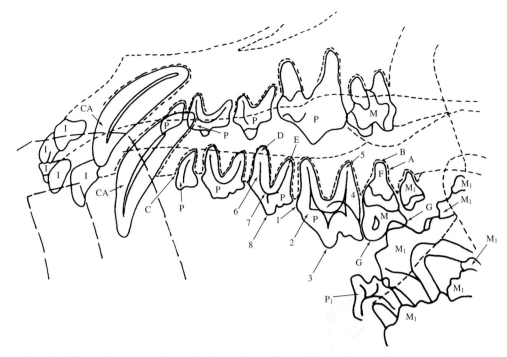

Figure 260   Ventrodorsal oblique (open mouth) projection of maxilla right lateral recumbency.

The drawing and labelling have been kept to a minimum to demonstrate teeth details.

I   Upper incisor. Total of six.

CA   Upper canine. Total of two.

P   Upper premolar. Total of eight.

M   Upper molar. Total of four. (In this dog left 2nd. molar is missing.)

P_1 Lower premolar. Total of eight.

M_1 Lower molar. Total of six.

Note that the term 'upper' can be replaced by 'superior' and 'lower' by 'inferior'.

Teeth are anchored in bony sockets or alveoli. Parallel to each tooth root is a region of clearly defined bony radiopacity called the lamina dura (A). With age the alveolar bone has radiopaque linear changes making the lamina dura less obvious in radiographs.

Between the lamina dura and the tooth root is a radiolucent shadow of the periodontal membrane (B).

A sharp angle is present at the junction of the lamina dura and the alveolar crest (C) adjacent to the dental cemento-enamel junction. With age, some vertical bone resorption can occur, reducing this sharp angle.

Anatomy of teeth
1   Neck
2   Crown
3   Tubercle

4   Root
5   Apex of root
6   Dentine. The periodontal membrane is attached on its dental surface to a thin layer of cement, but this is not radiographically distinguishable from the dentine.
7   Pulp cavity. In young dogs this is very large, reducing in size until 2 to 3 years of age and then slowly decreasing.
8   Enamel

D   Rostral or mesial root of 3rd. premolar (upper right)

E   Distal root of 3rd. premolar (upper right)

F   Lingual surface root of 1st. molar (upper right). The apex of this root appears to have some increased lucency which would indicate resorption. However, idiopathic resorption of roots in this region has been noted in mature dogs.

G   Vestibular surface roots of 1st. molar (upper right)

In young dogs (under 1 year of age) root apices are normally open.

To avoid confusion all roots have not been labelled. The 1st. premolar has only one root, the 2nd. and 3rd. have two roots (rostral and distal) while the 4th. upper premolar, or carnassial tooth, has three roots. Of the latter two roots are long and found on the vestibular surface, and the other is much shorter on the lingual surface. The 4th. lower premolar is similar to premolars 2 and 3.

Considering the molars, the upper have two small vestibular surface roots and one larger lingual surface roots. The lower molars all have two roots but the 1st. is very large and forms the lower carnassial tooth.

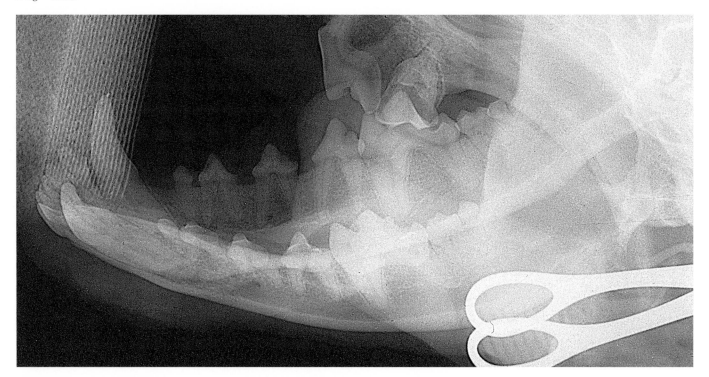

Figure 261 Dorsoventral oblique (open mouth) projection of mandible right lateral recumbency. Beagle dog 2.5 years old, entire male.

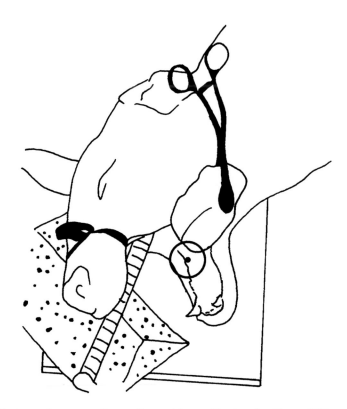

Figure 262 Line drawing of photograph representing radiographic positioning for Figure 261.

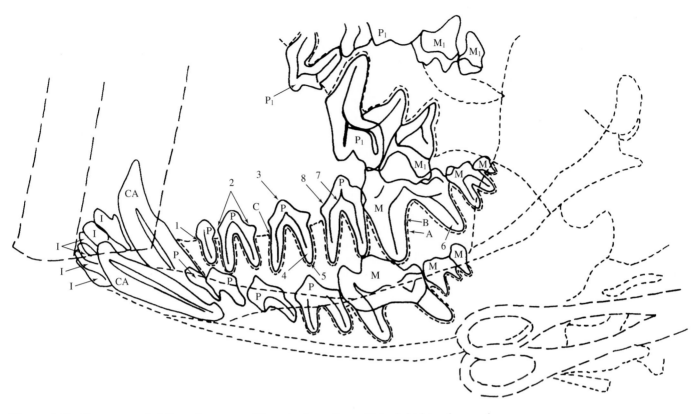

Figure 263 Dorsoventral oblique (open mouth) projection of mandible right lateral recumbency.

The drawing and labelling have been kept to a minimum to demonstrate teeth details.

I   Lower incisor. Total of six.

CA Lower canine. Total of two.

P   Lower premolar. Total of eight.

M   Lower molars. Total of six.

P1   Upper premolar. Total of eight.

M1   Upper molar. Total of four. (In this dog left 2nd. molar is missing.)

Note that the term 'lower' can be replaced by 'inferior' and 'upper' by 'superior'.

A   Lamina dura

B   Periodontal membrane

C   Cementoenamel junction

Please refer to ventrodorsal oblique (open mouth) projection of maxilla, Figure 260, for details of A, B and C.

Anatomy of teeth
1   Neck
2   Crown
3   Tubercle
4   Root
5   Apex of root
6   Dentine
7   Pulp cavity
8   Enamel

Please refer to ventrodorsal oblique (open mouth) projection of maxilla, Figure 260, for details of 1 to 8.

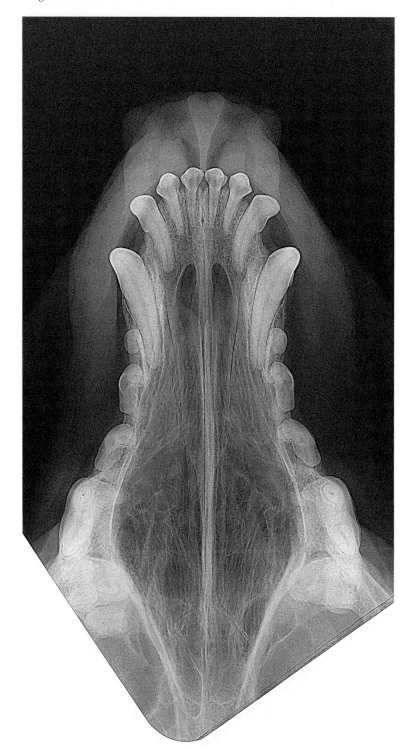

Figure 264 Dorsoventral intraoral projection of maxillary bones. Beagle dog 2.5 years old, entire male.

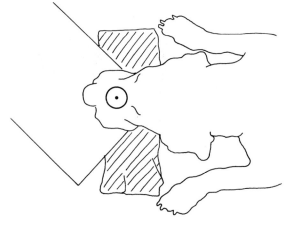

Figure 265 Line drawing of photograph representing radiographic positioning for Figure 264.

An Atlas of Interpretative Radiographic Anatomy of the Dog and Cat

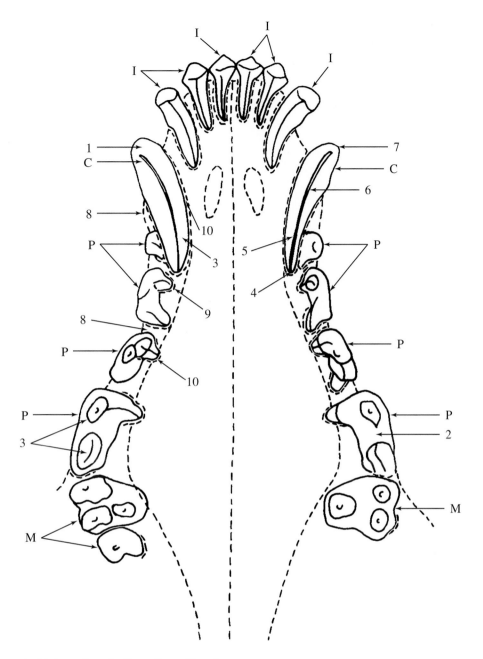

Figure 266   Dorsoventral intraoral projection of maxillary bones.

The drawing and labelling are to illustrate teeth details.

I   Upper incisors. Total of six.

C   Upper canines. Total of two.

P   Upper premolars. Total of eight.

M   Upper molars. Total of four. (In this dog left 2nd. molar is missing)

Note that the term 'upper' can be replaced by 'superior'.

Anatomy of teeth
  1   Crown
  2   Tubercle

3   Root
4   Apex of root
5   Dentine
6   Pulp cavity
7   Enamel

Anatomy of alveoli
  8   Alveolar crest
  9   Lamina dura
  10   Periodontal membrane (seen as a radiolucent line between the lamina dura and tooth root)

Please refer to ventrodorsal oblique (open mouth) projection of maxilla, Figure 260, for details of 1 to 10.

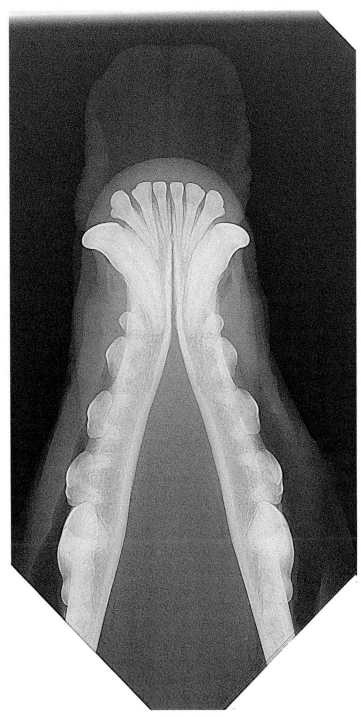

Figure 267 Ventrodorsal intraoral projection of mandibular bodies. Beagle dog 2.5 years old, entire male.

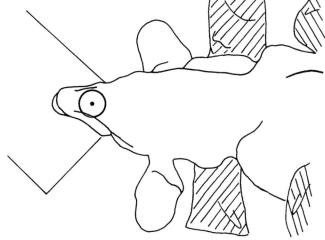

Figure 268 Line drawing of photograph representing radiographic positioning for Figure 267.

An Atlas of Interpretative Radiographic Anatomy of the Dog and Cat

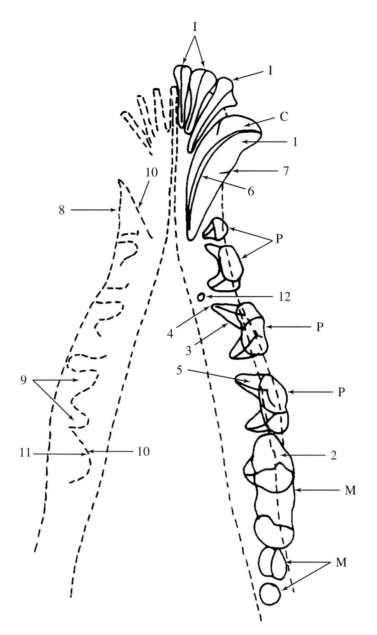

Figure 269 Ventrodorsal intraoral projection of mandibular bodies.

The teeth have been excluded from the drawing of the right mandible so that bony features are more easily identified.

I   Lower incisors. Total of six.

C   Lower canine. Total of two.

P   Lower premolars. Total of eight.

M Lower molars. Total of six.

    Note that the term 'lower' can be replaced by 'inferior'.

Anatomy of teeth
  1 Crown
  2 Tubercle
  3 Root

  4 Apex of root
  5 Dentine
  6 Pulp cavity
  7 Enamel

Anatomy of alveoli
  8 Alveolar crest
  9 Bony sockets or alveoli
 10 Lamina dura
 11 Periodontal membrane (seen as a radiolucent line between the lamina dura and tooth root)

    Please refer to ventrodorsal oblique (open mouth) projection of maxilla, Figure 260, for details of 1 to 11.

 12 Mental foramen

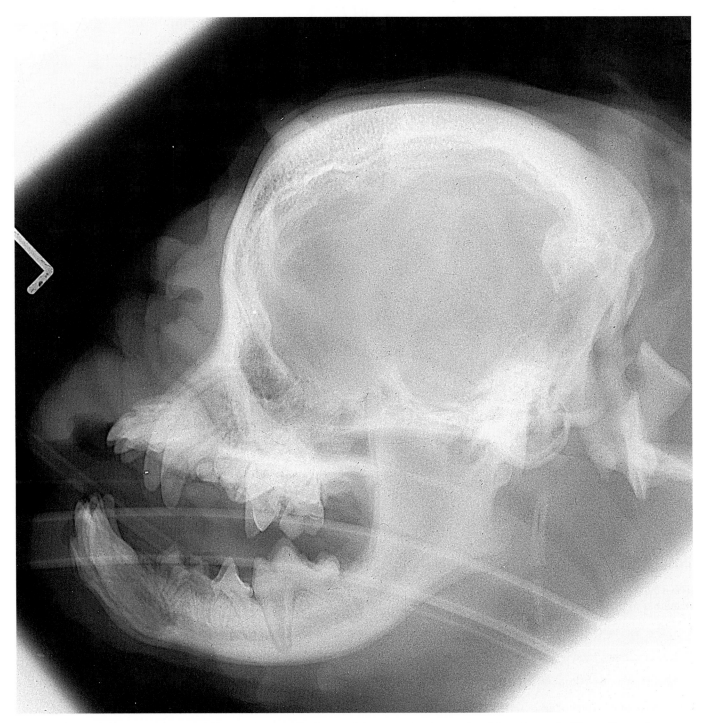

Figure 270 Lateral projection of skull. Brachycephalic breed of dog. Pug dog 9 months old, entire male. The radiograph demonstrates the short nasal chambers of the brachycephalic breed of dog. In addition the extreme dome shape of the cranium in this Pug breed has resulted in a reduction of the frontal sinuses shadow.

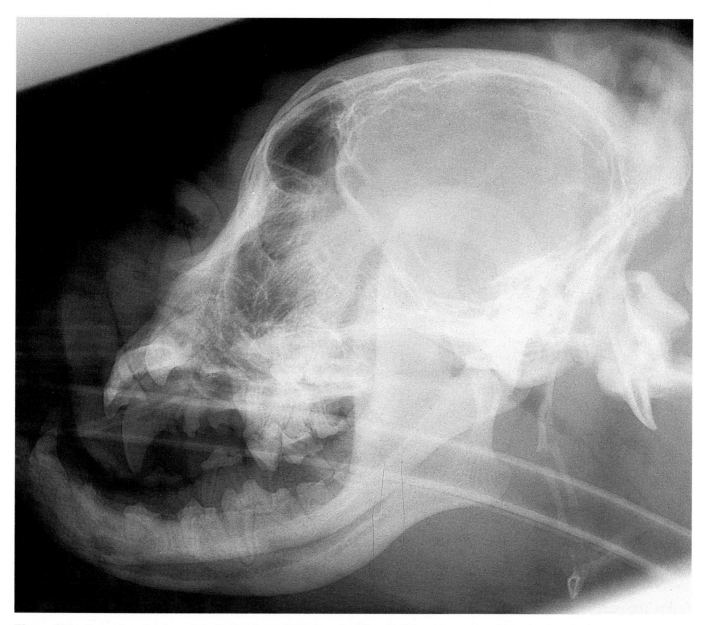

Figure 271   Lateral projection of skull. Brachycephalic breed of dog. Bulldog 18 months old, entire female (same dog as in dorsoventral projection of skull, Figure 276). The radiograph demonstrates the short nasal chambers of the brachycephalic breed. Prognathism of the mandible is also present, a condition commonly seen in this type of breed.

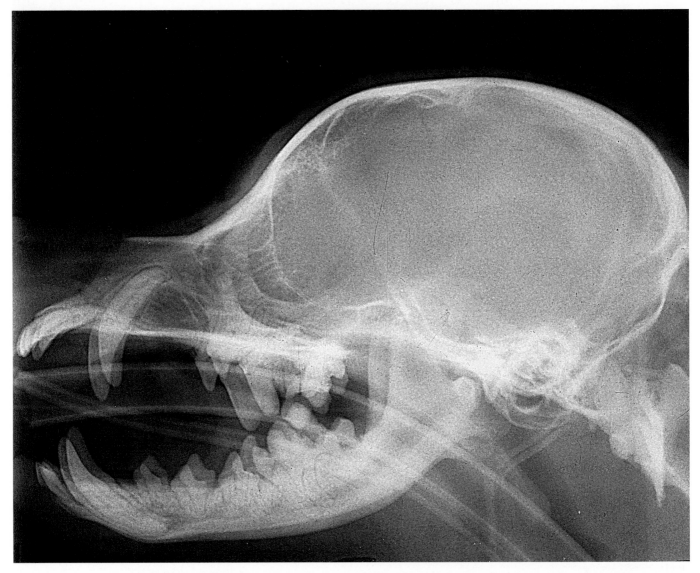

Figure 272 Lateral projection of skull. Toy breed of dog. Yorkshire Terrier dog 2 years old, entire female. The radiograph has been included to show doming of the cranium in toy breeds with the consequential reduction of the frontal sinuses shadow. The sinuses in this particular dog are almost entirely lost.

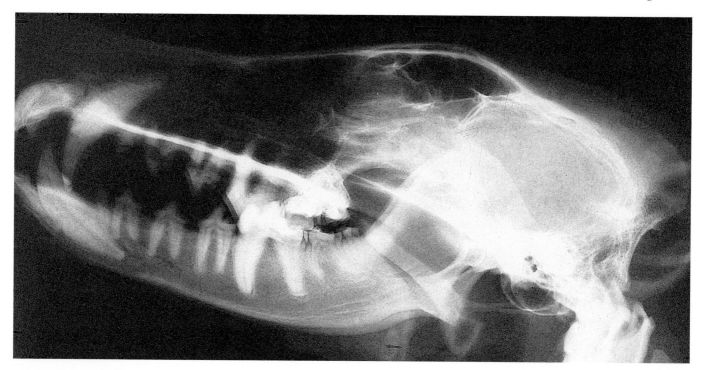

Figure 273   Lateral projection of skull. Dolichocephalic breed of dog. Radiograph includes all skull bones. Rough Collie dog 7 years old, entire male.

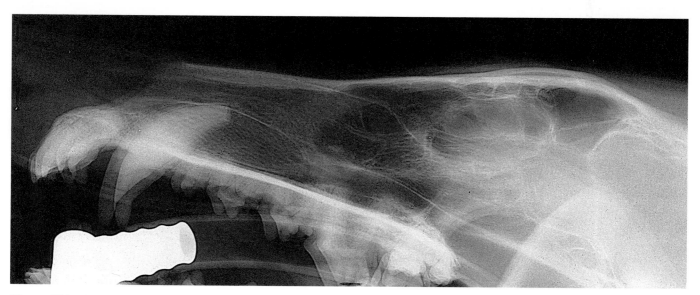

Figure 274   Lateral projection of skull. Dolichocephalic breed of dog. The primary beam has been coned down and centred on the nasal chambers. Rough Collie dog 6 years old, neutered female.

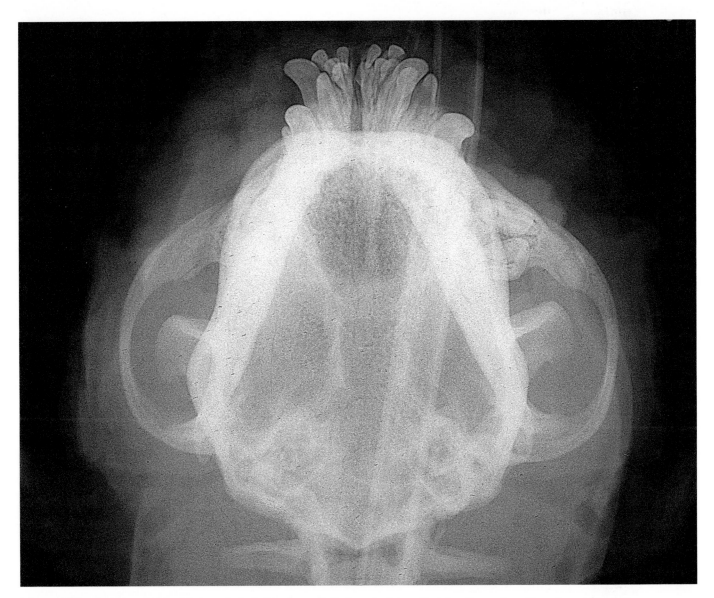

Figure 275   Dorsoventral projection of skull. Brachycephalic breed of dog. Pug dog 9 months old, entire male.

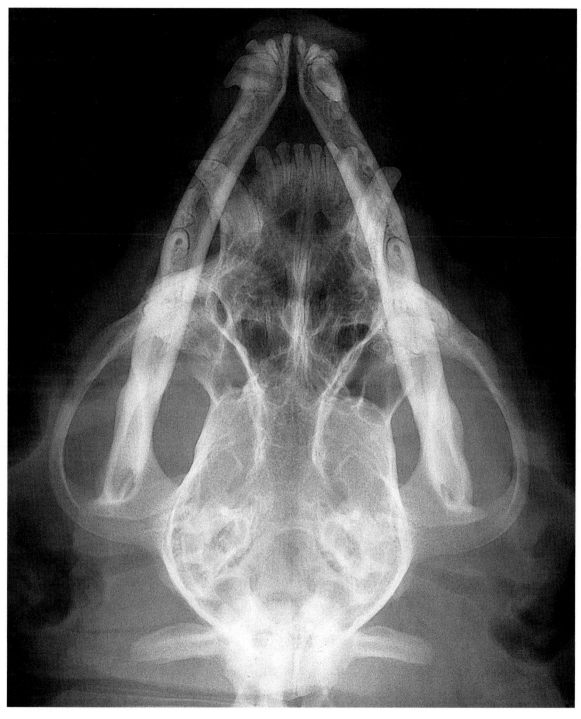

Figure 276 Dorsoventral projection of skull. Brachycephalic breed of dog. Bulldog 18 months old, entire female (same dog as in lateral projection of skull, Figure 271). Prognathism of the mandibles is present, a condition commonly seen in the brachycephalic breed of dog.

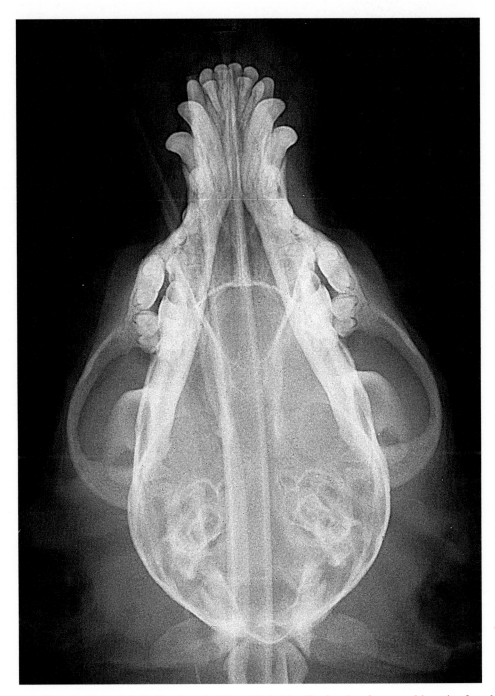

Figure 277   Dorsoventral projection of skull. Toy breed of dog. Yorkshire Terrier dog 2 years old, entire female.

An Atlas of Interpretative Radiographic Anatomy of the Dog and Cat

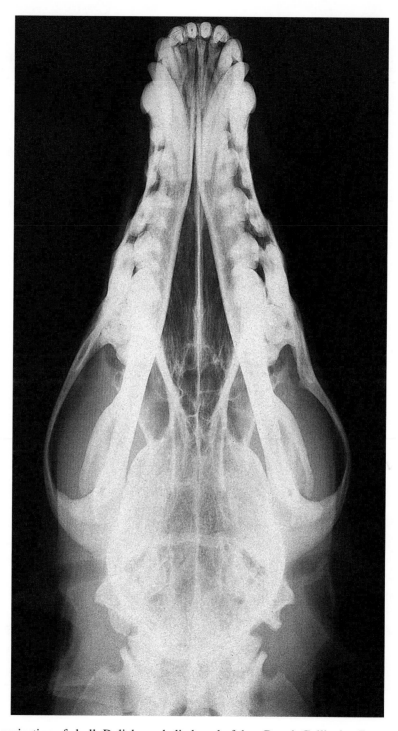

Figure 278 Dorsoventral projection of skull. Dolichocephalic breed of dog. Rough Collie dog 7 years old, entire male.

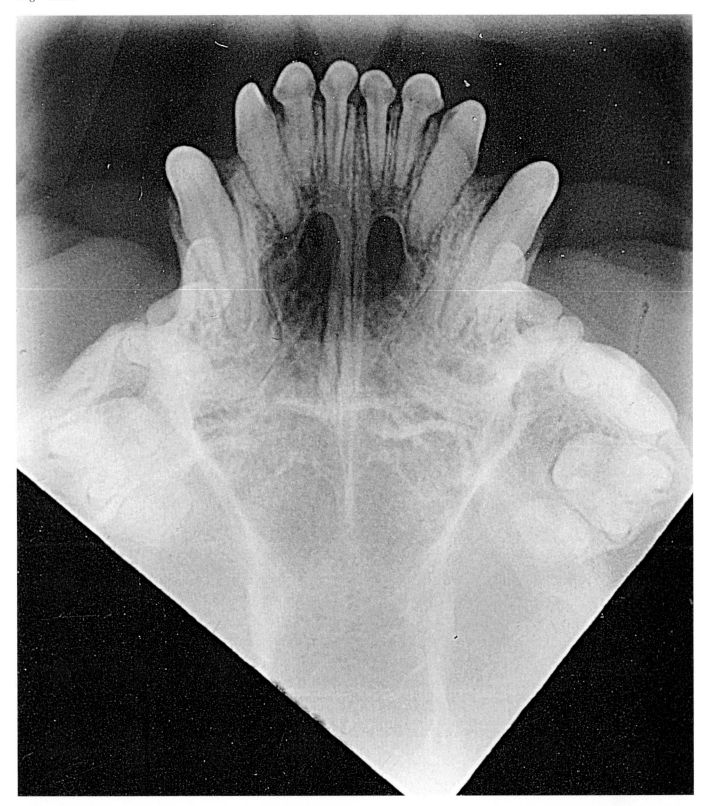

Figure 279   Dorsoventral intraoral projection of nasal chambers. Brachycephalic breed of dog. Boston Terrier dog 20 months old, entire female.

The radiograph demonstrates the severe reduction in the size of the nasal chambers found in this breed of dog. The right 4th. premolar tooth is congenitally absent in this particular dog. Such an abnormality is not uncommon in the brachycephalic breed of dog where the upper premolar teeth are usually affected. Lower molar teeth can also be congenitally absent.

An Atlas of Interpretative Radiographic Anatomy of the Dog and Cat

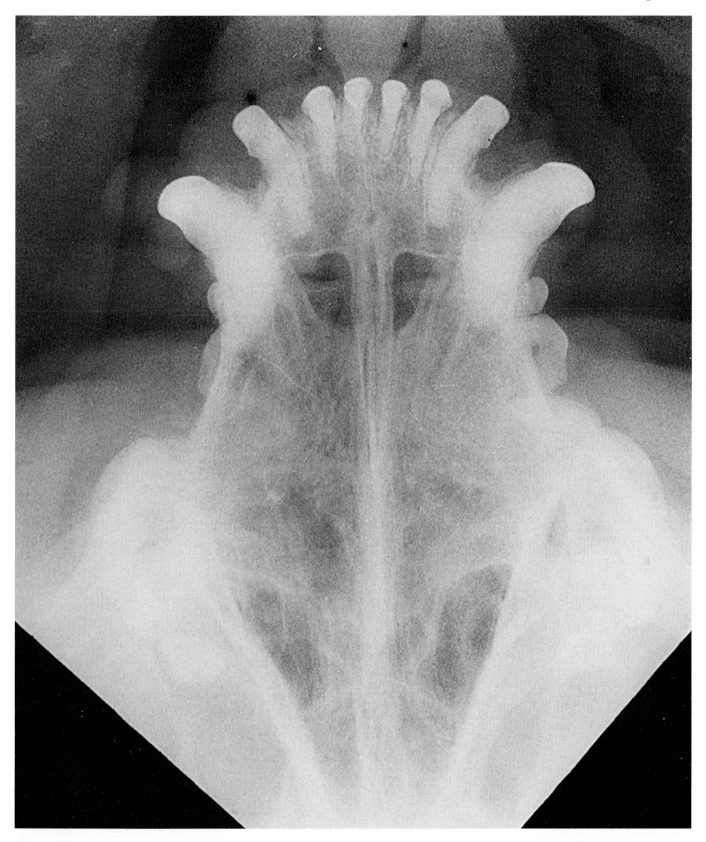

Figure 280 Dorsoventral intraoral projection of nasal chambers. Brachycephalic breed of dog. Boxer dog 9.5 years old, entire male. Note that the right 3rd. premolar is missing in this dog. This was a result of extraction and not a congenital absence. The reduction of nasal chamber shadows is not as great as in the Boston Terrier (Figure 279).

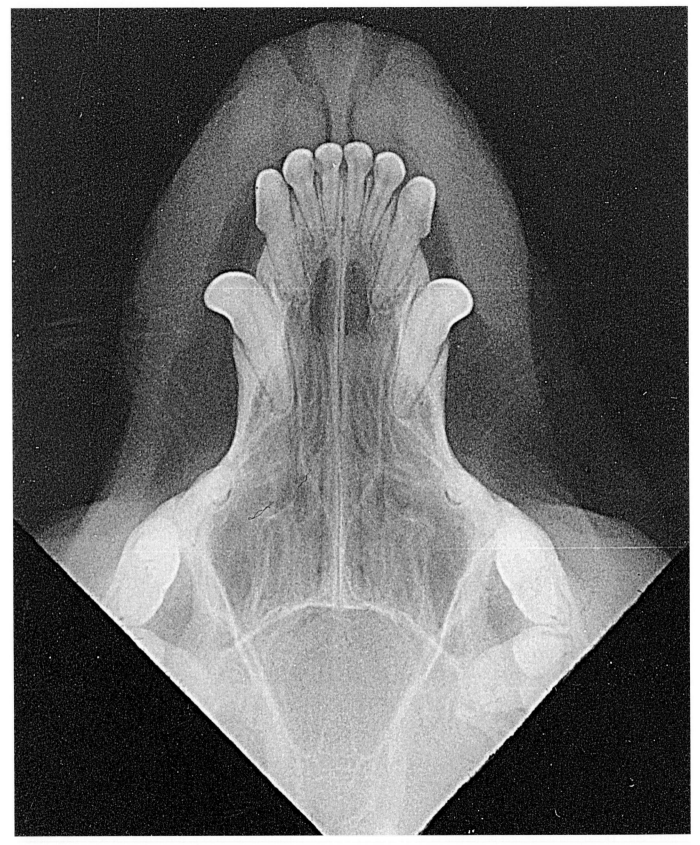

Figure 281 Dorsoventral intraoral projection of nasal chambers. Toy breed of dog. Yorkshire Terrier dog 2 years old, entire female.

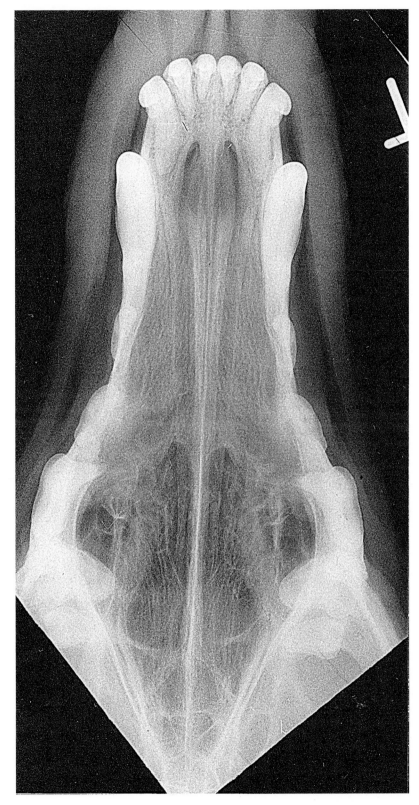

Figure 282 Dorsoventral intraoral projection of nasal chambers. Dolichocephalic breed of dog. Greyhound dog 2 years old, entire male.

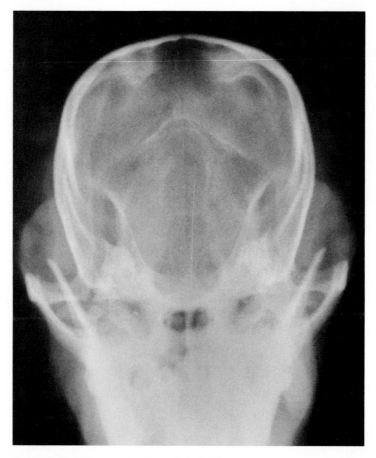

Figure 283 Caudodorsal–rostroventral oblique projection of skull. Foramen magnum variant in toy breed of dog. Yorkshire Terrier dog 5 years old, entire female.

The radiograph demonstrates a dorsal extension of the foramen magnum. Such an extension is very common in the toy breed of dog, but has been termed 'occipital dysplasia', and hence an abnormality, by some authorities.

As 'occipital dysplasia' it has been linked to congenital or developmental neurological dysfunction. However, the appearance of the foramen magnum, as seen in this radiograph, can be found extensively in clinically normal dogs and its presence in dogs exhibiting abnormal neurological signs is not conclusive for a diagnosis. Hence great care must be taken with the interpretation of this radiographic shadow as it often reflects only a variant and other conditions must be eliminated.

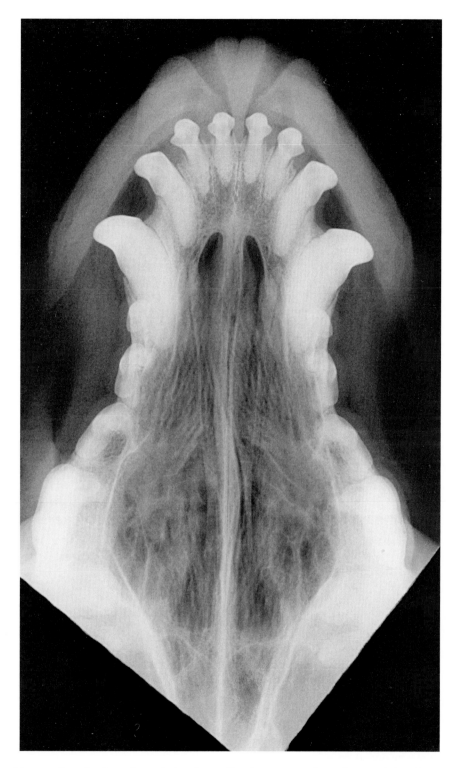

Figure 284   Dorsoventral intraoral projection of nasal chambers. Nasal septum variant. Samoyed dog 6 years old, entire female.
    The radiograph shows curvature of the nasal septum, to the left nasal chamber, at the mid chamber level. The bony shadows dividing the two nasal chambers can be seen midline and are intact. Positional variation of the nasal septum, and the vomer (also see Figure 653, Siamese cat), are sometimes seen and analysis of surrounding shadows must be made to ensure that the deviation is not part of a disease process such as neoplasia.
    The left and right nasal chambers are symmetrical in this dog, i.e. are normal.

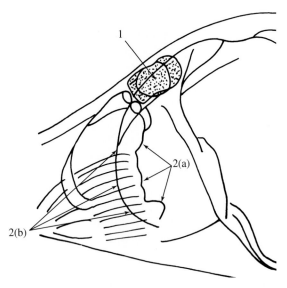

Figure 285a

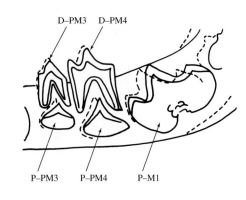

Figure 285b

Figures 285, 286, 287, 288   Lateral projection of skull. Samoyed crossbred dog entire male at 13, 25, 38, and 52 weeks of age. Correlating line drawings for 13, 25 and 38 weeks of age.

Figures 285a, 286a, 287a   Drawings to demonstrate frontal sinuses and ethmoidal region.

  1   Frontal sinuses (region shaded)
  2   Cribriform plate
    2(a) Caudal limit
    2(b) Rostral limit

Figures 285b, 286b, 287b   Drawings to demonstrate lower or inferior teeth within the central mandible. Deciduous teeth seen at 13 weeks of age only.

D–PM Premolars 3 and 4

Permanent teeth seen only as germs at 13 weeks of age

P–PM Premolars 3 and 4
P–M   Molars 1, 2 and 3

Note the narrowing of pulp cavities in permanent teeth, with age. Overlying shadows of corresponding teeth in opposing mandibular bone are shown by dotted lines.

Dental formulae for the dog:

Deciduous teeth	I 3	C 1	PM 3	
	3	1	3	
Permanent teeth	I 3	C 1	PM 4	M 2
	3	1	4	3

An Atlas of Interpretative Radiographic Anatomy of the Dog and Cat

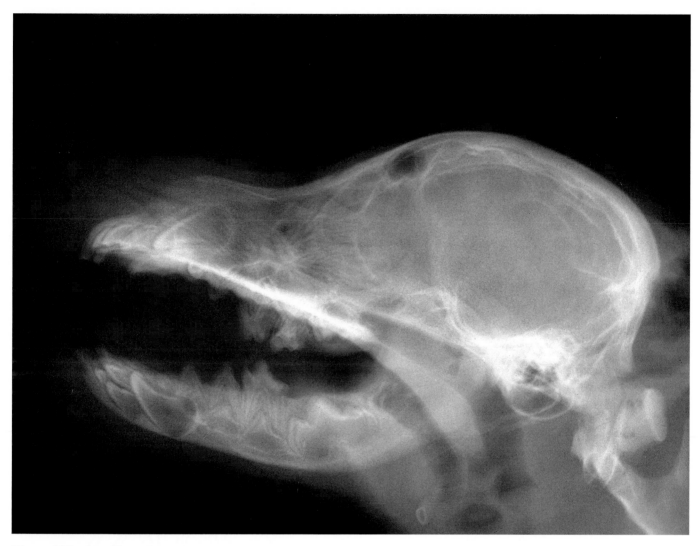

Figure 285   Age 13 weeks

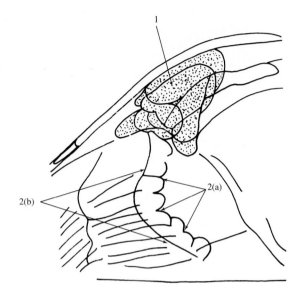

Figure 286a

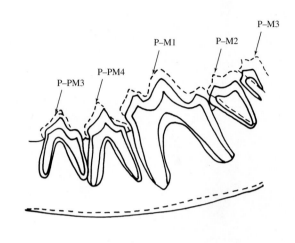

Figure 286b

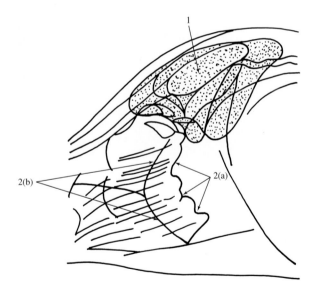

Figure 287a

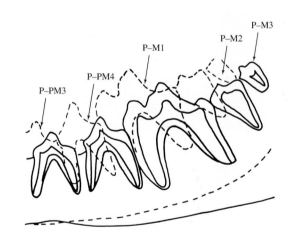

Figure 287b

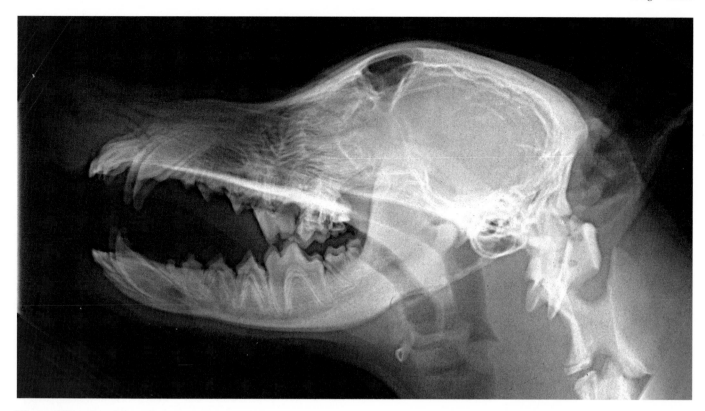

Figure 286   Age 25 weeks

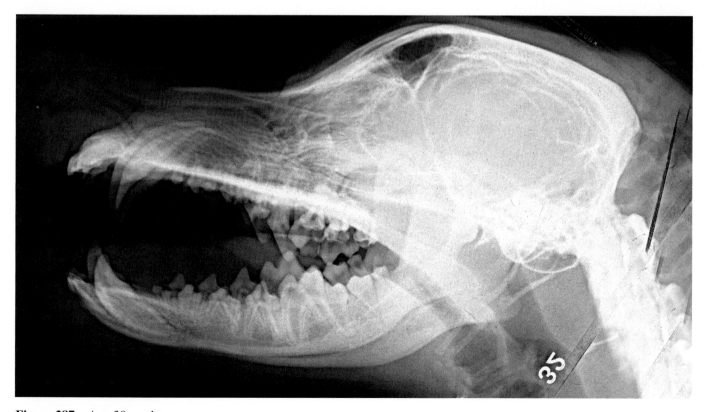

Figure 287   Age 38 weeks

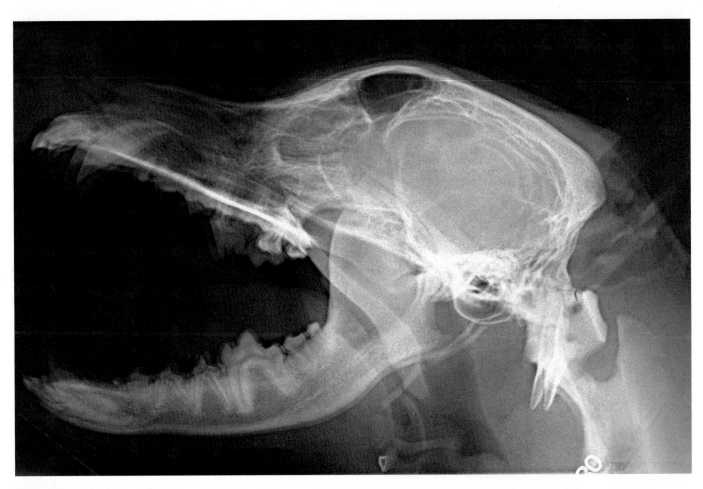

Figure 288   Age 52 weeks

An Atlas of Interpretative Radiographic Anatomy of the Dog and Cat

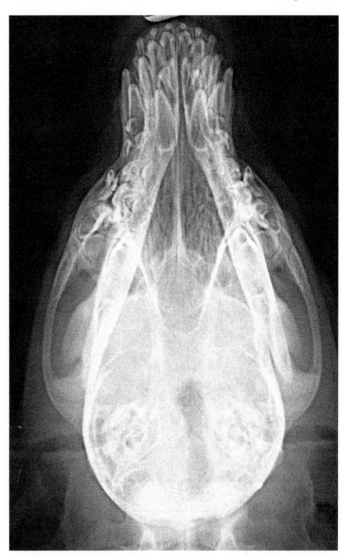

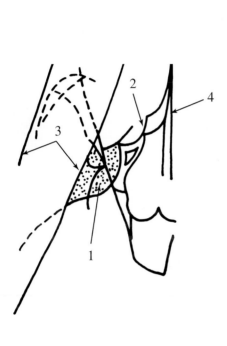

Figure 289

Figure 289   Age 13 weeks

Figures 289, 290, 291, 292   Ventrodorsal projection of skull. Samoyed crossbred dog entire male at 13, 25, 38 and 52 weeks of age. Correlating line drawings at 13, 25 and 38 weeks of age. Drawings to demonstrate frontal sinuses (right side).

1   Frontal sinuses (region shaded)

2   Cribriform plate

3   Mandible

4   Vomer (midline)

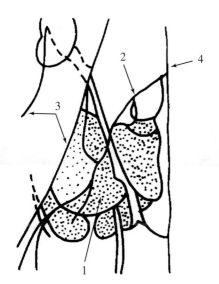

Figure 290

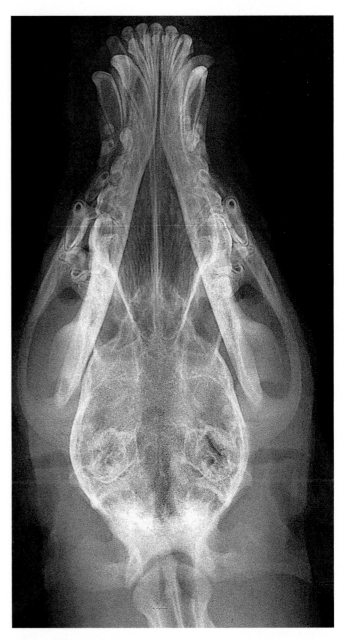

Figure 290   Age 25 weeks

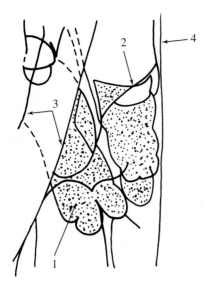

Figure 291

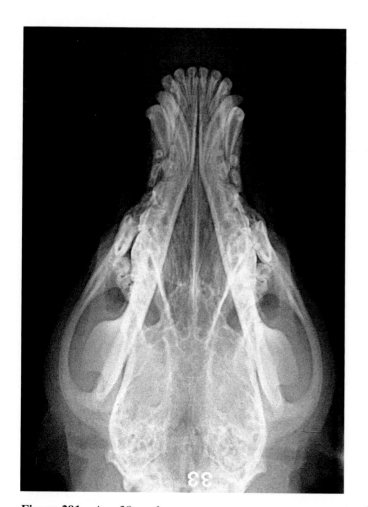

Figure 291   Age 38 weeks

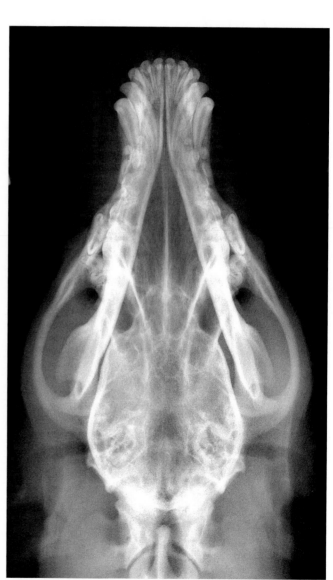

Figure 292   Age 52 weeks

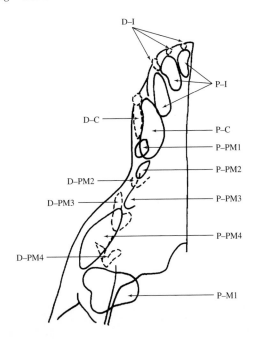

Figure 293

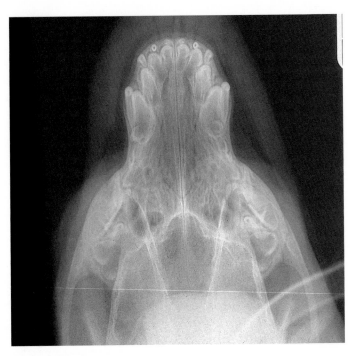

Figure 293 Age 13 weeks

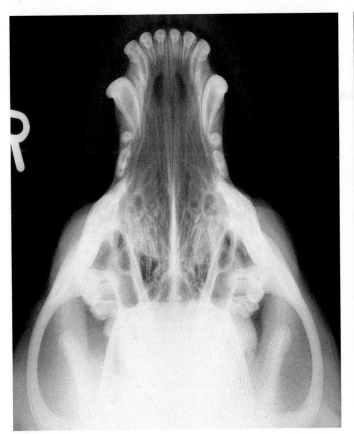

Figure 294 Age 38 weeks

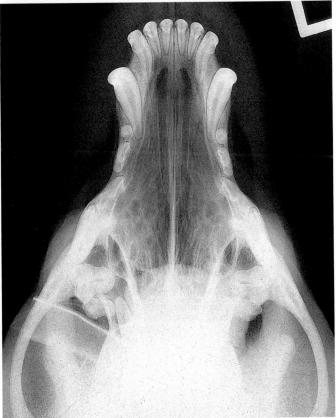

Figure 295 Age 52 weeks

Figures 293, 294, 295 Ventrodorsal oblique (open mouth) projection of maxilla. Samoyed crossbred dog entire male at 13, 38 and 52 weeks of age.

An Atlas of Interpretative Radiographic Anatomy of the Dog and Cat

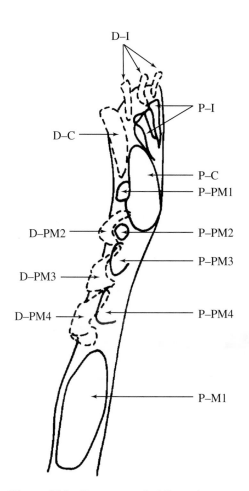

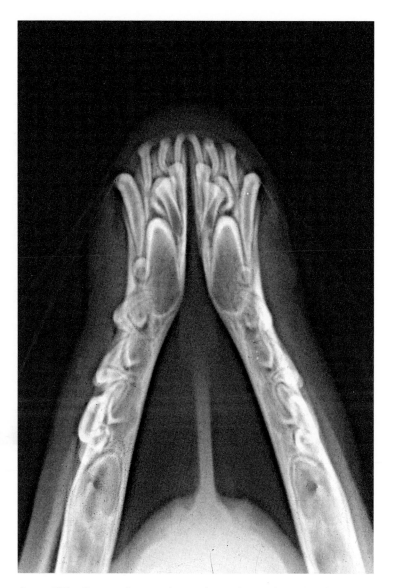

Figure 296 Dorsoventral oblique (open mouth) projection of mandible. Samoyed cross, dog entire male, at 13 weeks of age. Correlating line drawings at 13 weeks of age.

Deciduous teeth

D–I   Incisors

D–C   Canine

D–PM   Premolars 2, 3 and 4. Note no deciduous PM 1.

Permanent teeth

P–I   Incisors

P–C   Canine

P–PM   Premolars 1, 2, 3 and 4

P–M   Molar 1 (other molar teeth not easily seen in these projections)

Note the narrowing of pulp cavities of permanent teeth with age.

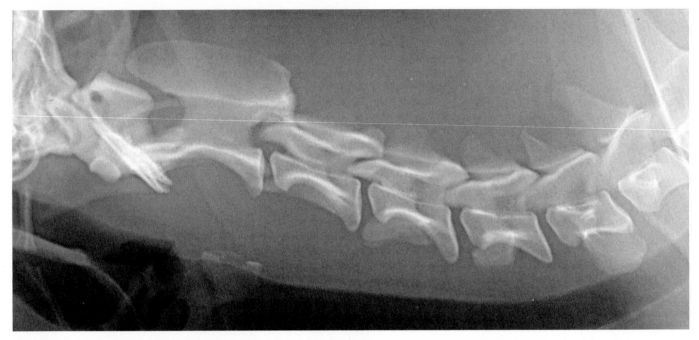

Figure 297   Extended lateral projection of cervical vertebrae. Beagle dog 2.5 years old, entire male.

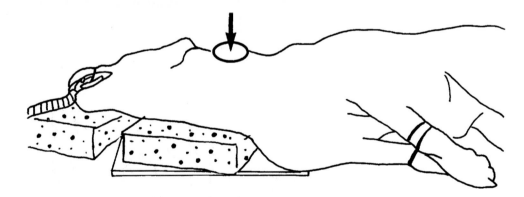

Figure 298   Line drawing of photograph representing radiographic positioning for Figure 297.

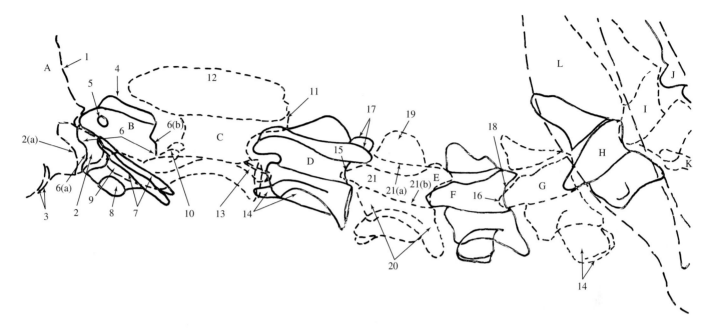

Figure 299   Extended lateral projection of cervical vertebrae.

A Skull
  1 Occipital bone
  2 Occipital condyle
    2(a) Rostral edge
  3 Tympanic bullae

B Atlas
  4 Dorsal arch
  5 Lateral vertebral foramen
  6 Articular surfaces
    6(a) Cranial articular surface or fovea
    6(b) Caudal articular surface or fovea
  7 Wings. Transverse processes.
  8 Body

C Axis
  9 Dens or odontoid peg
  10 Cranial articular surface
  11 Caudal articular surface
  12 Spinous process
  13 Transverse processes

D 3rd. cervical vertebra

E 4th. cervical vertebra

F 5th. cervical vertebra

G 6th. cervical vertebra

H 7th. cervical vertebra
  14 Transverse processes
  15 Cranial articular surface of 4th. cervical vertebra
  16 Cranial articular surface of 6th. cervical vertebra
  17 Caudal articular surface of 3rd. cervical vertebra
  18 Caudal articular surface of 5th. cervical vertebra
  19 Spinous process
  20 Body
  21 Vertebral foramen
    21(a) Dorsal margin
    21(b) Ventral margin
I 1st. thoracic vertebra
J 2nd. thoracic vertebra
K 1st. rib
L Scapula

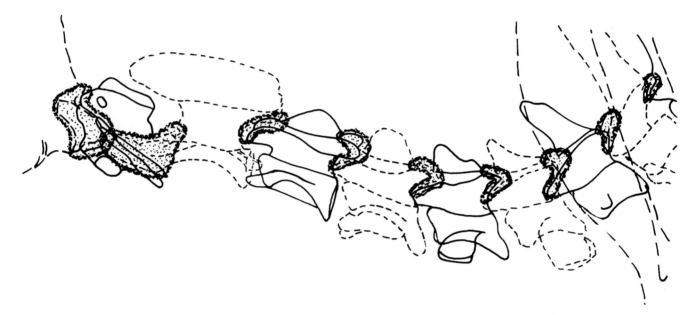

Figure 300 Schematic drawing of extended lateral projection of cervical vertebrae to demonstrate the extent of joint capsules of vertebrae.

= Joint capsule

= Synovial space. With the exception of the first two capsules this space is smaller than drawn.

The first two joint capsules communicate; atlanto-occipital with atlantoaxial.

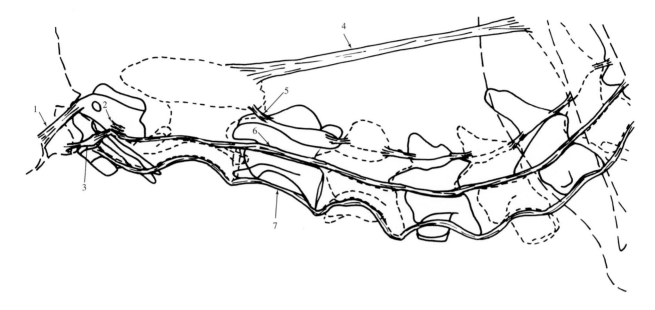

Figure 301 Schematic drawing of extended lateral projection of cervical vertebrae to demonstrate vertebral ligaments.

1 = Lateral atlanto-occipital ligament. Extends to jugular process of occipital bone.

2 = Transverse atlantal ligament. Connects both sides of atlantic ventral arch and so serves to hold dens against atlantic ventral arch.

3 = Apical ligament of dens. In three sections. Middle section to ventral part of foramen magnum with two lateral pillars. Lateral sections are heavier and attach to occipital bone medially at the caudal parts of occipital condyles.

4 = Nuchal ligament

5 = Yellow ligament

6 = Dorsal longitudinal ligament

7 = Ventral longitudinal ligament. Thinner than dorsal ligament.

Intervertebral discs are not shown but are found between the longitudinal ligaments in the intervertebral spaces from 2nd. to 3rd. cervical vertebrae caudally.
Dorsal atlanto-occipital and ventral atlanto-occipital membranes are not shown but act to reinforce the atlanto-occipital joint dorsally and ventrally.
Dorsal atlantoaxial membrane is not shown but it is the dorsal fibrous layer of the atlantoaxial joint capsule.

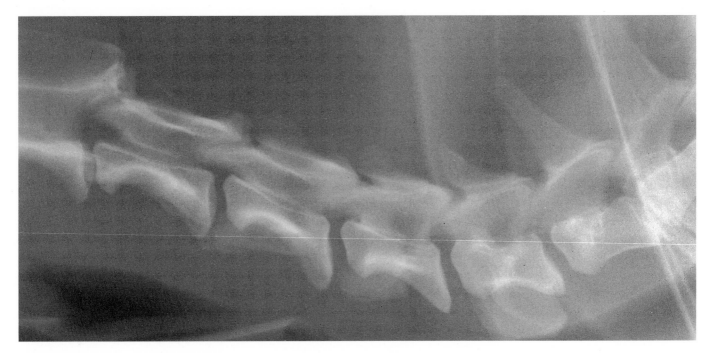

Figure 302 Extended lateral projection of cervical vertebrae in clinically normal dog. Beagle 2.5 years old, entire male (same dog as in Figures 305 and 308).

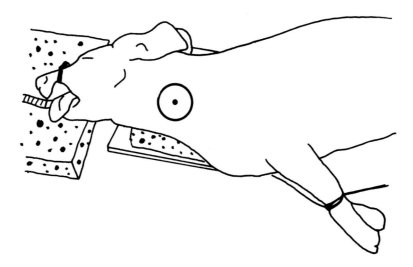

Figure 303 Line drawing of photograph representing radiographic positioning for Figure 302.

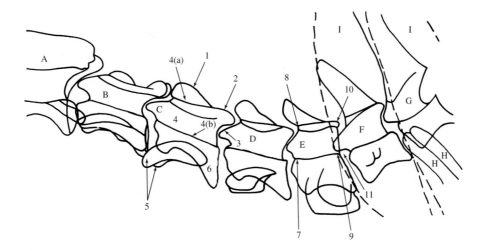

Figure 304 Extended lateral projection of cervical vertebrae in clinically normal dog.

A Axis

B 3rd. cervical vertebra

C 4th. cervical vertebra

D 5th. cervical vertebra

E 6th. cervical vertebra

F 7th. cervical vertebra

  1 Spinous process. (Process on 3rd. cervical vertebra ill defined.)
  2 Caudal articular surface
  3 Cranial articular surface
  4 Vertebral foramen
    4(a) Dorsal margin
    4(b) Ventral margin
  5 Transverse processes
  6 Body
  7 Cranial ventral margin of foramen
  8 Cranial dorsal margin of foramen

Distance between numbers 7 and 8 is the cranial sagittal diameter of the vertebral foramen.

  9 Caudal ventral margin of foramen
  10 Caudal dorsal margin of foramen

Distance between numbers 9 and 10 is the caudal sagittal diameter of the vertebral foramen.

Sagittal diameter measurements are used to evaluate possible stenosis of foramen. Note that measurements must always be compared cranially to cranially, caudally to caudally, as cranial diameters are often smaller than caudal ones in the normal dog. This is especially true for the more caudal cervical vertebrae.

Evaluation of the relationship between adjacent ventral foramen margins is also valuable. Measuring angles between the margins is important to determine whether stenosis is present. Where gross radiographic abnormality is present an obvious dorsal elevation of the cranial margin with respect to the caudal margin is seen.

Note that changes in lateral projection positions of the cervical vertebrae will alter the relationship of all foramina margins, as seen in the radiographs and line drawings, Figures 305 to 310.

  11 Dorsal extremity of intervertebral disc space.

G 1st. thoracic vertebra

H 1st. rib

I Scapula

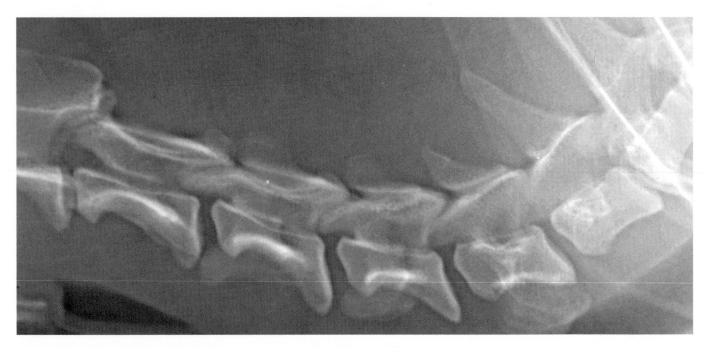

Figure 305 Hyperextended lateral projection of cervical vertebrae in clinically normal dog. Beagle dog 2.5 years old, entire male (same dog as in Figures 302 and 308).

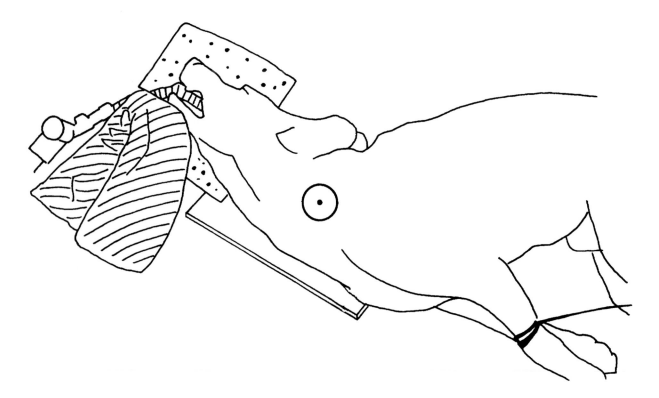

Figure 306 Line drawing of photograph representing radiographic positioning for Figure 305.

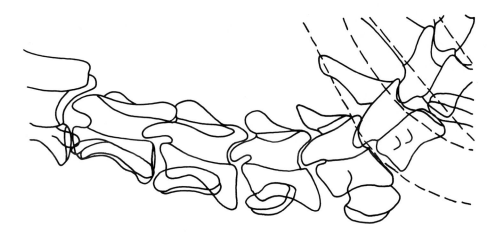

Figure 307   Hyperextended lateral projection of cervical vertebrae in clinically normal dog.

Cranial and caudal sagittal diameters are similar to the extended lateral projection of cervical vertebrae line drawing, Figure 304.

Cranial and caudal cervical ventral foramen margin angles are the same as in the extended lateral projection of cervical vertebrae line drawing, Figure 304.

There are no dorsal elevations of cranial ventral foramen margins.

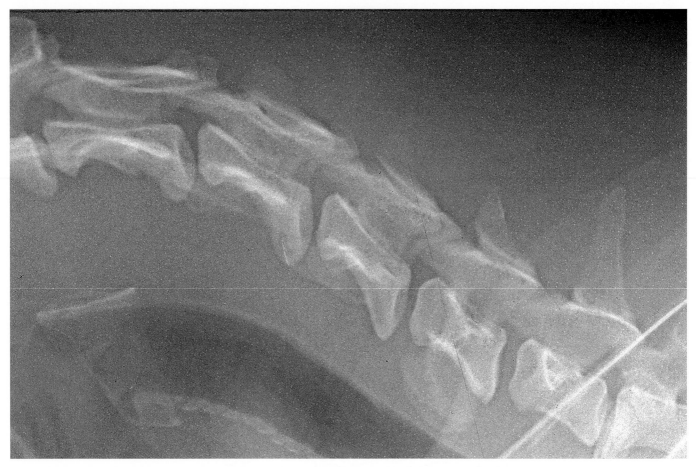

Figure 308 Hyperflexed lateral projection of cervical vertebrae in clinically normal dog. Beagle dog 2.5 years old, entire male (same dog as in Figures 302 and 305).

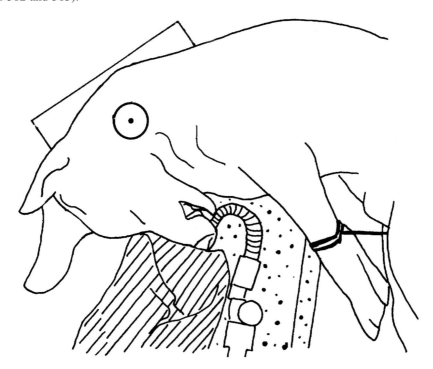

Figure 309 Line drawing of photograph representing radiographic positioning for Figure 308.

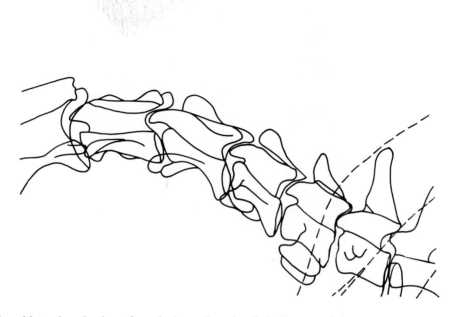

Figure 310   Hyperflexed lateral projection of cervical vertebrae in clinically normal dog.

Sagittal diameters and ventral foramen margin angles in extended and hyperextended lateral projections of cervical vertebrae were similar (see line drawings Figures 304 and 307). A marked change is now seen in the hyperflexed lateral projection of cervical vertebrae.

Cranial and caudal cervical ventral foramen margin angles have increased.

There are obvious dorsal elevations of cranial ventral foramen margins at 3rd., 4th., and 5th. cervical vertebrae. Dorsal elevations are less obvious at 6th. and 7th. cervical vertebrae.

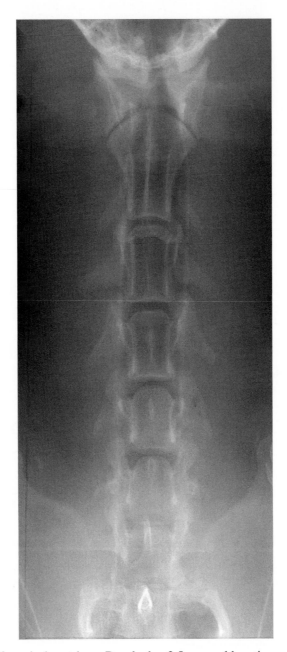

Figure 311   Ventrodorsal projection of cervical vertebrae. Beagle dog 2.5 years old, entire male.

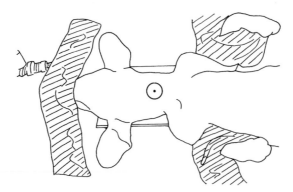

Figure 312   Line drawing of photograph representing radiographic positioning for Figure 311.

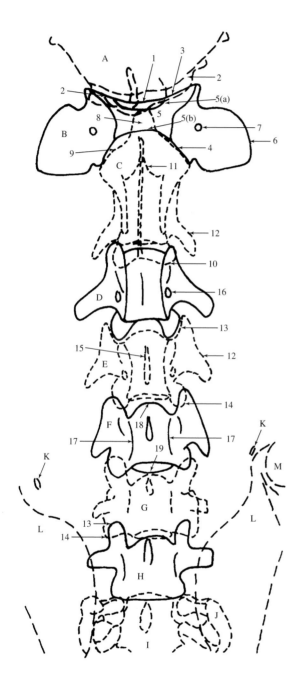

Figure 313   Ventrodorsal projection of cervical vertebrae.

A Skull
   1 Squamous part of occipital
      bone
   2 Occipital condyle

B Atlas
   3 Cranial articular fovea
   4 Caudal articular fovea
   5 Dorsal arch
      5(a) Cranial border
      5(b) Ventral arch caudal
          border
   6 Wing; transverse process
   7 Transverse foramen

C Axis
   8 Dens
   9 Cranial articular surface
  10 Caudal articular surface
  11 Spinous process
  12 Transverse process

D 3rd. cervical vertebra

E 4th. cervical vertebra

F 5th. cervical vertebra

G 6th. cervical vertebra

H 7th. cervical vertebra
  13 Cranial articular surface
  14 Caudal articular surface
  15 Spinous process
  16 Transverse foramen
  17 Lateral margin of vertebral
      foramen
  18 Dorsal cranial margin of
      body
  19 Ventral caudal margin of
      body

I 1st. thoracic vertebra

J 1st. rib

K Clavicle

L Scapula

M Humerus

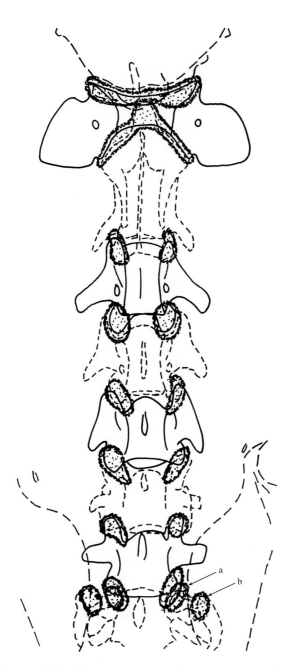

Figure 314 Schematic drawing of ventrodorsal projection of cervical vertebrae to demonstrate joint capsules.

⬤ = Joint capsule and synovial space of vertebral and costal articulations.

Atlanto-occipital joint capsule communicates ventromedially with atlantoaxial joint capsule.

a = Joint capsule of head of rib

b = Joint capsule of tubercle of rib

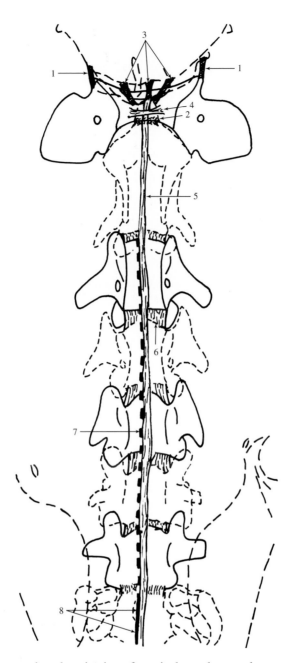

Figure 315 Schematic drawing of ventrodorsal projection of cervical vertebrae to demonstrate vertebral ligaments.

1 = Lateral atlanto-occipital ligament

2 = Dorsal atlantoaxial ligament

3 = Apical ligament of dens. Centrally attaches to ventral foramen magnum. Laterally attaches to occipital condyles.

4 = Transverse atlantal ligament. Passes dorsally over dens. A bursa separates ligament and dens.

5 = Positions of dorsal and ventral longitudinal ligaments

6 = Yellow ligament. Laterally extends as far as the joint capsules surrounding articular processes. Ventral to ligament is epidural space.

7 = Nuchal ligament. Ligament is anatomically in the midline but is illustrated to the right of midline to differentiate it from (5).

8 = Supraspinous ligament. Ligament is anatomically in the midline but is illustrated to the right of the midline to differentiate it from (5).

Rib ligaments and intervertebral discs not shown.

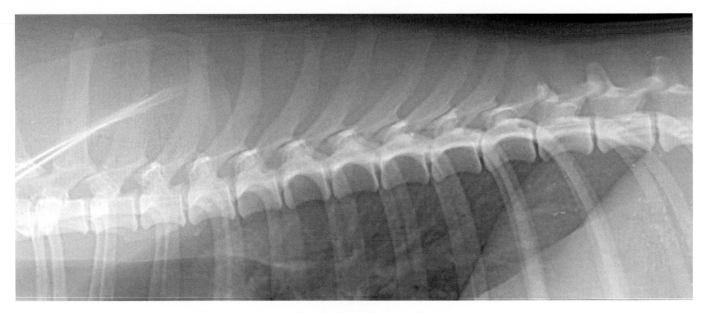

Figure 316 Lateral projection of thoracic vertebrae. Beagle dog 2.5 years old, entire male.

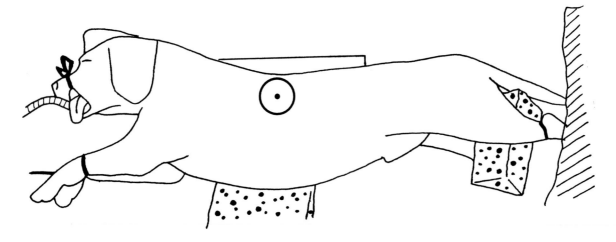

Figure 317 Line drawing of photograph representing radiographic positioning for Figure 316.

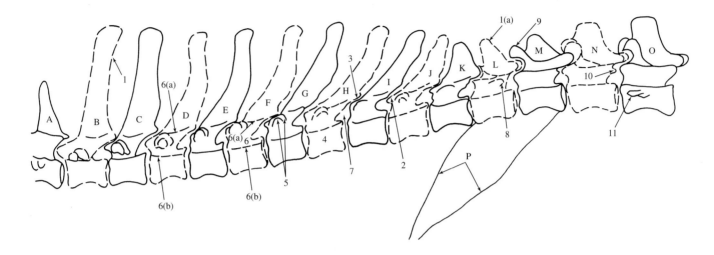

Figure 318 Lateral projection of thoracic vertebrae with rib shadows excluded for clarity.

A 7th. cervical vertebra

B 1st. thoracic vertebra

C 2nd. thoracic vertebra

D 3rd. thoracic vertebra

E 4th. thoracic vertebra

F 5th. thoracic vertebra

G 6th. thoracic vertebra

H 7th thoracic vertebra

I 8th. thoracic vertebra

J 9th. thoracic vertebra

K 10th. thoracic vertebra

L 11th. thoracic vertebra. Anticlinal vertebra.

M 12th. thoracic vertebra

N 13th. thoracic vertebra

1 Spinous process
 1(a) Spinous process of anticlinal vertebra. (Nearly perpendicular to axis)

2 Cranial articular process

3 Caudal articular process

4 Body

5 Transverse process. Includes mammillary process from 2nd. or 3rd. thoracic vertebra caudally.

6 Vertebral foramen
 6(a) Dorsal margin
 6(b) Ventral margin

7 Intervertebral foramen

8 First visible accessory process

9 Mammillary process

10 Accessory process

O 1st. lumbar vertebra

11 Transverse process

P Crura of diaphragm

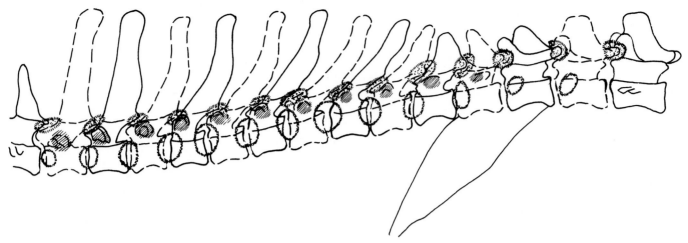

Figure 319 Schematic drawing of lateral projection of thoracic vertebrae to demonstrate the extent of joint capsules.

= Joint capsule and synovial space of vertebral articulation

= Joint capsule and synovial space of costovertebral joint. Head of rib.

= Joint capsule and synovial space of costovertebral joint. Tubercle of rib.

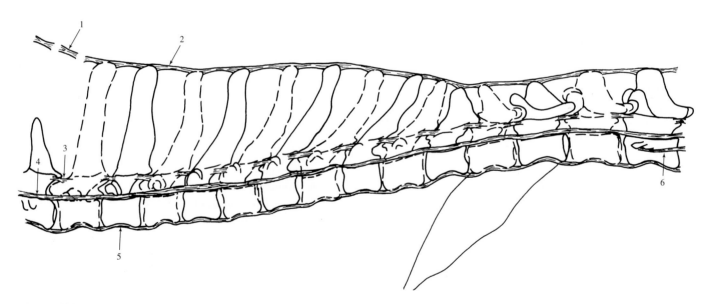

Figure 320 Schematic drawing of lateral projection of thoracic vertebrae to demonstrate vertebral ligaments.

1 = Nuchal ligament

2 = Supraspinous ligament

3 = Yellow ligament

4 = Dorsal longitudinal ligament

5 = Ventral longitudinal ligament

6 = Intertransverse ligament

Interspinous ligaments and intervertebral discs not shown.

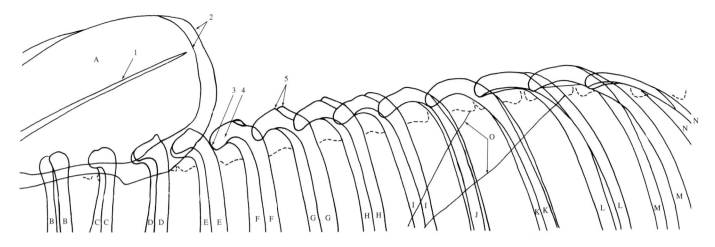

Figure 321   Lateral projection of thoracic vertebrae to demonstrate the rib shadows not seen in Figure 318.

A Scapula
  1 Spine
  2 Caudal margins of right and left

B 1st. rib

C 2nd. rib

D 3rd. rib

E 4th. rib

F 5th. rib

G 6th. rib

H 7th. rib

I 8th. rib

J 9th. rib

K 10th. rib

L 11th. rib

M 12th. rib

N 13th. rib
  3 Head
  4 Neck
  5 Tubercles (right and left)

O Crura of diaphragm

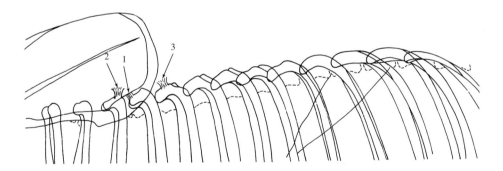

Figure 322   Schematic drawing of lateral projection of thoracic vertebrae to demonstrate rib ligaments.

1 = Ligament of head. Extends from head of rib to lateral part of intervertebral disc. Last three ribs are displaced and for these the ligament shifts to attach to the bodies of the vertebrae.

2 = Ligament of tubercle. Is distal to articular capsule. Crosses capsule and attaches to transverse process.

3 = Ligament of neck. Extends from neck to ventral surface of transverse process plus lateral body of vertebra.

Intercapital ligament not shown but is seen in a similar position to the head ligament. It runs across the ventral vertebral canal, at the level of the intervertebral disc, to attach to the head of the rib on the contralateral side. It is absent from 1st., 12th. and 13th. ribs.

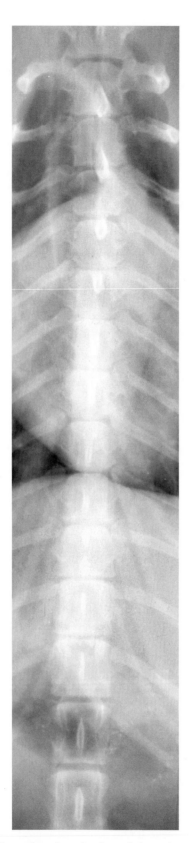

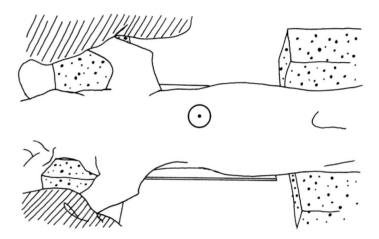

Figure 324 Line drawing of photograph representing radiographic positioning for Figure 323.

Figure 323 Ventrodorsal projection of thoracic vertebrae. Beagle dog 2.5 years old, entire male.

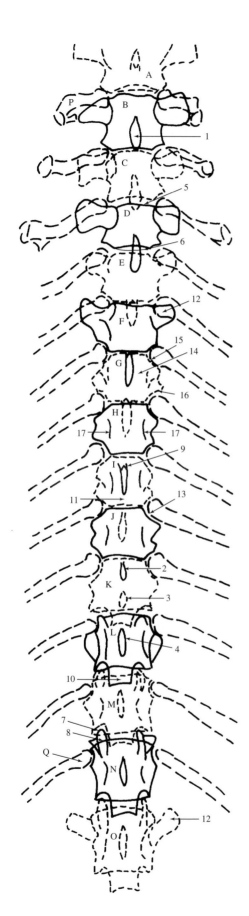

Figure 325   Ventrodorsal projection of thoracic vertebrae with ventral shadows of ribs excluded for clarity.

A   7th. cervical vertebra

B   1st. thoracic vertebra

C   2nd. thoracic vertebra

D   3rd. thoracic vertebra

E   4th. thoracic vertebra

F   5th. thoracic vertebra

G   6th. thoracic vertebra

H   7th. thoracic vertebra

I   8th. thoracic vertebra

J   9th. thoracic vertebra

K   10th. thoracic vertebra

L   11th. thoracic vertebra. Anticlinal vertebra.

M   12th. thoracic vertebra

N   13th. thoracic vertebra

O   1st. lumbar vertebra

1   Spinous process of 1st. thoracic vertebra. These processes incline caudally from 1st. to 10th. thoracic vertebrae.

2   Spinous process of 9th. thoracic vertebra

3   Spinous process of 10th. thoracic vertebra

4   Spinous process of 11th. thoracic vertebra

5   Cranial margin of body

6   Caudal margin of body

7   Cranial articular margin of 13th. thoracic vertebra

8   Mammillary process (seen as a distinct structure just caudal to the articular margin)

9   Cranial articular margin found near the median plane from thoracic vertebrae 2 to 10

10   Caudal articular margin of thoracic vertebra

11   Caudal articular margin found near the median plane from thoracic vertebrae 1 to 9

12   Transverse process

13   Costal fovea of transverse process

14   Body

15   Cranial costal fovea

16   Caudal costal fovea

17   Lateral margin of vertebral foramen

P   1st. rib

Q   13th. rib

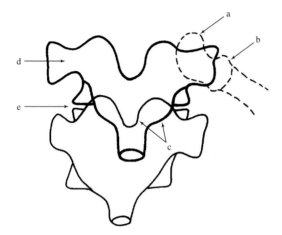

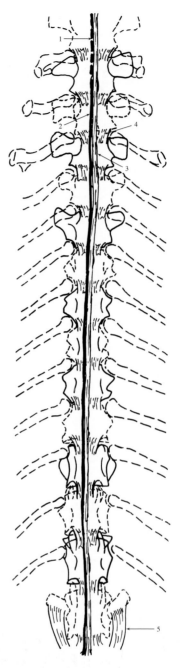

Figure 326 Sketch drawing of ventrodorsal thoracic vertebrae to demonstrate anatomically the joint articulations of vertebrae and ribs.

a = Costovertebral joint. Head of rib.

b = Costovertebral joint. Tubercle of rib.

c = Cranial and caudal articular facets of vertebral joint

d = Transverse process of thoracic vertebra

e = Intervertebral disc space for vertebral bodies

Only (a) and (e) are consistently visible in ventrodorsal projection of thoracic vertebrae, Figure 323, from 1st. to 13th. thoracic vertebrae.

The transverse processes (d) are very unclear throughout the thoracic vertebrae in Figure 323, so making (b) impossible to see.

The vertebral joint (c) is just seen from 11th. to 13th. thoracic vertebrae.

Figure 327 Schematic drawing of ventrodorsal projection of thoracic vertebrae to demonstrate vertebral ligaments.

1 = Nuchal ligament. Position is anatomically in the midline but it is drawn to the right side to differentiate it from (3).

2 = Supraspinous ligament. Position is anatomically the midline but it is drawn to the right side to differentiate it from (3).

3 = Position of dorsal and ventral longitudinal ligaments

4 = Yellow ligament

5 = Intertransverse ligament

Rib ligaments and intervertebral discs not shown.

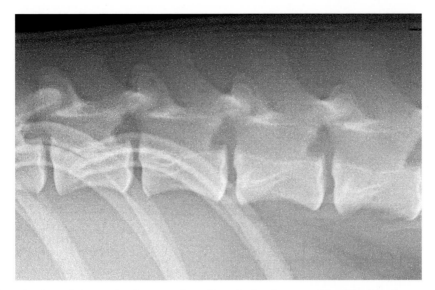

Figure 328   Lateral projection of thoracolumbar vertebrae. Beagle dog 2 years old, entire female.

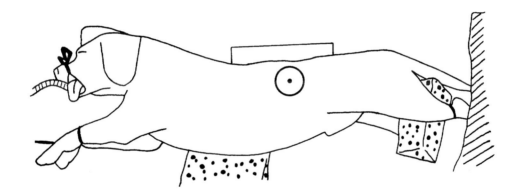

Figure 329   Line drawing of photograph representing radiographic positioning for Figure 328.

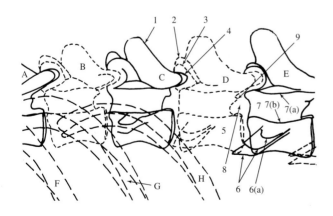

Figure 330   Lateral projection of thoracolumbar vertebrae.

A 12th. thoracic vertebra

B 13th. thoracic vertebra

C 1st. lumbar vertebra

D 2nd. lumbar vertebra

E 3rd. lumbar vertebra
  1 Spinous process
  2 Mammillary process
  3 Cranial articular process
  4 Caudal articular process
  5 Body

6 Transverse process
  6(a) Base
7 Vertebral foramen
  7(a) Dorsal margin
  7(b) Ventral margin
8 Intervertebral
   foramen
9 Accessory process

F 11th. rib

G 12th. rib

H 13th. rib

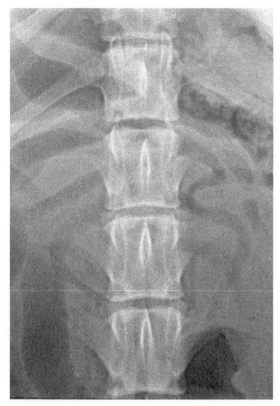

Figure 331 Ventrodorsal projection of thoracolumbar vertebrae. Beagle dog 2 years old, entire female.

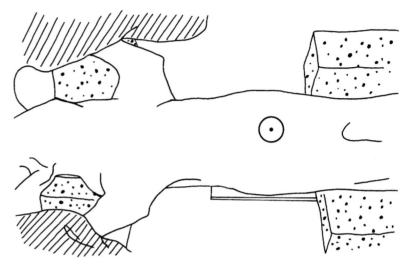

Figure 332 Line drawing of photograph representing radiographic positioning for Figure 331.

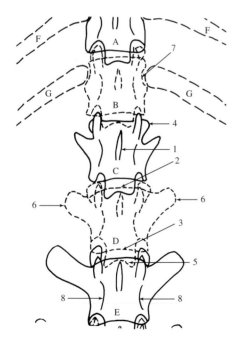

Figure 333 Ventrodorsal projection of thoracolumbar vertebrae.

A 12th. thoracic vertebra

B 13th. thoracic vertebra

C 1st. lumbar vertebra

D 2nd. lumbar vertebra

E 3rd. lumbar vertebra
  1 Spinous process
  2 Cranial margin of body
  3 Caudal margin of body

4 Cranial articular process including mammillary process

5 Caudal articular process

6 Transverse process

7 Costal fovea of vertebral body of 13th. thoracic vertebra

8 Lateral margin of vertebral foramen

F 12th. rib

G 13th. rib

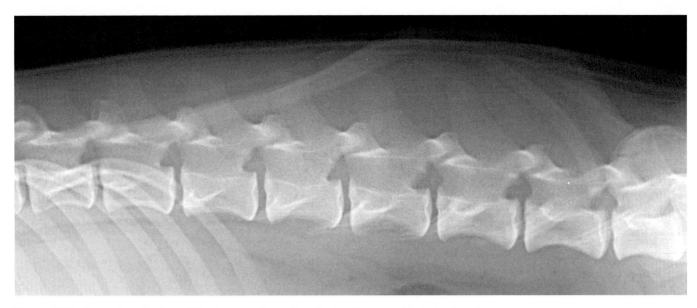

Figure 334   Lateral projection of lumbar vertebrae. Beagle dog 2 years old, entire female.

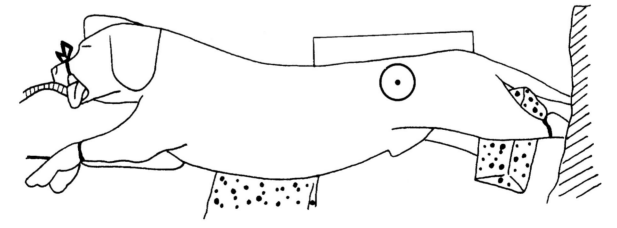

Figure 335   Line drawing of photograph representing radiographic positioning for Figure 334.

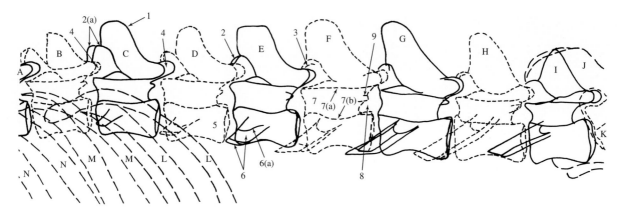

Figure 336 Lateral projection of lumbar vertebrae.

A 12th. thoracic vertebra

B 13th. thoracic vertebra

C 1st. lumbar vertebra

D 2nd. lumbar vertebra

E 3rd. lumbar vertebra

F 4th. lumbar vertebra

G 5th. lumbar vertebra

H 6th. lumbar vertebra

I 7th. lumbar vertebra
  1 Spinous process
  2 Mammillary process
    2(a) Both processes seen
  3 Cranial articular process

4 Caudal articular process
5 Body
6 Transverse process
  6(a) Base
7 Vertebral foramen
  7(a) Dorsal margin
  7(b) Ventral margin
8 Intervertebral foramen
9 Accessory process

J Ilium

K Sacrum

L 13th. rib

M 12th. rib

N 11th. rib

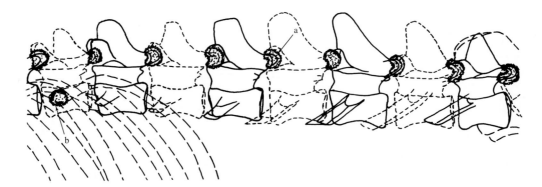

Figure 337 Schematic drawing of lateral projection of lumbar vertebrae to demonstrate the extent of joint capsules.

a = Joint capsule and synovial space of vertebral articulation

b = Joint capsule and synovial space of costovertebral joint. Head of rib.

An Atlas of Interpretative Radiographic Anatomy of the Dog and Cat

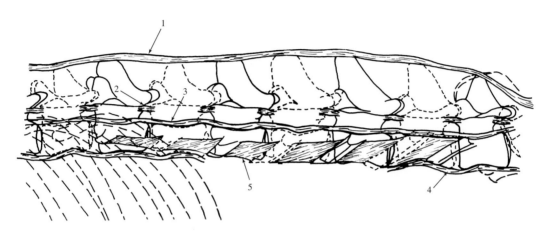

Figure 338 Schematic drawing of lateral projection of lumbar vertebrae to demonstrate vertebral ligaments.

1 = Supraspinous ligament. Extends to 3rd. coccygeal vertebra.

2 = Yellow ligament

3 = Dorsal longitudinal ligament

4 = Ventral longitudinal ligament

5 = Intertransverse ligament

Intervertebral discs interspinous and rib ligaments are not shown.

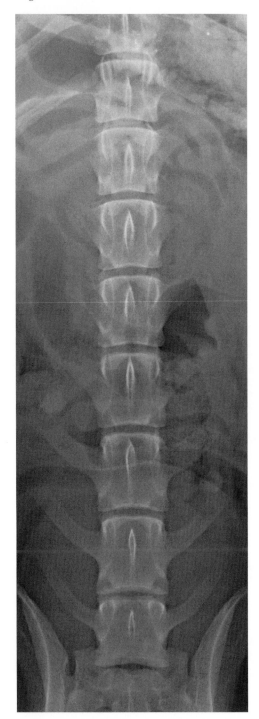

Figure 339 Ventrodorsal projection of lumbar vertebrae. Beagle dog 2 years old, entire female.

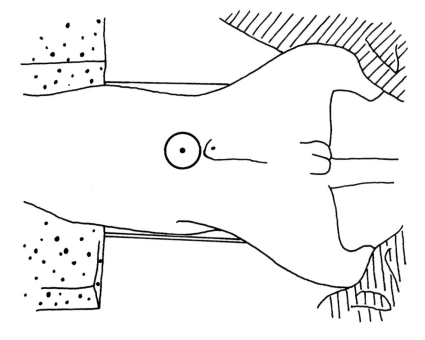

Figure 340 Line drawing of photograph representing radiographic positioning for Figure 339.

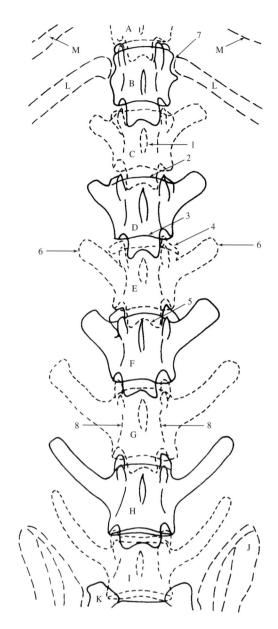

Figure 341   Ventrodorsal projection of lumbar vertebrae.

A 12th. thoracic vertebra

B 13th. thoracic vertebra

C 1st. lumbar vertebra

D 2nd. lumbar vertebra

E 3rd. lumbar vertebra

F 4th. lumbar vertebra

G 5th. lumbar vertebra

H 6th. lumbar vertebra

I 7th. lumbar vertebra
  1 Spinous process
  2 Cranial margin of body

3 Caudal margin of body
4 Cranial articular process including mammillary process
5 Caudal articular process
6 Transverse process (lateral aspects of some are obscured by soft tissue shadows making their appearance asymmetrical)
7 Costal fovea of vertebral body of 13th. thoracic vertebra
8 Lateral margin of vertebral foramen

J Ilium

K Sacrum

L 13th. rib

M 12th. rib

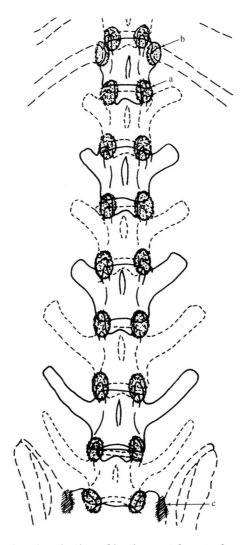

Figure 342   Schematic drawing of ventrodorsal projection of lumbar vertebrae to demonstrate extent of joint capsules.

a = Joint capsule of vertebral articulation

b = Joint capsule of costovertebral articulation. Head of rib.

c = Fibrocartilaginous joint of sacroiliac joint

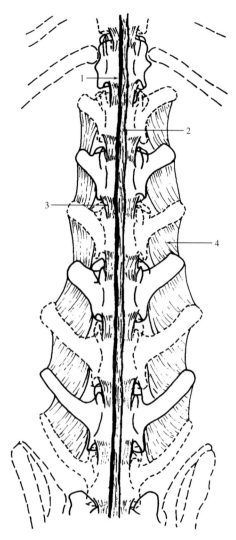

Figure 343   Schematic drawing of ventrodorsal projection of lumbar vertebrae to demonstrate vertebral ligaments.

1 = Supraspinous ligament. Shown drawn to the right of midline to separate it from longitudinal ligaments (2). True anatomical position is midline.

2 = Position of dorsal and ventral longitudinal ligaments.

3 = Yellow ligament

4 = Intertransverse ligament

Rib ligaments and intervertebral discs not shown.

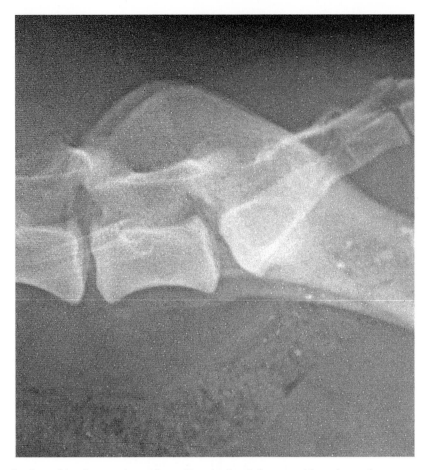

Figure 344   Lateral projection of lumbosacral vertebrae. Beagle dog 2.5 years old, entire male.

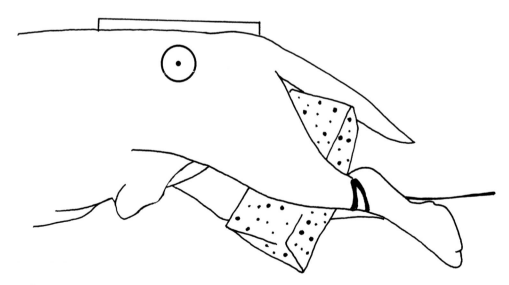

Figure 345   Line drawing of photograph representing radiographic positioning for Figure 344.

An Atlas of Interpretative Radiographic Anatomy of the Dog and Cat

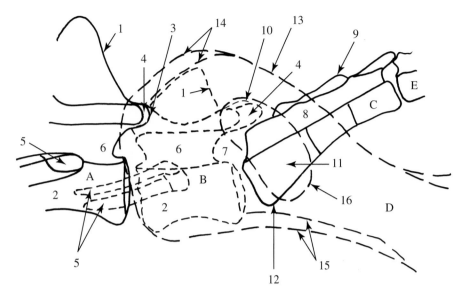

Figure 346 Lateral projection of lumbosacral vertebrae.

A 6th. lumbar vertebra

B 7th. lumbar vertebra
   1 Spinous process
   2 Body
   3 Cranial articular process
   4 Caudal articular process
   5 Transverse processes
   6 Vertebral foramen
   7 Intervertebral foramen

C Sacrum
   8 Sacral canal
   9 Intermediate sacral crest
  10 Mammillary process of cranial articular process
  11 Wing
  12 Promontory

D Ilium
  13 Dorsal margins
  14 Cranial margins
  15 Ventral margins
  16 Sacroiliac articulation

E Coccygeal or caudal vertebra

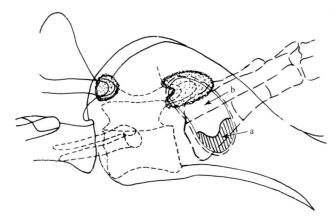

Figure 347 Schematic drawing of lateral projection of lumbosacral vertebrae to demonstrate joint capsules.

 = Joint capsule of vertebral articulation

—— = Joint capsule of sacroiliac articulation
    a Synovial part
    b Fibrocartilaginous part

 = Auricular surface of sacroiliac joint

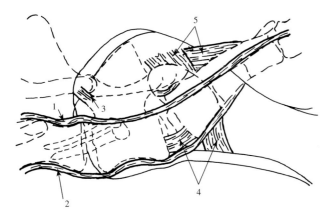

Figure 348 Schematic drawing of lateral projection of lumbosacral vertebrae to demonstrate vertebral ligaments.

1 = Dorsal longitudinal ligament. Stops at 5th. coccygeal vertebra.

2 = Ventral longitudinal ligament. Stops at midsacral level.

3 = Yellow ligament

4 = Ventral sacroiliac ligament

5 = Dorsal sacroiliac ligament. Dorsal ligament is thicker than ventral.

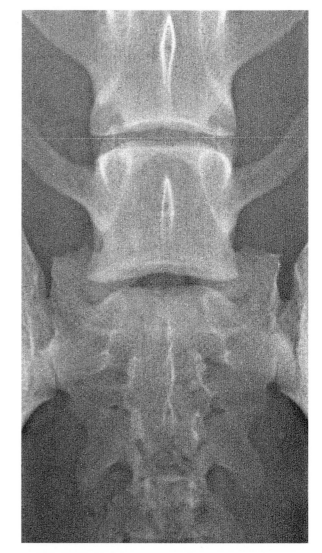

Figure 349 Ventrodorsal projection of lumbosacral vertebrae. Beagle dog 2 years old, entire female.

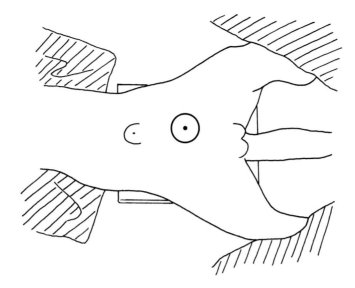

Figure 350   Line drawing of photograph representing radiographic positioning for Figure 349.

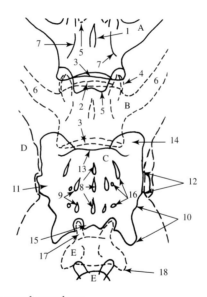

Figure 351   Ventrodorsal projection of lumbosacral vertebrae.

A 6th. lumbar vertebra

B 7th. lumbar vertebra
  1 Spinous process
  2 Cranial margin of body
  3 Caudal margin of body
  4 Cranial articular process including mammillary process
  5 Caudal articular process
  6 Transverse process
  7 Lateral margin of vertebral foramen

C Sacrum
  8 Median sacral crest
  9 Intermediate sacral crest

10 Lateral sacral crest
11 Wing
12 Position of synovial joint between bony articular margins
13 Base
14 Cranial articular process
15 Caudal articular process
16 Sacral foramina

D Ilium

E Coccygeal or caudal vertebra
  17 Cranial articular process
  18 Transverse process

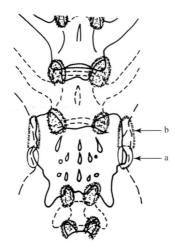

Figure 352   Schematic drawing of ventrodorsal projection of lumbosacral vertebrae to demonstrate the extent of joints.

= Joint capsule of vertebral articulation

Sacroiliac articulation

——   a = Synovial part of sacroiliac joint capsule

||||||||||||| b = Fibrocartilaginous part of sacroiliac joint capsule

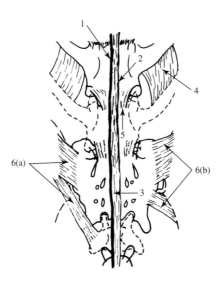

Figure 353   Schematic drawing of ventrodorsal projection of lumbosacral vertebrae to demonstrate vertebral ligaments.

1 = Position of supraspinous ligament. Shown drawn to the right of the midline to separate it from longitudinal ligaments (2). True anatomical position is midline.

2 = Position of dorsal and ventral longitudinal ligaments

3 = Continuation of dorsal longitudinal ligament

4 = Intertransverse ligament

5 = Yellow ligament

6 = Positions of sacroiliac ligaments

    6(a) Dorsal position shown on right side

    6(b) Ventral position shown on left side

An Atlas of Interpretative Radiographic Anatomy of the Dog and Cat

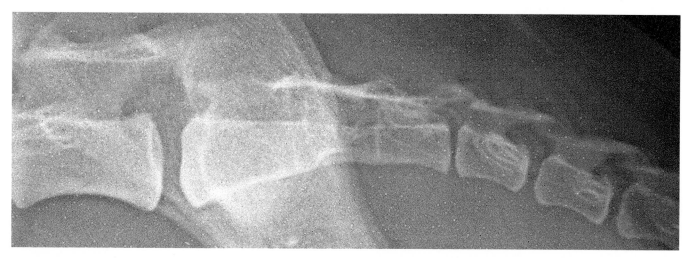

Figure 354 Hyperflexed lateral projection of lumbosacral vertebrae including proximal coccygeal vertebrae. Beagle dog 2.5 years old, entire male.

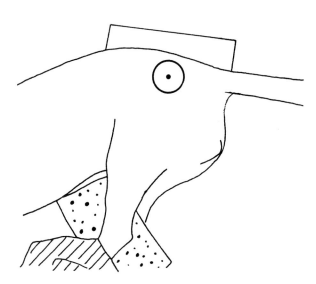

Figure 355 Line drawing of photograph representing radiographic positioning for Figure 354.

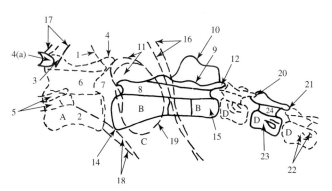

Figure 356 Hyperflexed lateral projection of lumbosacral vertebrae including proximal coccygeal vertebrae.

A 7th. lumbar vertebra
  1 Spinous process
  2 Body
  3 Cranial articular process
  4 Caudal articular process
    4(a) Process of 6th. lumbar vertebra
  5 Transverse processes
  6 Vertebral foramen
  7 Intervertebral foramen

B Sacrum
  8 Sacral canal
  9 Intermediate sacral crest
  10 Median sacral crest (only just visible)
  11 Cranial articular process

12 Caudal articular process
13 Wing
14 Promontory
15 Body of 3rd. sacral segment

C Ilium
16 Dorsal margins
17 Cranial margins
18 Ventral margins
19 Sacroiliac articulation

D Coccygeal or caudal vertebra
20 Cranial articular process
21 Caudal articular process
22 Transverse processes
23 Body
24 Vertebral foramen

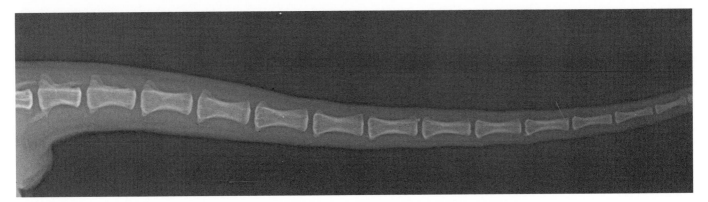

Figure 357   Lateral projection of coccygeal or caudal vertebrae. Beagle dog 2 years old, entire female.

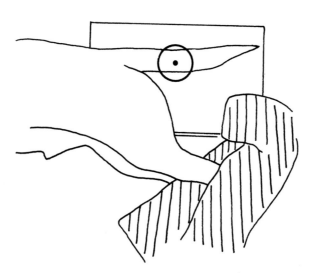

Figure 358   Line drawing of photograph representing radiographic positioning for Figure 357.

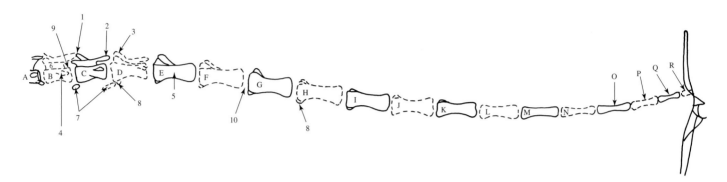

Figure 359 Lateral projection of coccygeal or caudal vertebrae.

A 2nd. coccygeal vertebra

B 3rd. coccygeal vertebra

C 4th. coccygeal vertebra

D 5th. coccygeal vertebra

E 6th. coccygeal vertebra

F 7th. coccygeal vertebra

G 8th. coccygeal vertebra

H 9th. coccygeal vertebra

I 10th. coccygeal vertebra

J 11th. coccygeal vertebra

K 12th. coccygeal vertebra

L 13th. coccygeal vertebra

M 14th. coccygeal vertebra

N 15th. coccygeal vertebra

O 16th. coccygeal vertebra

P 17th. coccygeal vertebra

Q 18th. coccygeal vertebra

R 19th. coccygeal vertebra

  1 Cranial articular process

  2 Caudal articular process

Both processes gradually disappear so that by the 12th. vertebra they are no longer present.

  3 Mammillary process

  4 Transverse process

  5 Body

  6 Vertebral foramen. Lumen gradually becomes smaller so that by the 6th. or 7th. vertebra it is only a groove.

  7 Haemal arches

  8 Haemal process

  9 Intervertebral foramen

 10 Position of intervertebral disc of the intervertebral symphysis

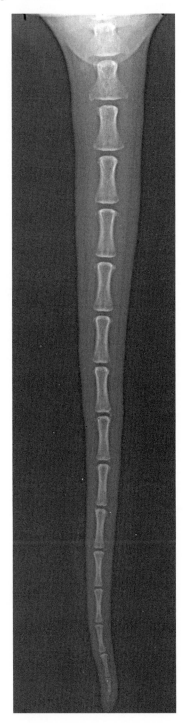

Figure 360 Ventrodorsal projection of coccygeal or caudal vertebrae. Beagle dog 2 years old, entire female.

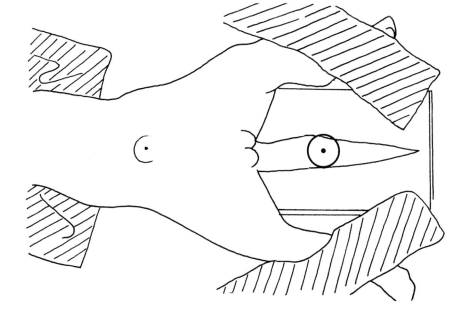

Figure 361 Line drawing of photograph representing radiographic positioning for Figure 360.

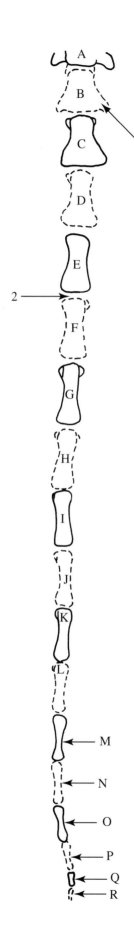

Figure 362 Ventrodorsal projection of coccygeal or caudal vertebrae.

A 3rd. coccygeal vertebra

B 4th. coccygeal vertebra

C 5th. coccygeal vertebra

D 6th. coccygeal vertebra

E 7th. coccygeal vertebra

F 8th. coccygeal vertebra

G 9th. coccygeal vertebra

H 10th. coccygeal vertebra

I 11th. coccygeal vertebra

J 12th. coccygeal vertebra

K 13th. coccygeal vertebra

L 14th. coccygeal vertebra

M 15th. coccygeal vertebra

N 16th. coccygeal vertebra

O 17th. coccygeal vertebra

P 18th. coccygeal vertebra

Q 19th. coccygeal vertebra

R 20th. coccygeal vertebra. Last vertebra.

1 Transverse process

2 Position of intervertebral disc of the intervertebral symphysis

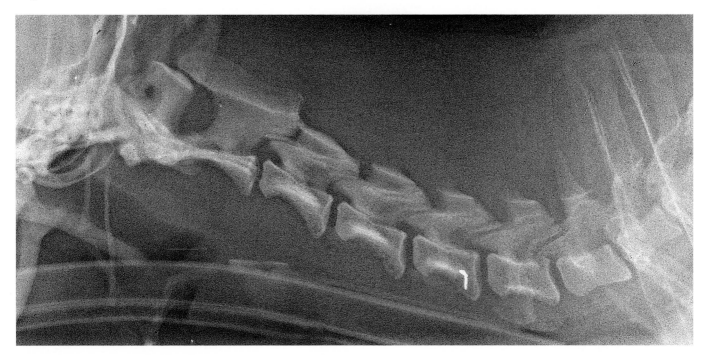

Figure 363 Extended lateral projection of cervical vertebrae. Toy breed of dog. Yorkshire Terrier dog 5 years old, entire female (same dog as in Figures 364 and 365).

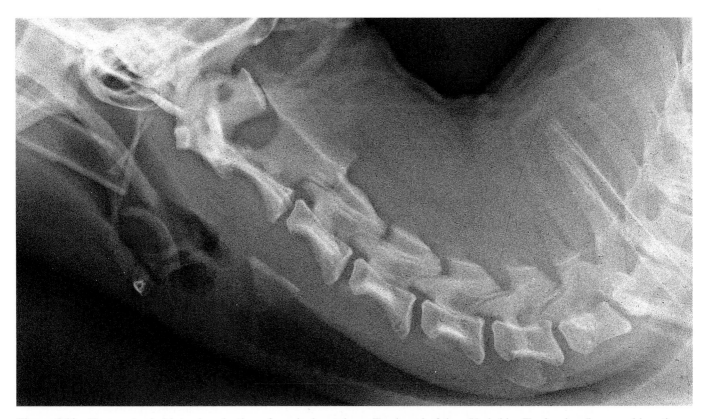

Figure 364 Hyperextended lateral projection of cervical vertebrae. Toy breed of dog. Yorkshire Terrier dog 5 years old, entire female (same dog as in Figures 363 and 365).

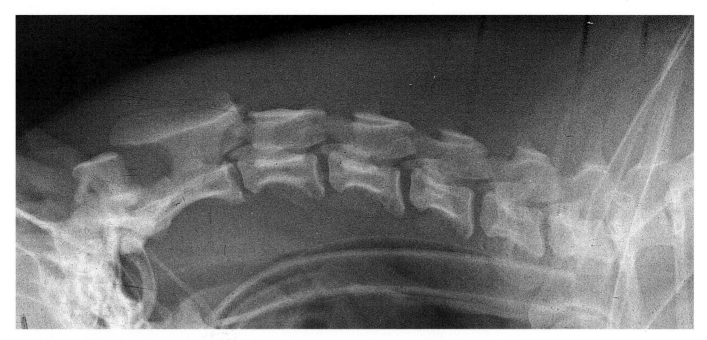

Figure 365   Hyperflexed lateral projection of cervical vertebrae. Toy breed of dog. Yorkshire Terrier dog 5 years old, entire female (same dog as in Figures 363 and 364).

This series of three radiographs has been included to demonstrate the normal relationship between the 1st. and 2nd. cervical vertebrae during extreme flexion and extension of the neck. Note the dorsal space between the 1st. and 2nd. cervical vertebrae, or atlas and axis, which shows little variation in the three projections. Also observe the dorsal borders of the first two vertebrae to be parallel to one another. The dens of the axis remains in a ventral position within the vertebral canal in all the projections.

The atlas, axis and occipital condyle of the skull are all of a normal size and conformation. Analysis of these anatomical characteristics is very important for this particular region as abnormalities of this area, in toy breeds, are well recognised. The atlas and the dens of the axis are not reduced in size. The occipital condyle can be seen to be a normal size and in the correct articular position.

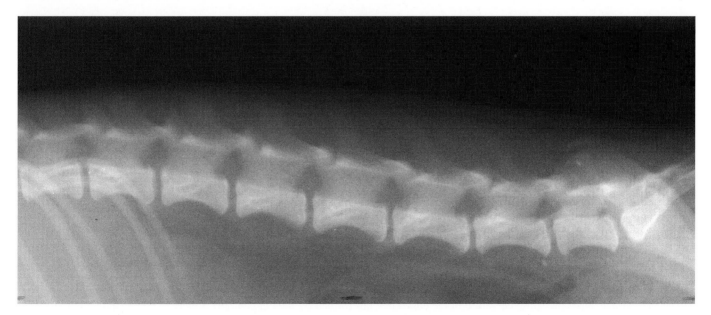

Figure 366   Lateral projection of lumbar vertebrae. Toy breed of dog. Yorkshire Terrier dog 1 year old, entire male. Note the appearance of the bodies of the lumbar vertebrae. They are comparatively long for a dog and could be mistaken for cat lumbar vertebrae.

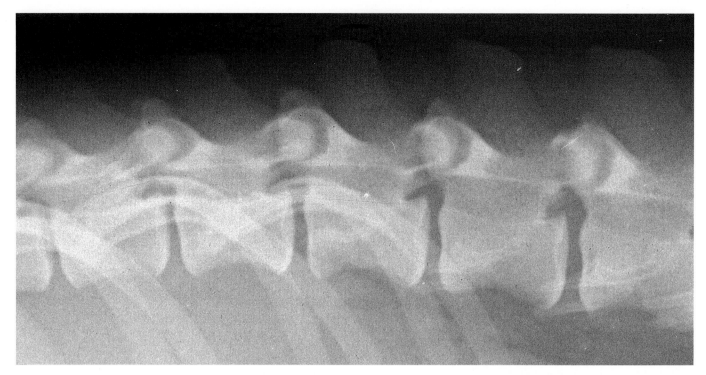

Figure 367 Lateral projection of lumbar vertebrae. Chondrodystrophic breed of dog. Standard Dachshund dog 7 years old, entire male.

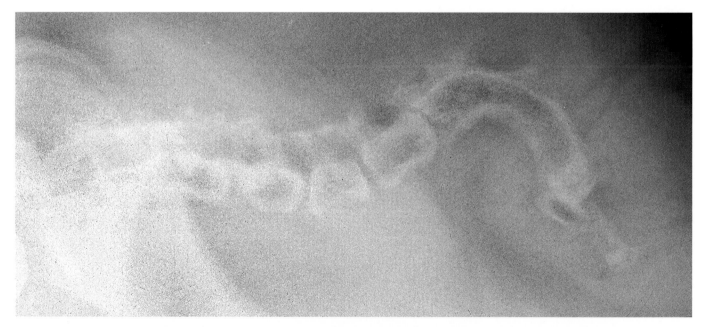

Figure 368 Lateral projection of sacrum and coccygeal vertebrae. Corkscrew tail. Bulldog 1 year old, entire female.
The radiograph shows the spiral curvature of the corkscrew tail formed by the congenitally abnormal coccygeal vertebrae. Distally there is fusion of the bodies (block vertebrae) as seen by the long length of these vertebrae. Proximally the 1st. and 2nd. coccygeal vertebrae are congenitally malformed having wedge-shaped bodies (hemivertebrae).
Incomplete fusion of the 3rd. sacral segment is also present.

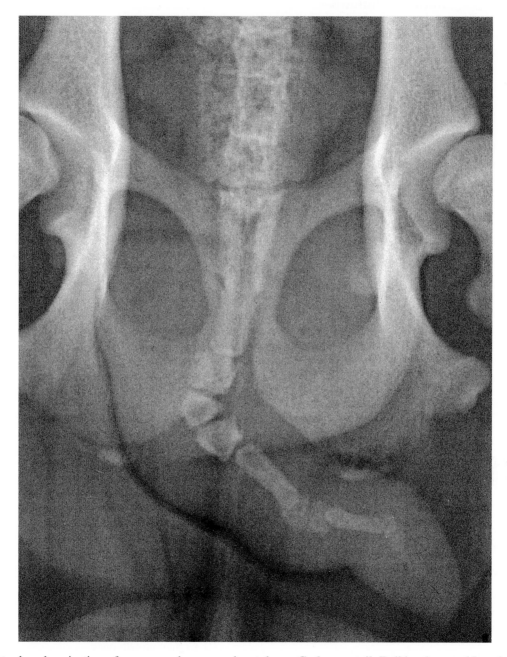

Figure 369   Ventrodorsal projection of sacrum and coccygeal vertebrae. Corkscrew tail. Bulldog 1 year old, entire female.

   The radiograph shows the spiral curvature of the corkscrew tail as formed by the congenitally deformed coccygeal vertebrae. Distally the vertebral bodies are fused (block vertebrae), while proximally the bodies are much shorter and broader. The body of the 2nd. coccygeal vertebra has a wedge shape (hemivertebra).

   Incomplete fusion of the 3rd. sacral segment is also seen.

   This particular Bulldog has severe hip dysplasia with secondary joint degeneration (see Figure 145 for normal chondrodys-trophic breed of dog hip joints).

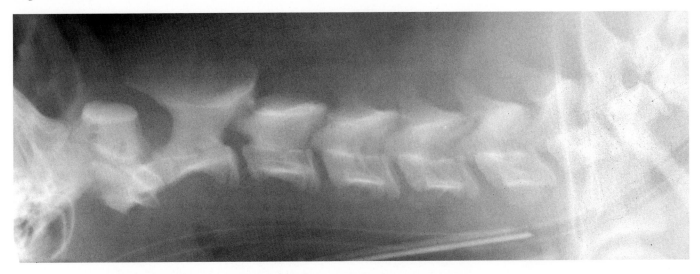

Figure 370   Age 13 weeks.

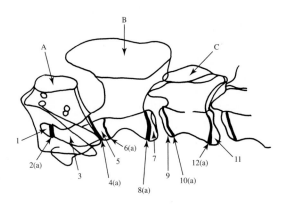

Figure 370

Figures 370, 371, 372, 373   Lateral projection of cervical vertebrae. Samoyed crossbred dog entire male at 13, 25, 38, and 52 weeks of age. Correlating line drawings for all ages except 52 weeks.

A Atlas; 1st. cervical vertebra

B Axis; 2nd. cervical vertebra
   1 Proatlas. Centrum for apex of dens
   2 Intercentrum
   2(a) Open
   3 Centrum for dens
   4 Intercentrum
   4(a) Open
   5 Centrum for cranial body equivalent to cranial epiphysis
   6 Cranial growth plate
   6(a) Open
   7 Caudal epiphysis
   8 Caudal growth plate

   8(a) Open
   8(b) Closing

C 3rd. cervical vertebra
   9 Cranial epiphysis
   10 Cranial growth plate
   10(a) Open
   10(b) Closing
   11 Caudal epiphysis
   12 Caudal growth plate
   12(a) Open
   12(b) Closing

For clarity transverse process shadows have been excluded from all drawings.

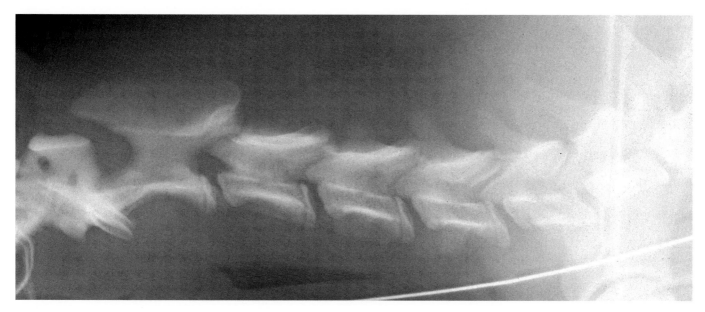

Figure 371 Age 25 weeks.

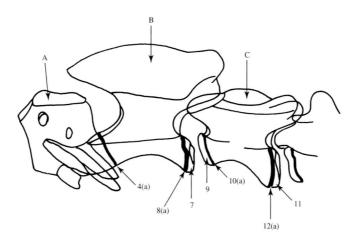

Figure 371

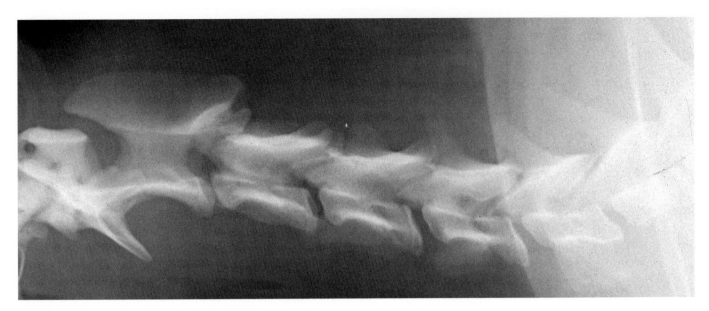

Figure 372   Age 38 weeks.

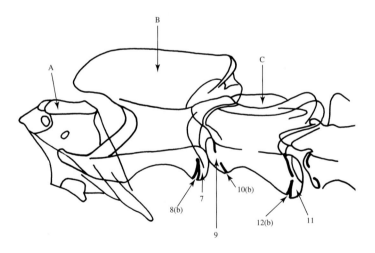

Figure 372

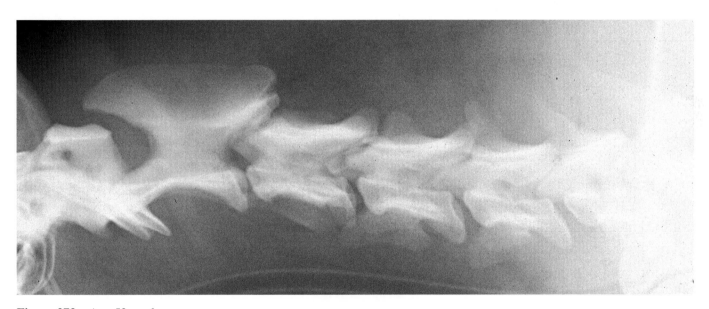

Figure 373   Age 52 weeks.

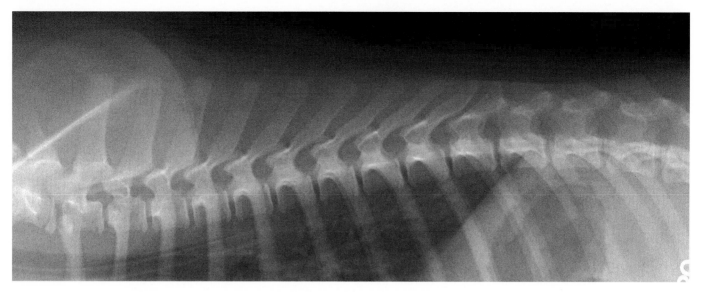

Figure 374   Age 13 weeks.

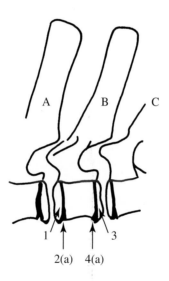

Figure 374

Figures 374, 375, 376, 377   Lateral projection of thoracic vertebrae. Samoyed crossbred dog entire male at 13, 25, 38 and 52 weeks of age. Correlating line drawings for all ages except 52 weeks.

A 2nd. thoracic vertebra

B 3rd. thoracic vertebra
  1 Cranial epiphysis
  2 Cranial growth plate
    2(a) Open
  3 Caudal epiphysis

4 Caudal growth plate
  4(a) Open
  4(b) Closing

C 4th. thoracic vertebra

  For clarity rib shadows have been excluded from all drawings.

An Atlas of Interpretative Radiographic Anatomy of the Dog and Cat

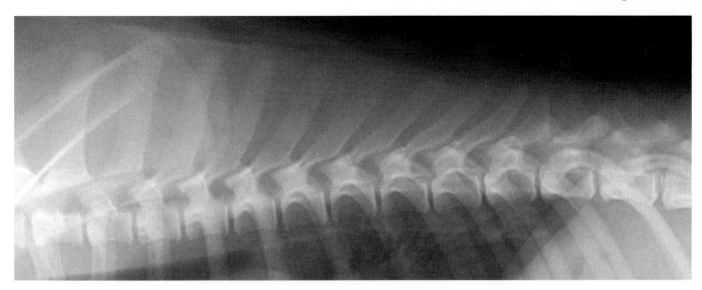

Figure 375 Age 25 weeks.

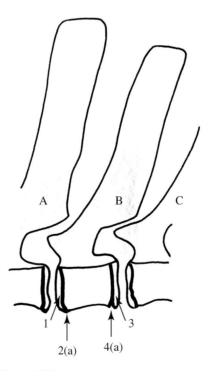

Figure 375

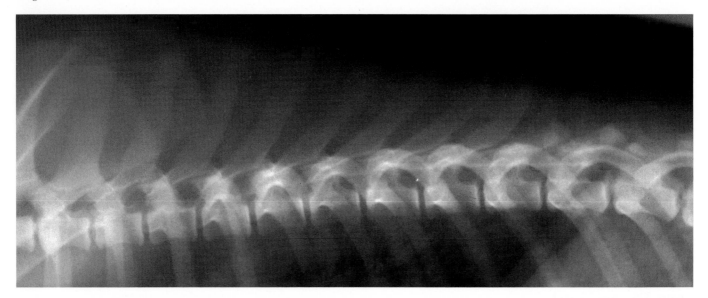

Figure 376 Age 38 weeks.

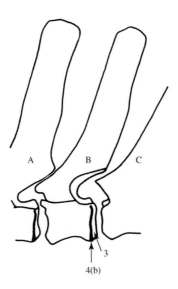

Figure 376

An Atlas of Interpretative Radiographic Anatomy of the Dog and Cat

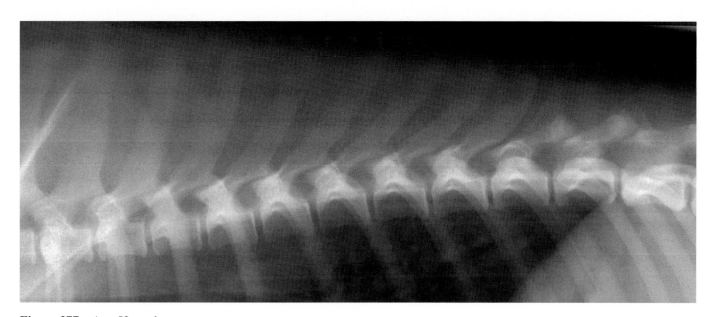

Figure 377   Age 52 weeks.

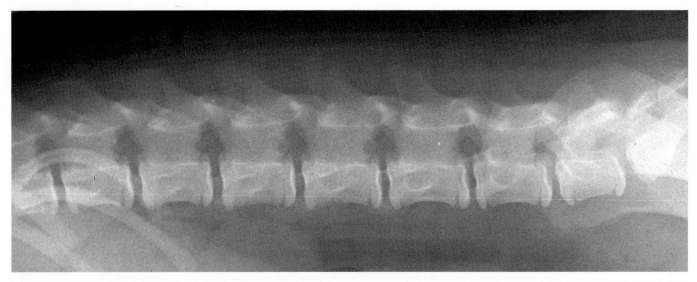

Figure 378 Age 13 weeks.

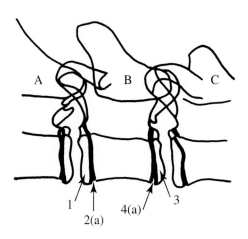

Figure 378

Figures 378, 379, 380, 381 Lateral projection of lumbar vertebrae. Samoyed crossbred dog entire male at 13, 25, 38 and 52 weeks of age. Correlating line drawings for all ages except 52 weeks.

A 3rd. lumbar vertebra

B 4th. lumbar vertebra
  1 Cranial epiphysis
  2 Cranial growth plate
    2(a) Open
  3 Caudal epiphysis
  4 Caudal growth plate
    4(a) Open
    4(b) Closing

C 5th. lumbar vertebra

For clarity transverse process shadows have been excluded from all drawings.

At 25 weeks of age the 3rd. sacral segment, or sacral vertebra, can be seen as a separate segment.

By 38 weeks of age fusion of the 3rd. sacral segment has taken place.

At 25, 38 and 52 weeks of age the iliac crest of the pelvis can be seen as a separate ossification centre. This ossification centre was not visible on the ventrodorsal projections of the pelvis.

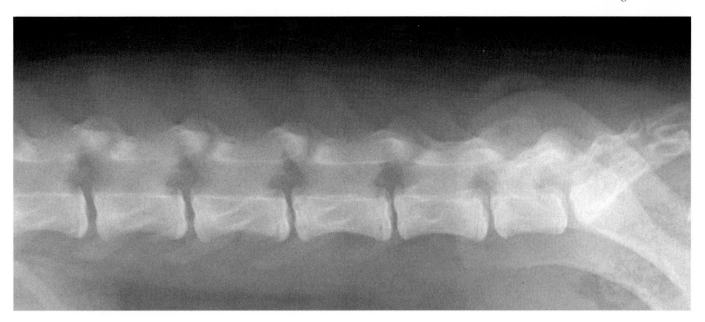

Figure 379   Age 25 weeks.

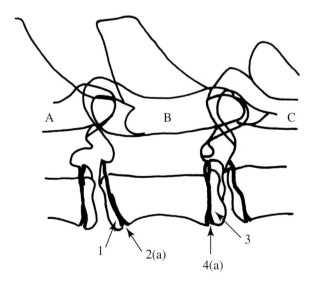

Figure 379

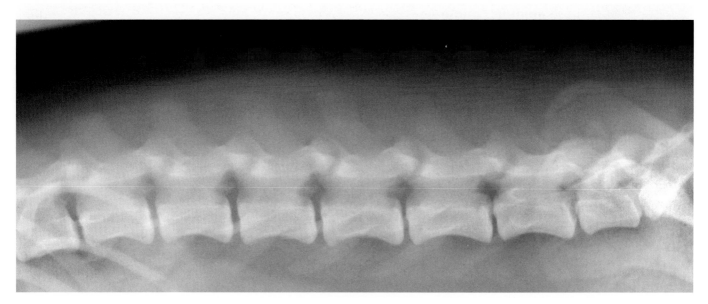

Figure 380   Age 38 weeks.

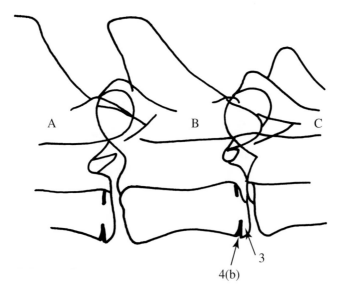

Figure 380

An Atlas of Interpretative Radiographic Anatomy of the Dog and Cat

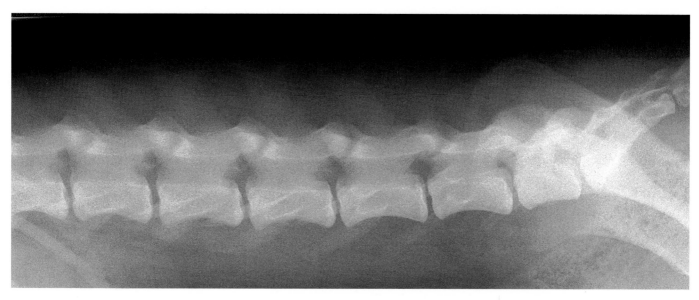

Figure 381   Age 52 weeks.

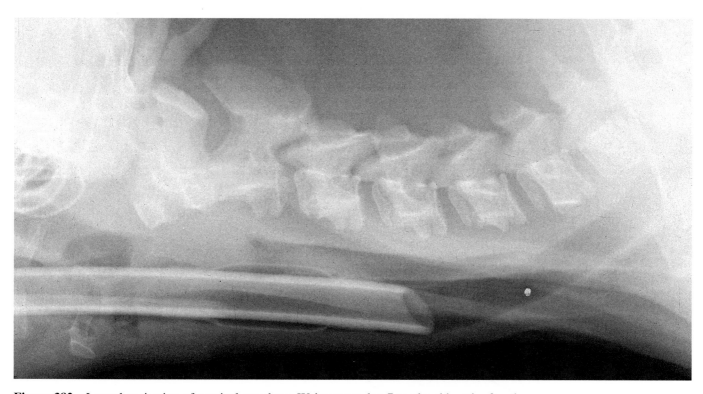

Figure 382   Lateral projection of cervical vertebrae. Weimaraner dog 7 weeks old, entire female.

The radiograph has been included to demonstrate the appearance of the atlas and axis after 1 week of age but before 13 weeks of age.

The atlas still has a distinct separate ossification centre for its body. This centre is not seen in the lateral projection of cervical vertebrae of the 13 week old Samoyed crossbred dog, Figure 370.

Great care must be taken with the interpretation of radiographs from young animals. Knowledge of ossification centres is essential. The ossification centre of the atlas body is sometimes misdiagnosed as a fracture causing neurological signs in dogs under 3 months of age.

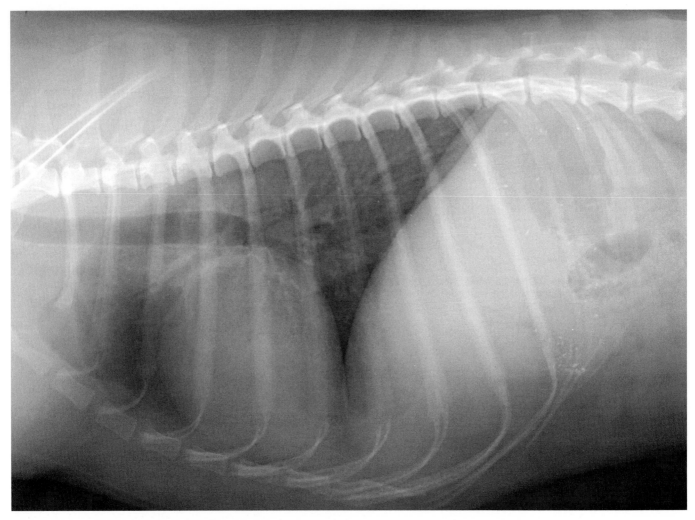

Figure 383   Lateral projection of thorax (exposure for ribs). Beagle dog 2.5 years old, entire male.

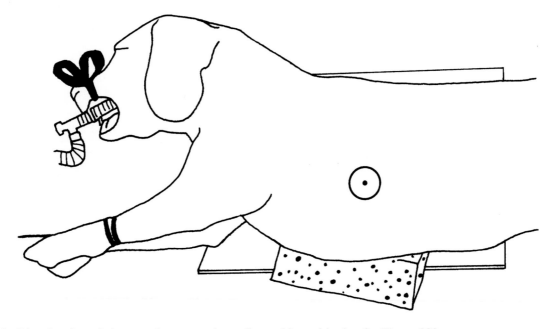

Figure 384   Line drawing of photograph representing radiographic positioning for Figure 383.

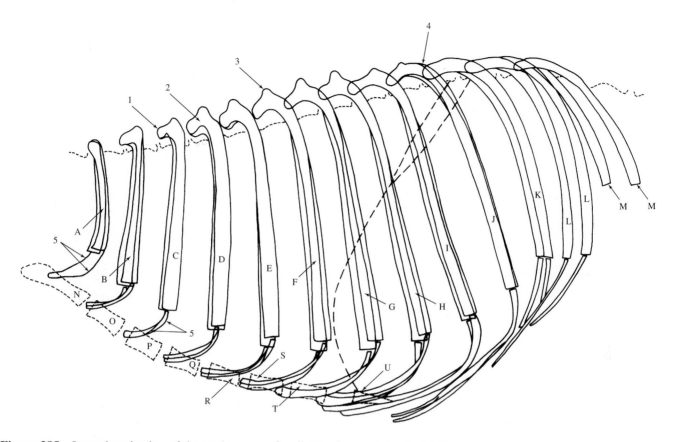

Figure 385   Lateral projection of thorax (exposure for ribs) to demonstrate rib details.

A   1st. pair of ribs

B   2nd. pair of ribs

C   3rd. pair of ribs

D   4th. pair of ribs

E   5th. pair of ribs

F   6th. pair of ribs

G   7th. pair of ribs

H   8th. pair of ribs

I   9th. pair of ribs
   A to I are sternal ribs

J   10th. pair of ribs

K   11th. pair of ribs

L   12th. pair of ribs

M 13th. pair of ribs

J to M are asternal ribs. 13th asternal ribs are the floating ribs.
1   Head of rib
2   Neck of rib
3   Tubercle of rib
4   Angle of rib
5   Costal cartilages. Cartilages are calcified except for their most dorsal aspects. 1st. rib cartilages are poorly calcified. Cartilages 10, 11 and 12 form the costal arch.

N Manubrium of sternum

O 2nd. sternebra

P   3rd. sternebra

Q   4th. sternebra

R   5th. sternebra

S   6th. sternebra

T   7th. sternebra

U   Xiphoid process

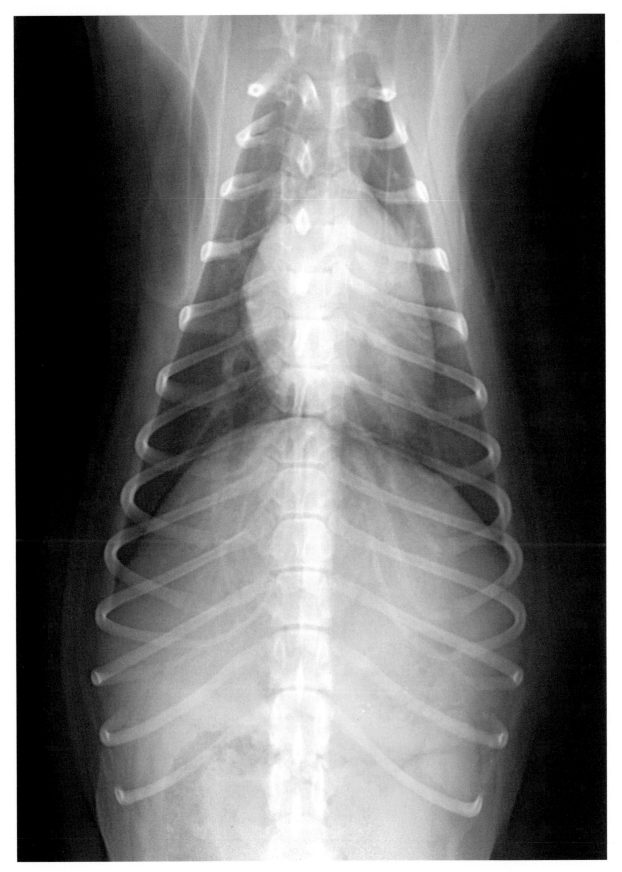

Figure 386   Dorsoventral projection of thorax (exposure for ribs). Beagle dog 2.5 years old, entire male.

An Atlas of Interpretative Radiographic Anatomy of the Dog and Cat

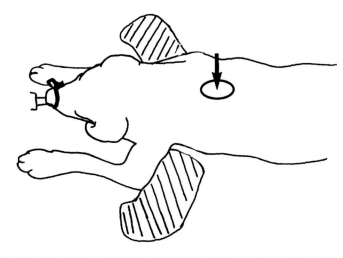

Figure 387 Line drawing of photograph representing radiographic positioning for Figure 386.

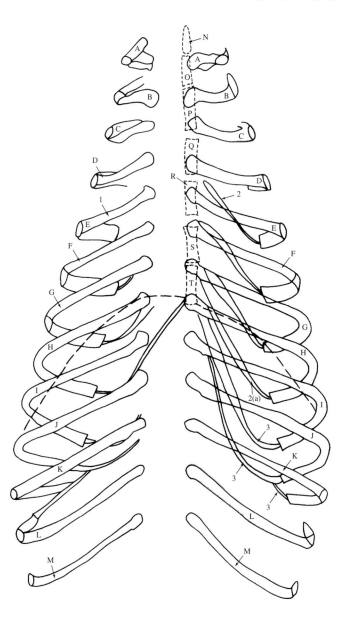

Figure 388 Dorsoventral projection of thorax (exposure for ribs) to demonstrate rib details.

A   1st. pair of ribs

B   2nd. pair of ribs

C   3rd. pair of ribs

D   4th. pair of ribs

E   5th. pair of ribs

F   6th. pair of ribs

G   7th. pair of ribs

H   8th. pair of ribs

I   9th. pair of ribs

A to I   are sternal ribs

J   10th. pair of ribs

K   11th. pair of ribs

L   12th. pair of ribs

M   13th. pair of ribs

J to M are asternal ribs. 13th. asternal ribs are the floating ribs.

1   Body of rib

2   Costal cartilage (calcified)

2(a) Costal cartilage of last 9th. sternal rib

3   Costal cartilages of asternal ribs 10, 11 and 12 which make up the costal arch.

Rotation of the thorax has allowed sternal shadows to be seen separately from vertebral shadows. See Figures 400, 414 and 420 for evaluation of thoracic structures in non-rotated films.

N   Manubrium of sternum

O   2nd. sternebra

P   3rd. sternebra

Q   4th. sternebra

R   5th. sternebra

S   6th. sternebra

T   7th. sternebra

Xiphoid process is not discernible.

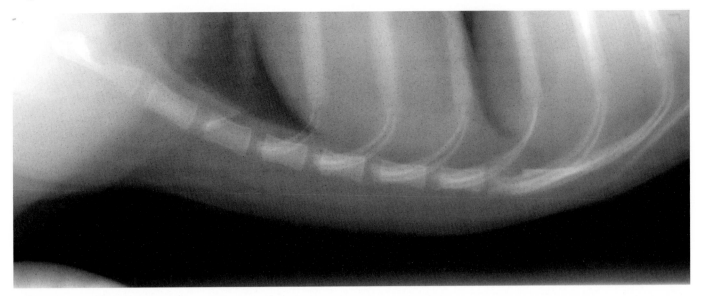

Figure 389   Lateral projection of sternum. Beagle dog 2.5 years old, entire male.

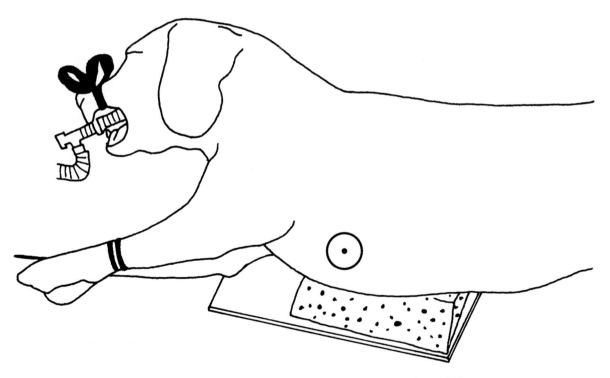

Figure 390   Line drawing of photograph representing radiographic positioning for Figure 389.

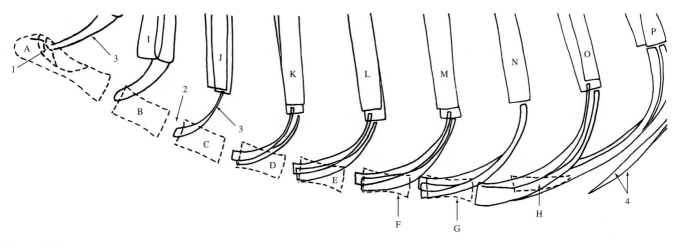

Figure 391 Lateral projection of sternum.

A Manubrium of sternum
  1 Lateral prominence. Site of articular facet for costal
     cartilages of 1st. rib.

B 2nd. sternebra

C 3rd. sternebra

D 4th. stenebra

E 5th. sternebra

F 6th. sternebra

G 7th. sternebra

H Xiphoid process. Xiphoid cartilage extending caudally is
  not calcified.

2 Intersternebral cartilage (non-calcified)
3 Costal cartilage (poorly calcified at 1st. and 2nd. ribs)
4 Costal cartilages of the asternal 10th. ribs

I 2nd. pair of ribs

J 3rd. pair of ribs

K 4th. pair of ribs

L 5th. pair of ribs

M 6th. pair of ribs

N 7th. pair of ribs

O 8th. pair of ribs

P 9th. pair of ribs

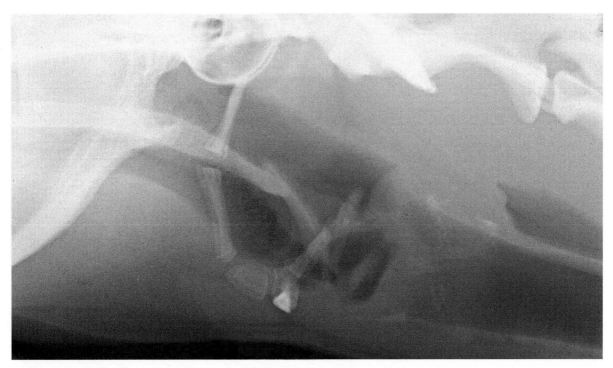

Figure 392   Lateral projection of pharynx and larynx. Beagle dog 2.5 years old, entire male. (See Figure 424 for brachycephalic breed of dog)

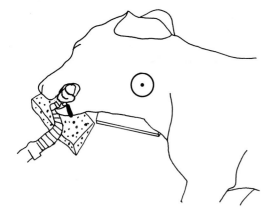

Figure 393   Line drawing of photograph representing radiographic positioning for Figure 392.

Notes for Figure 394

A Mandibles
   1 Angular processes
B Temporomandibular joints
C Tympanic bullae
D Occipital condyle
E Atlas
F Axis
G 3rd. cervical vertebra
H Stylohyoid bones
I Epihyoid bones
J Ceratohyoid bones
K Basihyoid bone

L Thyrohyoid bones
   2 Soft palate
   3 Epiglottis
   4 Arytenoid cartilage
     4(a) Cuneiform process
     4(b) Corniculate process
   5 Thyroid cartilage. (Some calcification of cartilage is present at ventral aspect (5(a).)
   6 Cricoid cartilage. (Some calcification of cartilage is seen especially at dorsal aspect (6(a).)

Calcification of laryngeal cartilages is a normal ageing process in the dog but can be present as early as 6 to 12 months of age. The calcification pattern and opacity vary between the different cartilages and individual dogs. As in this dog, thyroid and cricoid cartilages are the most commonly affected and opacity will increase with age.

   7 Tracheal cartilages
   8 Tracheal lumen
   9 Lateral ventricle of larynx
  10 Nasopharynx
  11 Oropharynx
  12 Laryngopharynx
  13 Laryngeal vestibule
  14 Laryngeal glottis
  15 Infraglottic cavity
  16 Thyro- and cricopharyngeal muscles obliterating the lumen of laryngopharynx dorsal to the arytenoid and cricoid cartilage regions
  17 Oesophageal lumen

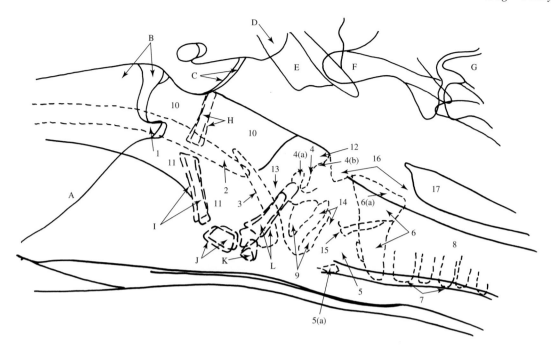

Figure 394   Lateral projection of pharynx and larynx.

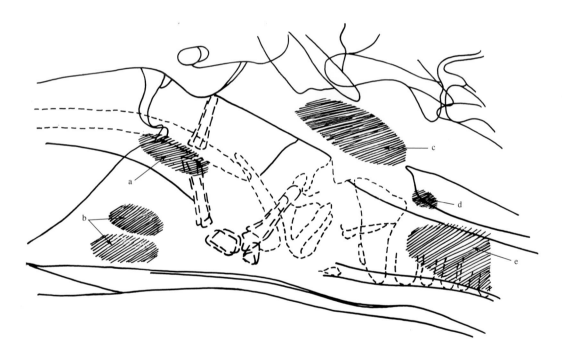

Figure 395   Schematic drawing of lateral projection of pharynx and larynx to illustrate positions of lymphatic structures and thyroid gland.

a = Palatine tonsil

b = Mandibular lymph nodes

c = Medial retropharyngeal lymph node

d = Cranial deep cervical lymph node

e = Thyroid gland

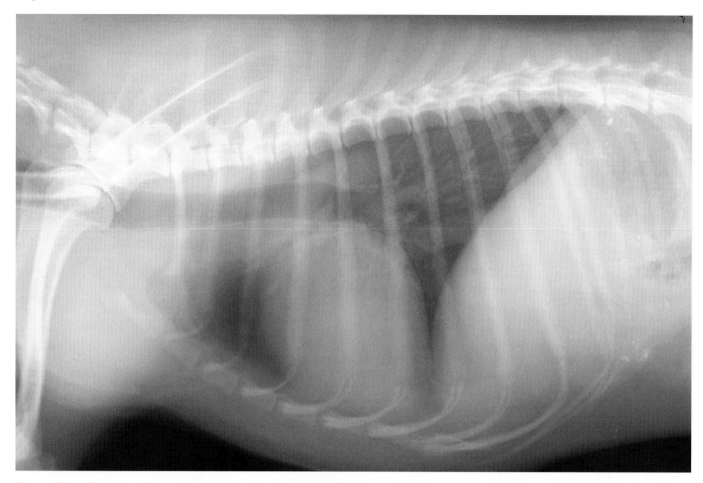

Figure 396 Right lateral recumbent projection of thorax. Projection to highlight cardiovascular system. Radiograph taken during general anaesthesia with full inflation of lung lobes. Beagle dog 2.5 years old, entire male (same dog as in dorsoventral projection of thorax, Figure 400).

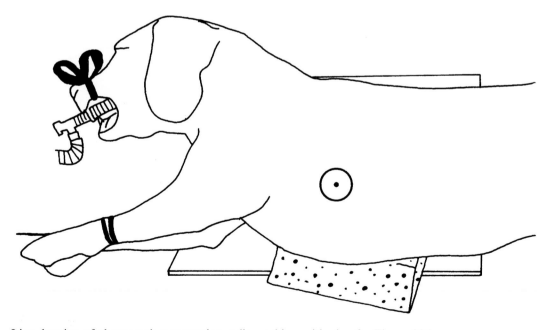

Figure 397 Line drawing of photograph representing radiographic positioning for Figure 396.

An Atlas of Interpretative Radiographic Anatomy of the Dog and Cat

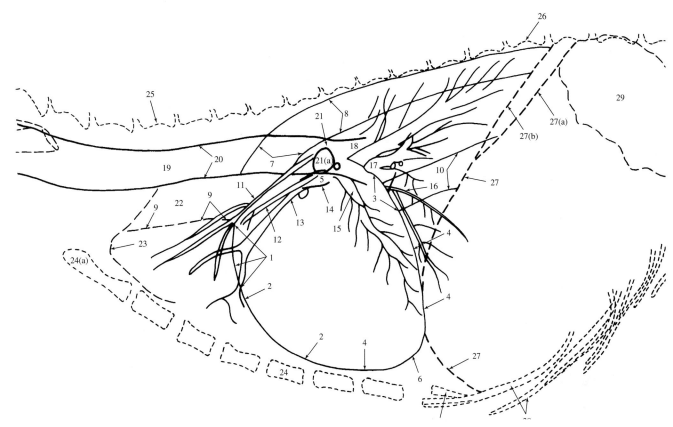

Figure 398   Right lateral recumbent projection of thorax. Drawing to highlight cardiovascular system.

Pericardium and heart

Cranial border
  1 Right auricle
  2 Right ventricle

In this radiograph the aortic arch is not visible but it can often be seen as a separate structure. Very rarely the cranial border of the pulmonary artery is seen.

Note that the aortic arch can be seen in the respiratory system radiographs and drawings, Figures 404 and 406.

A small indentation can sometimes be seen in the craniodorsal border of the cardiac shadow representing the junction of the cranial vena cava and the cranial border. This is known as the cranial waistline. In this radiograph the pulmonary vessels are obscuring the waistline level.

Caudal border
  3 Left atrium. Dorsally obscured by pulmonary vessels.
  4 Left ventricle

The junction between the atrium and ventricle is marked by a definite sulcus in the caudal border as it curves cranially. This is known as the caudal waistline and is found at the level of the ventral border of the caudal vena cava. Unlike the cranial waistline it is a consistent finding in the normal cardiac shadow.
  5 Dorsal base
  6 Apex

The pericardium, the fibroserous sac surrounding the heart, is not seen as a separate structure. In very obese dogs fat can accumulate within the sac and the middle mediastinum. Even so, the fat density may not be readily interpreted as a different tissue and without careful evaluation of the cardiac shadow a misdiagnosis of 'cardiac enlargement' can be made.

Note that the right lateral recumbent projection of thorax is preferred for the cardiac shadow as the phrenicopericardial ligament acts to anchor the apex. Although small there are noticeable differences in the cardiac, caudal vena cava and aortic silhouettes in right and left lateral recumbencies (see respiratory system radiographic Figures 404 and 408).

Vascular
  7 Aortic arch. Occasionally an ill-defined shadow representing an outflow vessel from this arch is seen in the right lateral recumbent projection of thorax (not present in this radiograph).

8   Thoracic aorta
9   Level of cranial vena cava

The cranial vena cava cannot be seen as a separate structure but will be found at the ventral level of the cranial mediastinal shadow. It is formed at a level cranial to the thoracic inlet.

10   Caudal vena cava. (In this projection it is seen entering the central tendon of the diaphragm just right of the midline.) In most right lateral recumbent projections of thorax the entry is clearly defined as right sided and can be used to confirm recumbency.
11   Right cranial lobe artery
12   Right cranial lobe vein
13   Left cranial lobe vein

The left cranial lobe artery cannot be clearly seen in this radiograph but it will be present just ventral to the right cranial lobe vein.

Radiolucent shadows between the paired cranial vessels are the corresponding lobe bronchial lumen. These should not be mistaken for the abnormal air bronchograms. Often the bronchial walls are also visible and in this radiograph the most dorsal portions are just seen as fine radiopaque lines (14).

15   Artery and vein of caudal segment of left cranial lobe cranially
16   Artery and vein of right middle lobe caudally
17   Right pulmonary artery and veins. Right pulmonary artery, when seen as a separate structure, passes ventral to the tracheal bifurcation and is a round/oval soft tissue opacity in its end-on projection.
18   Left pulmonary artery and veins. Left pulmonary artery crosses the trachea, passing cranial to the tracheal bifurcation.

The left vascular trees are located just dorsal to the right but identification is very difficult. Also, differentiating between artery and vein is hard. However, arteries usually are more opaque, often slightly curved and are more well defined. Veins are usually shorter and stubbier. In addition arteries are located following the bronchial tree whereas veins travel to the left atrium via the shortest route.

Non-cardiovascular structures

19   Tracheal lumen
20   Tracheal walls
21   Level of tracheal bifurcation; carina
      21(a) Left cranial bronchus at bifurcation into bronchi for cranial and caudal segments. This shadow is often incorrectly named 'carina'.
22   Cranial mediastinum occupied by large veins and arteries cranial to the heart, especially the cranial vena cava and brachiocephalic trunk
23   Pleural cupola. Area of lung extending cranial to 1st. rib
24   Sternum
      24(a) Manubrium of sternum
      24(b) Xiphoid process
25   1st. thoracic vertebra
26   11th. thoracic vertebra
27   Diaphragmatic shadow
      27(a) Left 'crus'
      27(b) Right 'crus'
28   Calcified costal cartilages
29   Gas-filled gastric fundus

Fluid-filled oesophagus can often be seen in the caudodorsal thoracic cavity in the right lateral recumbent projection of thorax. (Not present in this radiograph but can be seen in the mediastinal structures section, Figures 417 and 418.)

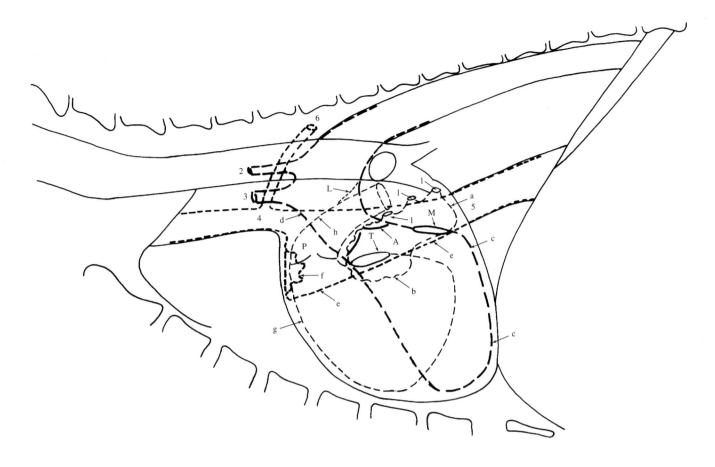

Figure 399   Schematic drawing of right lateral recumbent projection of thorax to illustrate cardiac chambers and major vessels (corresponds to line drawing Figure 398 but with the exclusion of some thoracic cavity details seen in the radiograph).

Left side with associated vessels

   a = Left atrium with pulmonary veins (1)

   b = Left auricle

   c = Left ventricle (drawing does not indicate wall thickness)

   d = Aorta with left subclavian artery (2) and brachiocephalic trunk (3)

   M = Left atrioventricular valve; mitral

   A = Aortic valve

Right side with associated vessels

   e = Right atrium with cranial vena cava (4), and caudal vena cava (5), plus azygous vein (6)

   f = Right auricle

   g = Right ventricle (drawing does not indicate wall thickness)

   h = Pulmonary trunk. Main pulmonary artery or pulmonary artery segment.

   L = Ligamentum arteriosum. Remnant of foetal ductus arteriosus.

   P = Valve of pulmonary trunk

   T = Right atrioventricular valve; tricuspid.

An Atlas of Interpretative Radiographic Anatomy of the Dog and Cat

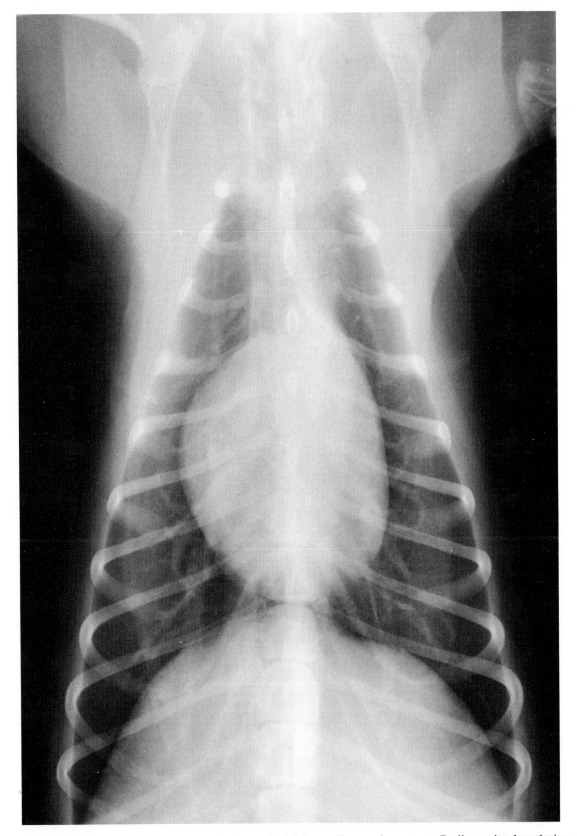

Figure 400 Dorsoventral projection of thorax. Projection to highlight cardiovascular system. Radiograph taken during general anaesthesia with full inflation of lung lobes. Beagle dog 2.5 years old, entire male (same dog as in right lateral recumbent projection of thorax, Figure 396).

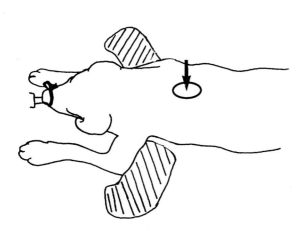

Figure 401 Line drawing of photograph representing radiographic positioning for Figure 400.

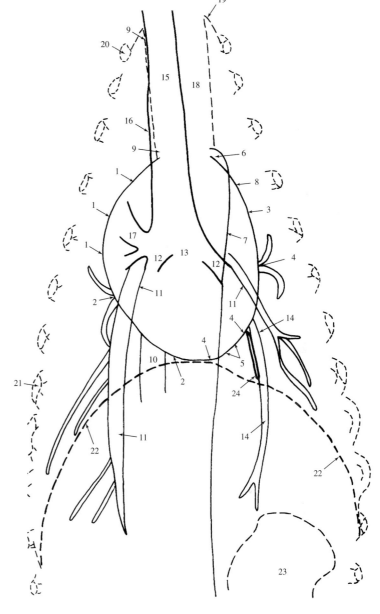

Figure 402 Dorsoventral projection of thorax. Drawing to highlight cardiovascular system.

Pericardium and heart

Right side
1 Right atrium
2 Right ventricle. Shadow of ventricle just crosses the midline.

Left side
3 Left auricle
4 Left ventricle
5 Apex. Formed by the wall of left ventricle.

Please see right lateral recumbent projection of thorax to highlight cardiovascular system, Figure 398, for more details.

Vascular

6 Aortic arch
7 Aorta
8 Pulmonary trunk. Main pulmonary artery or pulmonary artery segment.
9 Level of cranial vena cava within cranial mediastinum soft tissue shadow.
10 Caudal vena cava
11 Arteries to caudal lung lobes. Originate cranial to tracheal bifurcation level, carina, and travel lateral to principal caudal lobe bronchus (12).
  The carina is not clearly seen in this radiograph but will be located at (13).

(402 continued.)

14 Veins to caudal lung lobes. Located caudal to tracheal bifurcation level, carina, and travel medial to main caudal lobe bronchi. In this radiograph the right vein is obscured by the shadow of the caudal vena cava. Veins are slightly smaller than arteries.

Care must be taken in identifying arteries and veins in this projection as the calcified costal cartilage shadows 'mimic' vessels. To distinguish between the two sets of shadows one must trace the full course of the shadows. Shadows of the calcified costal cartilages will be seen to travel caudally then curve cranially at, or near, the costochondral junctions.

To avoid confusion the calcified costal cartilages and bony rib shadows have been excluded from the drawing but the reader should now identify these shadows. A line drawing of the calcified cartilages and ribs, Figure 388, can be found in the axial skeleton section.

Non-cardiovascular structures

15 Tracheal lumen
16 Tracheal wall
17 Right cranial bronchial lumen
18 Cranial mediastinum. The right border is formed by the cranial vena cava while the left is formed by the left subclavian artery. In addition, both the trachea and oesophagus lie within the cranial mediastinum.
19 Pleural cupola
20 1st. rib
21 8th. rib
22 Diaphragmatic shadow
23 Gas-filled lumen of gastric fundus
24 Phrenicopericardial ligament. Ligament is a fibrous thickening of the ventral portion of caudal mediastinum.

Although the phrenicopericardial ligament is usually seen at the cardiac apex a more lateral position can sometimes occur, as in this radiograph. The attachment of the ligament is pericardial not heart.

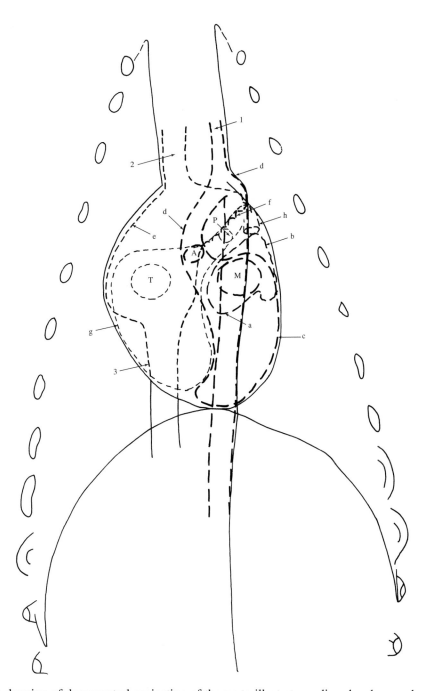

Figure 403 Schematic drawing of dorsoventral projection of thorax to illustrate cardiac chambers and major vessels. (corresponds to line drawing Figure 402 but with the exclusion of some thoracic cavity details seen in radiograph).

Left side with associated vessels

   a = Left atrium

   b = Left auricle

   c = Left ventricle (drawing does not indicate wall thickness)

   d = Aorta, root plus arch, with brachiocephalic trunk (1)

   A = Aortic valve

   M = Left atrioventricular valve; mitral

Right side with associated vessels

   e = Right atrium with cranial vena cava (2) and caudal vena cava (3)

   f = Right auricle

   g = Right ventricle (drawing does not indicate wall thickness)

   h = Main pulmonary artery

   P = Valve of pulmonary trunk

   T = Right atrioventricular valve; tricuspid

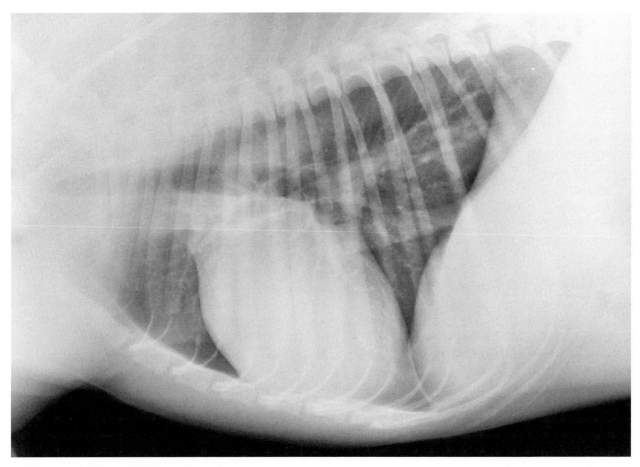

Figure 404   Left lateral recumbent projection of thorax. Projection to highlight respiratory system. Radiograph taken during general anaesthesia with full inflation of lung lobes. Beagle dog 7 years old, entire male (same dog as in all projections of thorax to highlight respiratory system, Figures 408, 411 and 414).

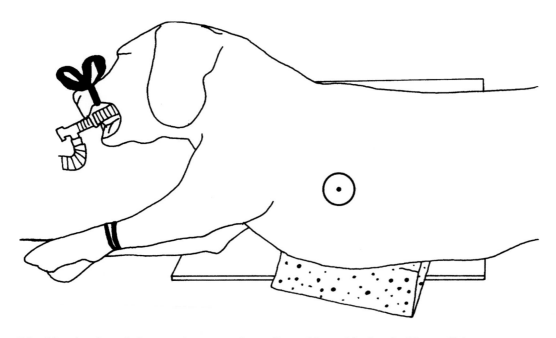

Figure 405   Line drawing of photograph representing radiographic positioning for Figure 404.

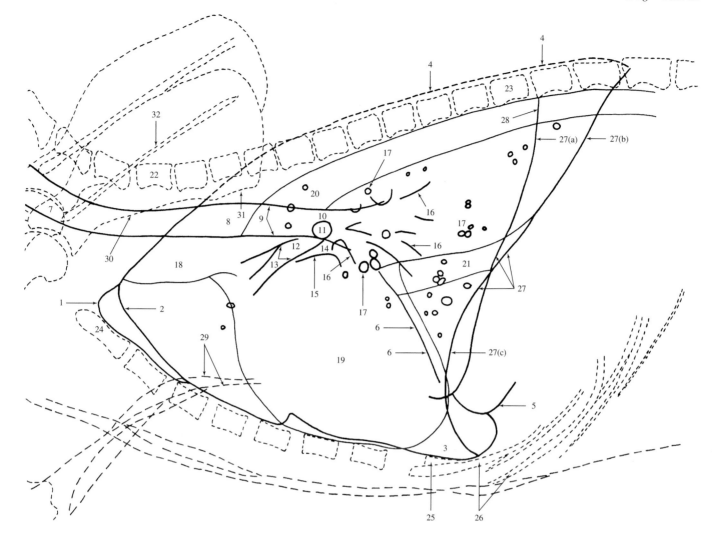

Figure 406 Left lateral recumbent projection of thorax.
Drawing to highlight respiratory system.

1 Cranial limit of the left cranial lung lobe. Extends beyond
  the 1st. pair of ribs into pleural cupola in well-inflated
  lung lobes.
2 Cranial limit of the right cranial lung lobe
3 Lucent shadow created by right middle lung lobe. This
  lung lobe is larger than the corresponding caudal segment
  of the left cranial lung lobe. Its presence at full inflation
  between the cardiac and sternal shadows should not be
  mistaken for free pleural gas. Pulmonary opacities
  can be seen in the lucent region, so confirming lung
  tissue.

Note that there is no left middle lung lobe in the dog.

4 Dorsal limit of caudal lung lobes. (The limit is more dorsal than normal, caused by positional rotation of the dog
  during radiographic exposure, as seen by rib shadows
  superimposed over vertebral canal.)

In a non-rotated lateral projection of the thorax the limit is at
the level of the dorsal edge of vertebral body.

5 Ventral border of caudal lung lobe

From plain radiographs of the thorax it is not possible to identify many individual lung lobes due to extensive superimposition.
The above labels the peripheral extents of some of the lobes
which can be recognised and the schematic drawing attempts to
demonstrate the areas covered by the individual lobes.

6 Pleural fissure line between middle and caudal lobes
7 Cervical tracheal lumen
8 Thoracic tracheal lumen
9 Tracheal walls
10 Level of tracheal bifurcation into right and left principal
   bronchi; carina
11 Radiolucent circular shadow demonstrating end-on
   projection of left cranial lobe bronchus at bifurcation into
   bronchus for cranial and caudal segments

(406 continued.)

This shadow is often incorrectly labelled 'carina'. The carina cannot be seen as a distinct shadow on lateral thorax projections.

12   Right cranial bronchial lumen
13   Right cranial bronchial wall
14   Left cranial bronchial lumen
15   Left cranial bronchial wall
16   Linear opacities representing bronchial walls
17   Circular opacities representing bronchial walls seen end on

    Bronchial markings, as labelled above, are a normal feature in older dogs. Also, the appearance of the pleura is not uncommon. In addition nodular, linear and circular interstitial opacities will be found, as in this 7-year-old dog. The lung shadows in this figure should be compared with the ones found in the cardiovascular system right lateral recumbent radiograph, Figure 396. In the latter the dog is 2.5 years old.

    Opacity changes will start to appear from approximately 4 years of age but environmental factors have to be considered e.g. town versus country (urban/rural). The opacity changes represent fibrous tissue and/or calcification of bronchial and interstitial tissues. They are more pronounced, and occur at a younger age, in the chondrodystrophic breeds.

    Note that this radiograph has been taken at full inflation to avoid radiographic error of 'increased lung opacity'.

18   Cranial mediastinum occupied by large veins and arteries cranial to the heart, especially cranial vena cava and brachiocephalic trunk
19   Cardiac shadow including aortic arch at cranial border and at dorsal and ventral extremities the extensions of the pericardium
20   Aorta
21   Caudal vena cava seen entering the central tendon of the diaphragm at a level just right of the midline
22   1st. thoracic vertebra
23   11th. thoracic vertebra
24   Manubrium of sternum
25   Xiphoid process
26   Calcified costal cartilages
27   Diaphragmatic shadow
     27(a) Left 'crus'
     27(b) Right 'crus'
     27(c) Cupola
28   Lumbodiaphragmatic recess
29   Ventral skin folds superimposed on thorax shadows
30   Caudal border of scapula
31   Caudal angle of scapula
32   Spine of scapula

An Atlas of Interpretative Radiographic Anatomy of the Dog and Cat

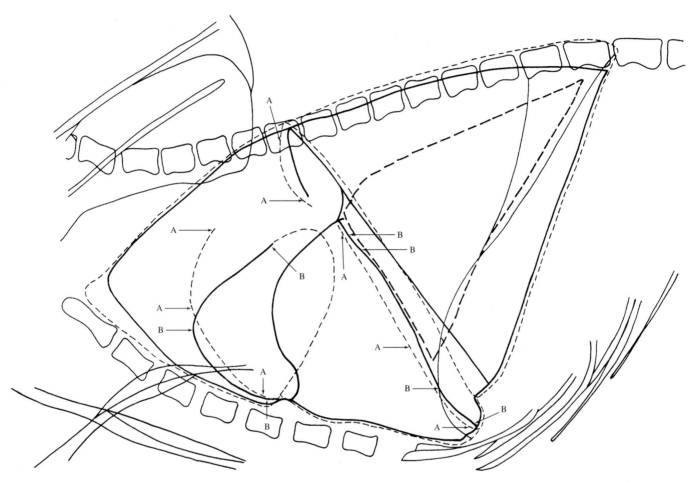

Figure 407 Schematic drawing of left lateral recumbent projection of thorax to illustrate lung lobes (corresponds to line drawing Figure 406 but with the exclusion of thoracic cavity details seen in the radiograph).

- - - = Left lung. Cranial (cranial and caudal segments) and caudal lobes

A = Medial borders of the lobes of the left lung

━━ = Right lung. Cranial, middle and caudal lobes

B = Medial borders of the lobes of the right lung

── = Accessory lobe of right lung obscured by caudal lung lobe

The terms apical, cardiac, diaphragmatic and intermediate lung lobes are no longer in common usage.

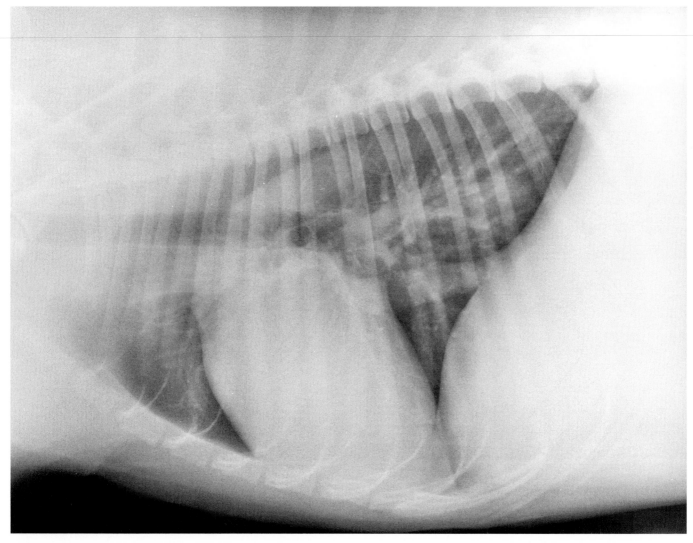

Figure 408   Right lateral recumbent projection of thorax. Projection to highlight respiratory system. Radiograph taken during general anaesthesia with full inflation of lung lobes. Beagle dog 7 years old, entire male (same dog as in all projections of thorax to highlight respiratory system, Figures 404, 411 and 414).

The right lateral recumbent projection has been included in this section to illustrate the subtle but definite difference of the right and left recumbencies. Notice the obvious diaphragmatic shadow changes but also the more obvious oesophageal fluid in the right lateral and the pleural fissure line seen in the left lateral (labelled (6) on line drawing Figure 406).

Both left and right recumbent laterals should be performed for full evaluation of lung tissue. Radiographic changes in the more recumbent lobes can easily be overlooked or even be not evident on one recumbent projection.

Cardiac shadow also changes depending on the recumbency. As rotation is present in both of these projections the cardiac shadow cannot be critically analysed but as a routine the right lateral recumbency is superior for cardiac shadow evaluation.

If lung pathology is suspected in one hemithorax, radiography must ensure that in the lateral projection that hemithorax is uppermost. To perform both recumbencies may prove impractical if respiratory distress is severe.

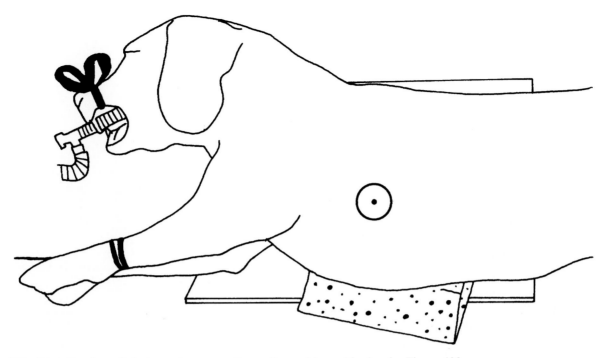

Figure 409   Line drawing of photograph representing radiographic positioning for Figure 408.

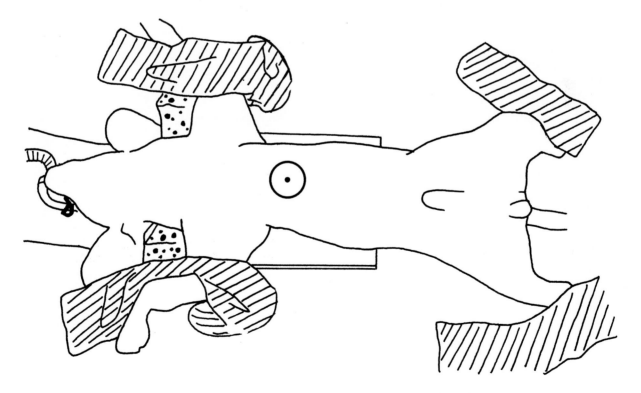

Figure 410   Line drawing of photograph representing radiographic positioning for Figure 411.

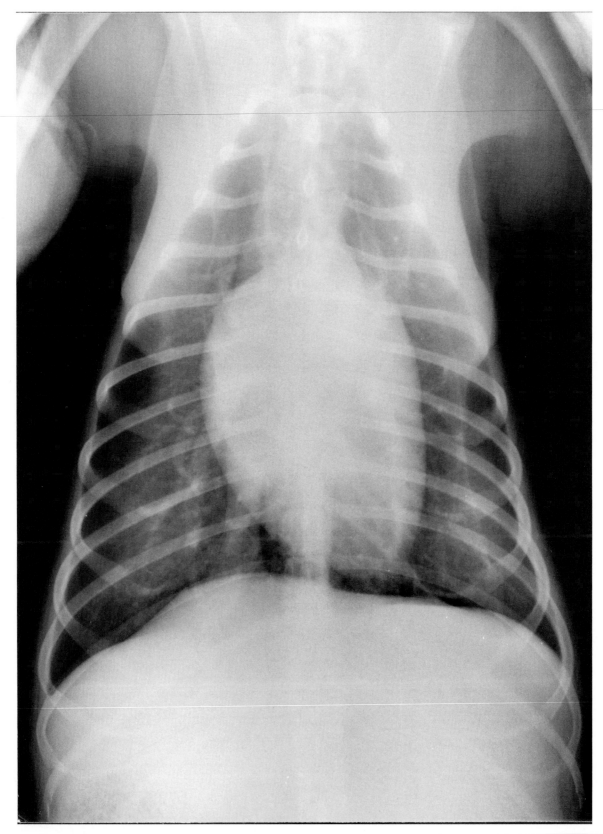

Figure 411 Ventrodorsal projection of thorax. Projection to highlight respiratory system. Radiograph taken during general anaesthesia with full inflation of lung lobes. Beagle dog 7 years old, entire male (same dog as in all projections of thorax to highlight respiratory system, Figures 404, 408 and 414).

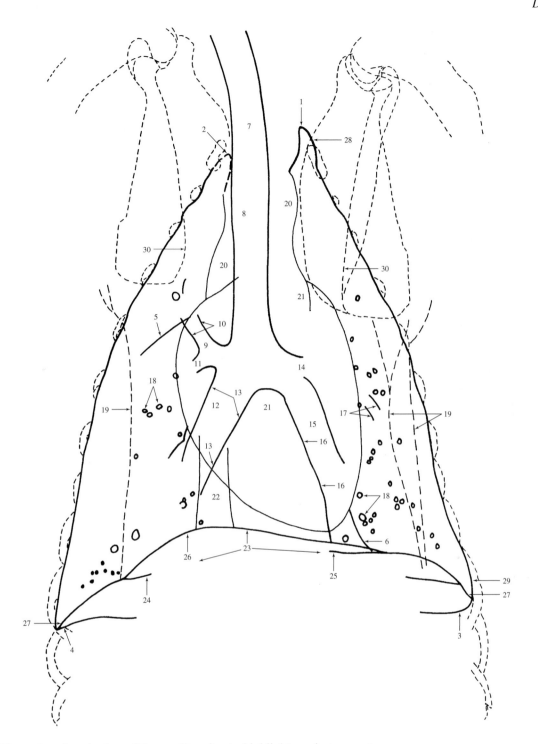

Figure 412   Ventrodorsal projection of thorax. Drawing to highlight respiratory system.

1 Cranial limit of the left cranial lung lobe. Extends beyond the 1st. pair of ribs into pleural cupola in well-inflated lung lobes. Just visible in this radiograph.

2 Cranial limit of the right cranial lung lobe

3 Caudal limit of the left caudal lung lobe

4 Caudal limit of the right caudal lung lobe

5 Thickened, fibrotic, pleural tissue at caudal border of right cranial lung lobe. Medially more distinct and demonstrates the pleural fissure line between right cranial and right middle lung lobes.

6 Phrenicopericardial ligament. Represents ventral portion of the caudal mediastinum.

7 Tracheal lumen at thoracic inlet

(412 continued.)

8 Tracheal lumen within the cranial mediastinum just right of the midline

9 Right cranial bronchial lumen

10 Right cranial bronchial walls

11 Right middle bronchial lumen

12 Right caudal bronchial lumen

13 Right caudal bronchial walls

14 Caudal segment of left cranial bronchial lumen

Note that there is no left middle lung lobe.

15 Left caudal bronchial lumen

16 Left caudal bronchial walls

17 Linear opacities representing a portion of the bronchial walls to the caudal segment of the left cranial lung lobe

18 Circular opacities representing bronchial walls seen end-on

The same comments on bronchial markings apply to this projection as in the left lateral recumbent projection of thorax, Figure 406.

   In addition, with the ventrodorsal projection the more lateral areas often appear more opaque due to the presence of skin folds (19). Skin folds are distinguished from thoracic cavity structures by following their continuous shadows beyond the cavity limits. Folds must not be mistaken for abnormal lung lobes.

20 Cranial mediastinum

21 Cardiac shadow including aortic arch at cranial border. (Shadow is narrower, with an elongated shape, in this ventrodorsal projection than in the corresponding dorsoventral projection, Figure 414.)

22 Caudal vena cava

23 Diaphragmatic shadow. (Triple shadow in this ventro-dorsal projection compared to the corresponding dorsoventral projection, Figure 414.)

24 Right 'crus' of diaphragm

25 Left 'crus' of diaphragm

26 Cupola of diaphragm

27 Costodiaphragmatic recess

28 1st. rib

29 10th. rib

30 Spine of scapula

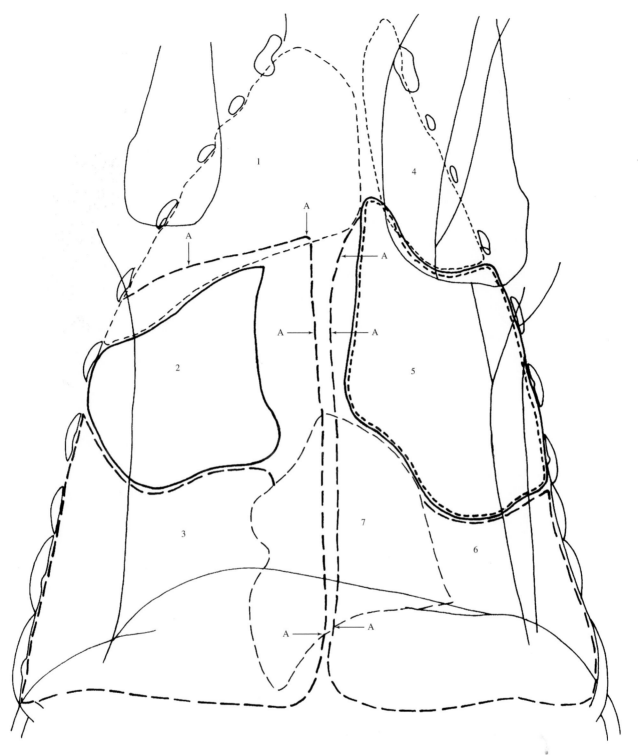

Figure 413 Schematic drawing of ventrodorsal projection of thorax to illustrate lung lobes (corresponds to line drawing Figure 412 but with the exclusion of thoracic cavity details seen in the radiograph).

--- 1 = Right cranial lung lobe

— 2 = Right middle lung lobe

—— 3 = Right caudal lung lobe

----- 4 = Left cranial lung lobe, cranial segment

===== 5 = Left cranial lung lobe, caudal segment

—— 6 = Left caudal lung lobe

—— 7 = Accessory lung lobe

A = Dorsal border of caudal lung lobes

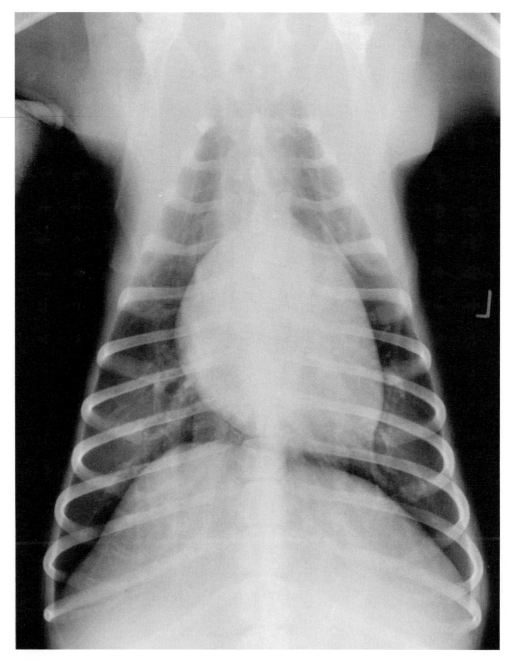

Figure 414   Dorsoventral projection of thorax. Projection to highlight respiratory system. Radiograph taken during general anaesthesia with full inflation of lung lobes. Beagle Dog 7 years old, entire male (same dog as in all projections of thorax to highlight respiratory system, Figures 404, 408 and 411).

The dorsoventral projection has been included in this section to show that even with fully inflated lungs, the area of lung exposed is less in this projection compared with the ventrodorsal. This effect is smaller in the cat but with this species the thoracic cavity is greatly reduced, and appears more triangular, when the front limbs are not extended forwards.

The dorsoventral projection should always be used for cardiovascular evaluation as cardiac position is not altered. Also the caudal pulmonary vessels are more clearly defined.

The ventrodorsal projection is preferable for lung tissue evaluation. It also shifts pleural fluid dorsally and cranial mediastinal shadows are clearer. However, this position may be clinically contraindicated.

It must also be remembered that the ventrodorsal and/or dorsoventral projection(s) should be performed first, before the recumbent lateral projections. Hypostatic congestion/lung lobe collapse occurs rapidly in recumbent animals suffering from cardiovascular or respiratory problems. Even in clinically normal animals hypostatic congestion will develop during lateral recumbency (see Figure 432).

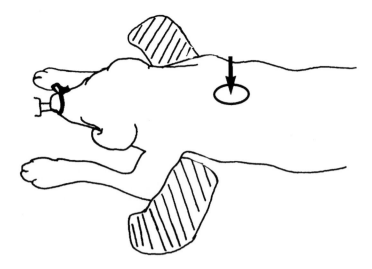

Figure 415   Line drawing of photograph representing radiographic positioning for Figure 414.

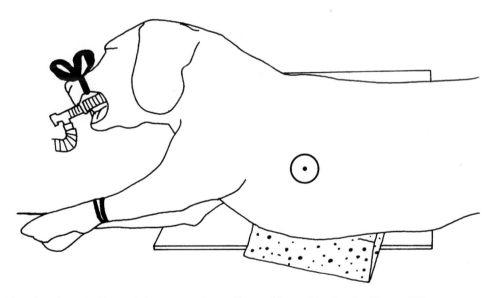

Figure 416   Line drawing of photograph representing radiographic positioning for Figure 417.

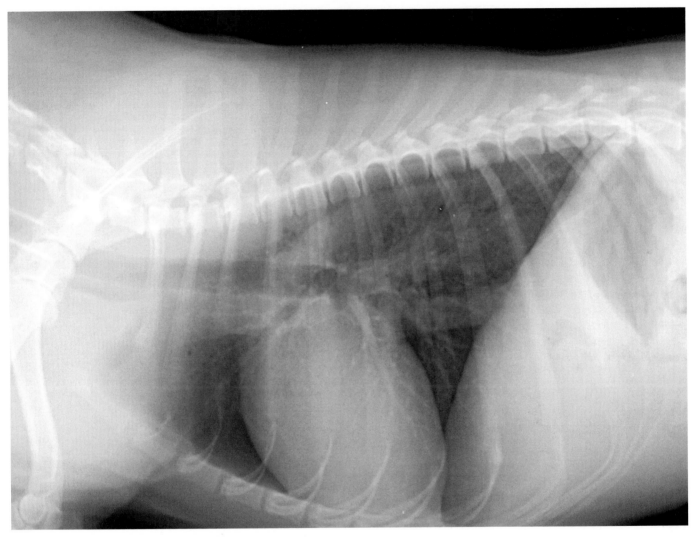

Figure 417   Right lateral recumbent projection of thorax. Projection to highlight mediastinal structures. Radiograph taken during general anaesthesia with full inflation of lung lobes. Beagle dog 2 years old, entire female (same dog as in dorsoventral projection of thorax, Figure 421).

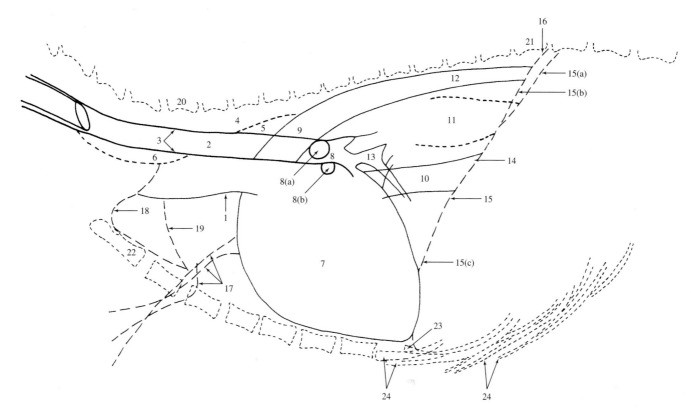

Figure 418   Right lateral recumbent projection of thorax.
Line drawing to highlight mediastinal structures (pleura
excluded and diaphragm included in respiratory system
drawings).

Cranial mediastinum. Portion cranial to cardiac shadow.

1 Ventral border of cranial vena cava. (Seen in this dog but
   often it is not present as a distinct shadow.)
2 Tracheal lumen
3 Tracheal walls
4 Longus colli muscle shadow
5 Gas-filled oesophagus extending caudally. Gas filled
   oesophagus is also seen at thoracic inlet (6).
6 Gas-filled oesophagus

Middle mediastinum. Portion containing cardiac shadow.

7 Cardiac shadow
8 Level of tracheal bifurcation; carina. Note that the carinal
   shadow cannot be seen on lateral projections.
   8(a) Origin of right cranial lobe bronchus
   8(b) Origin of left cranial lobe bronchus

   Slight rotation of this lateral recumbent projection has
allowed both cranial lobe bronchi to be seen. Often only one
radiolucent circular shadow can be seen at this level, the end-
on projection of left cranial lobe bronchus at bifurcation into
bronchi for cranial and caudal segments. This shadow is often
incorrectly named the 'carina'.

9 Aortic arch

Caudal mediastinum

10 Caudal vena cava
11 Fluid-filled lumen of oesophagus
12 Descending aorta

   The mediastinum can be further subdivided into dorsal and
ventral portions. The dorsal portion is simple from 1st. rib to
diaphragm, but the ventral portion contains the pericardium
and the heart. In the dog the mediastinum is incomplete but
the pleural coating is non-fenestrated.

13 Pulmonary vessels
14 Caudal vena cava seen entering diaphragm at caval
    foramen
15 Diaphragmatic shadow
    15(a) Left 'crus'
    15(b) Right 'crus'
    15(c) Cupola
16 Lumbodiaphragmatic recess
17 Ventral skin folds superimposed on thoracic cavity
    shadows
18 Cranial limit of left cranial lung lobe
19 Cranial limit of right cranial lung lobe
20 1st. thoracic vertebra
21 12th. thoracic vertebra
22 Manubrium of sternum
23 Xiphoid process

(418 continued.)

24 Calcified costal cartilages

The presence of fat within the middle mediastinum has been noted in the cardiovascular drawing, Figure 398. Large fat deposits can also be found in the cranial mediastinum in obese old dogs. Dogs of the smaller breeds, and especially the brachycephalic breeds, are prone to accumulate fat in the cranial mediastinum. Fat may also develop in the cranio-ventral mediastinum resulting in a dorsal elevation of the cardiac shadow.

Fat accumulation, as referenced above, must not be misdiagnosed as a pathological condition. Knowledge of breed variation, plus radiographic opacity evaluation, is required for correct interpretation of thoracic radiographs.

A number of radiographs follow the 'normal' dog radiographs to illustrate the above comments.

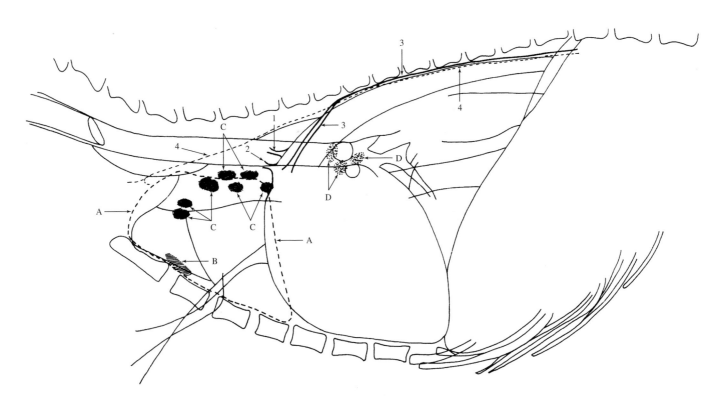

Figure 419   Schematic drawing of right lateral recumbent projection of thorax to illustrate mediastinal structures.

—— A = Thymus seen in young dog. As dog ages glandular tissue reduces and is replaced by fat.

///// B = Sternal lymph nodes. Usually one each side of thoracic cavity.

● C = Cranial mediastinal lymph nodes. Left side: one to six in number. Right side: two to three, maximum of six.

⋰ D = Tracheobronchial lymph nodes. Right and left lie in the angle between the lateral surface of each cranial principal bronchus and the trachea. Middle (V shaped) is dorsally at the angle of tracheal bifurcation.

1 = Left subclavian artery

2 = Brachiocephalic trunk

3 = Azygous vein

——— 4 = Thoracic duct

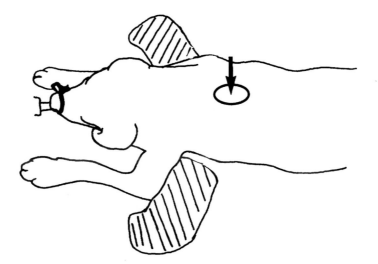

Figure 420   Line drawing of photograph representing radiographic positioning for Figure 421.

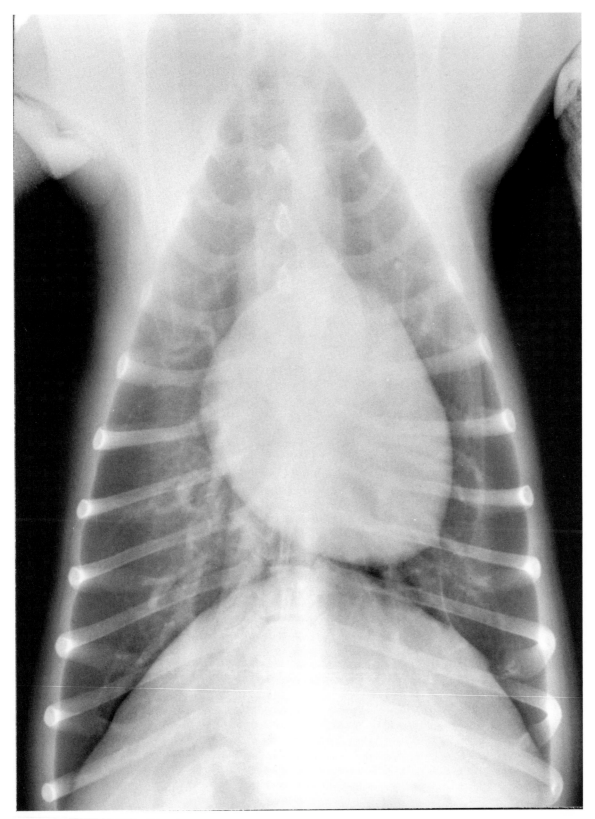

Figure 421   Dorsoventral projection of thorax. Projection to highlight mediastinal structures. Radiograph taken during general anaesthesia with full inflation of lung lobes. Beagle dog 2 years old, entire female (same dog as in right lateral recumbent projection of thorax, Figure 417).

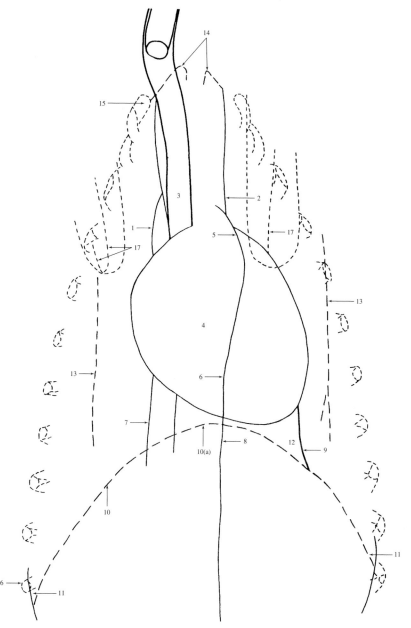

Figure 422 Dorsoventral projection of thorax. Drawing to highlight mediastinal structures (pleura excluded and diaphragm included in respiratory system drawings).

Cranial mediastinum. Portion cranial to cardiac shadow.

1 Right border of cranial vena cava
2 Left border of left subclavian artery
3 Tracheal lumen. Thoracic portion lies slightly to the right until its termination when it is midline.

Middle mediastinum. Portion containing cardiac shadow.

4 Cardiac shadow
5 Aortic arch
6 Descending aorta

Caudal mediastinum. Portion caudal to cardiac shadow.

7 Caudal vena cava

8 Descending aorta
9 Phrenicopericardial ligament. Ligament is a fibrous thickening in the ventral portion of the caudal mediastinum.
10 Diaphragmatic shadow
   10(a) Cupola
11 Costodiaphragmatic recess
12 Cardiodiaphragmatic angle
13 Skin folds superimposed on thoracic cavity shadows
14 Cranial limit of cranial lung lobes
15 1st. rib
16 11th. rib
17 Spine of scapula

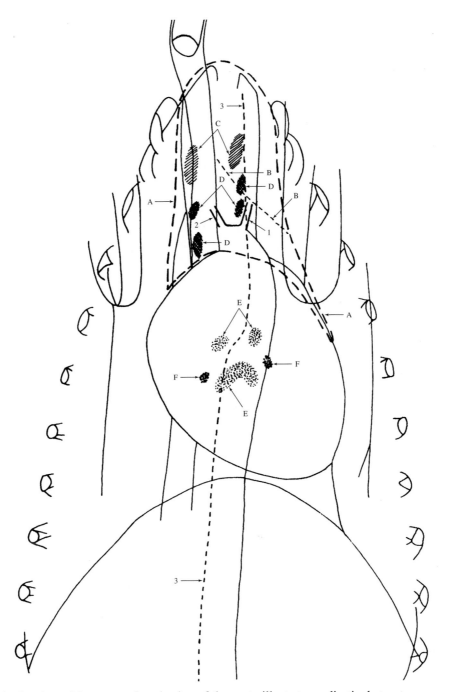

Figure 423   Schematic drawing of dorsoventral projection of thorax to illustrate mediastinal structures.

—— A = Thymus seen in young dogs. As dog ages, lymphoid tissue reduces but in older dogs a vestigial thymus is often seen (B). This shadow is known as the 'sail sign'.

///// C = Sternal lymph nodes

⬤ D = Cranial mediastinal lymph nodes. Ventral and dorsal positions.

⠢ E = Tracheobronchial lymph nodes

⣿ F = Pulmonary lymph nodes. Often absent.

   1 = Left subclavian artery

   2 = Brachiocephalic trunk

------ 3 = Thoracic duct

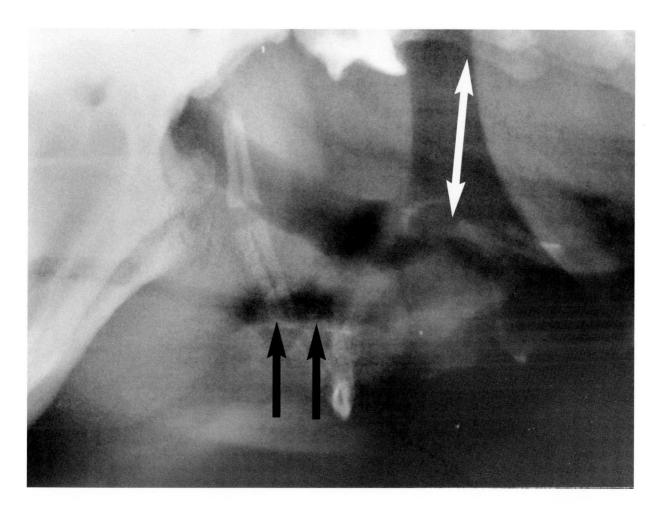

Figure 424 Lateral projection of larynx and pharynx. Brachycephalic breed of dog. Radiograph taken during general anaesthesia with endotracheal tube removed for clarity of radiographic shadows. Bulldog 5 years old, entire female.

The radiograph shows the vertical position of the hyoid bones together with a much reduced oropharynx and very large soft palate shadow. The nasopharynx is also small and the endotracheal intubation has caused the epiglottis (closed arrow) to lie ventrocranially.

On recovery from the general anaesthetic, when swallowing reflexes return, the epiglottis will rotate dorsocranially and come to rest just ventrocranially to the soft palate.

Note the large retropharyngeal space (open arrow) which is normal in this type of breed but does create an apparent ventral displacement of the laryngeal cartilages.

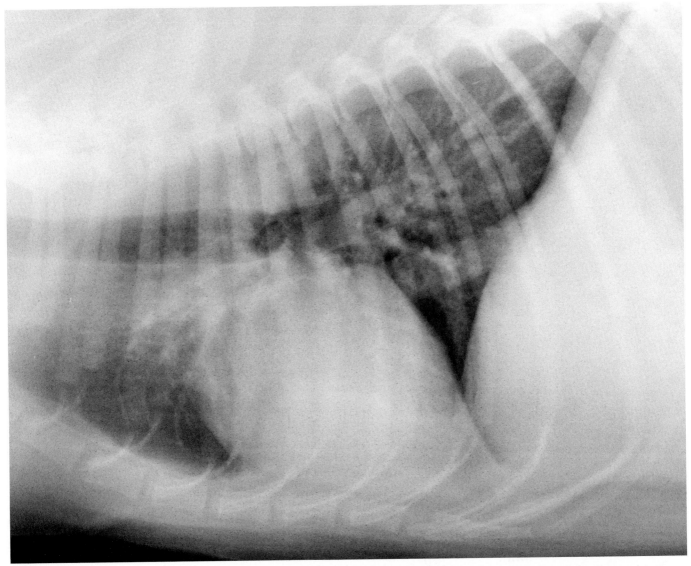

Figure 425   Right lateral recumbent projection of thorax. Short, barrel chested breed of dog. Radiograph taken during general anaesthesia with full inflation of lung lobes. Samoyed dog 6 years old, entire female (same dog as in Figure 427)

The radiograph demonstrates the rounded cardiac shadow, with increase in sternal contact, caused by the horizontal position of the heart within the thoracic cavity. Cardiac measurements, when compared to a normal or intermediate chested breed of dog, are greater in the craniocaudal direction.

The comparatively large craniocaudal measurement together with rounding of cranial cardiac border and increase in sternal contact must not be misdiagnosed as right-sided cardiac enlargement (atrial and ventricular).

The lung opacities in this dog are due to 'age' changes within the bronchial walls and interstitial tissue (see Figure 433 for 'age' changes).

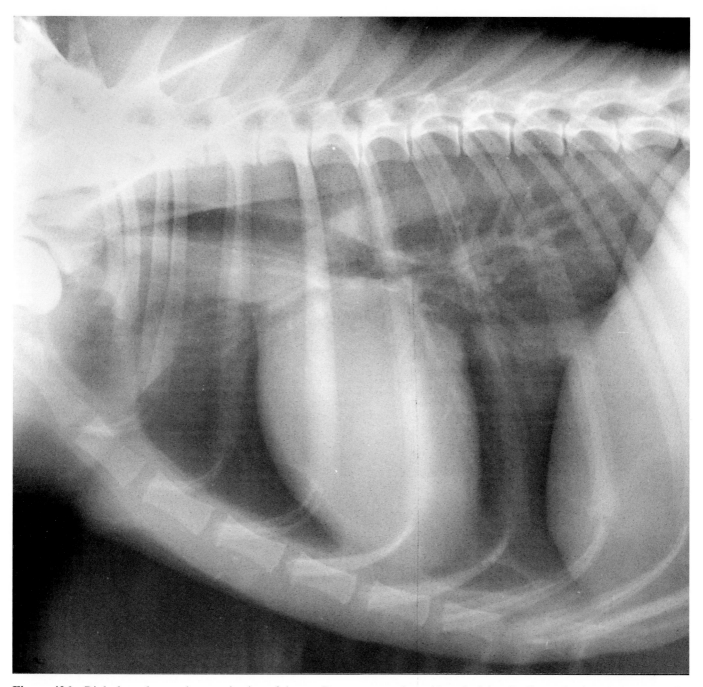

Figure 426 Right lateral recumbent projection of thorax. Deep, narrow chested breed of dog. Radiograph taken during general anaesthesia with full inflation of lung lobes. Afghan Hound dog 2 years old, entire female.

The radiograph shows the 'upright' appearance of the cardiac shadow. This is caused by the position of the heart within the thoracic cavity being almost perpendicular to the thoracic spine. Cardiac measurements, compared to a normal or intermediate chested breed of dog, are less in the craniocaudal direction and greater in the dorsoventral direction.

Care must be taken when analysing this type of cardiac shadow as the upright appearance, especially of the caudal border, may be misdiagnosed as left-sided cardiac enlargement. In particular, an enlarged left atrium could be interpreted.

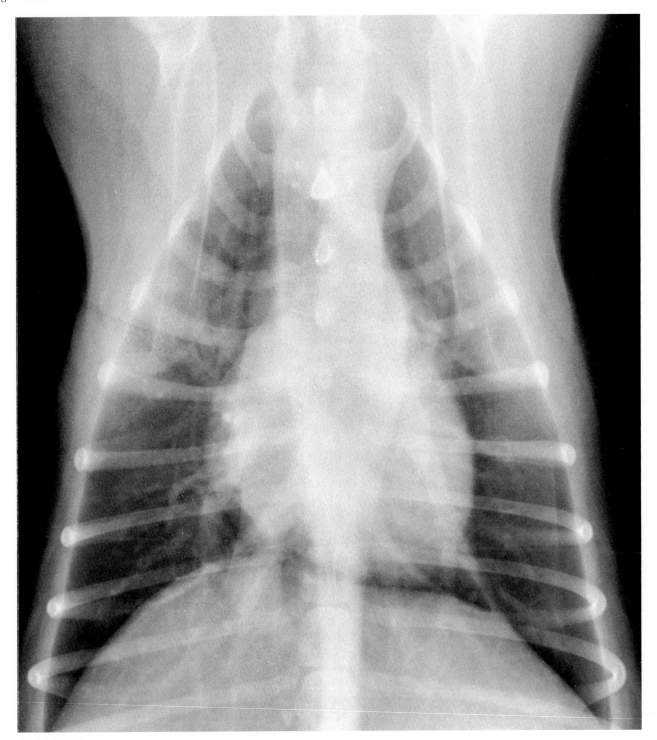

Figure 427   Dorsoventral projection of thorax. Short, barrel chested breed of dog. Radiograph taken during general anaesthesia with full inflation of lung lobes. Samoyed dog 6 years old, entire female (same dog as in Figure 425).

The radiograph shows the rounded left and right cardiac borders seen in this type of chested breed of dog.

Rounded cardiac apex is more left of the midline compared to the normal or intermediate chested breed of dog. The apical level is due to the oblique position of the heart across the thoracic cavity's midline.

As with the right lateral recumbent projection of thorax, the appearance of the cardiac shadow in the short, barrel chested breed of dog must not be confused with right-sided cardiac enlargement (atrial and ventricular).

Also note the fat deposition mimicking a wide cranial mediastinum and right-sided cardiac enlargement (see fat deposition within thoracic cavity, Figure 435).

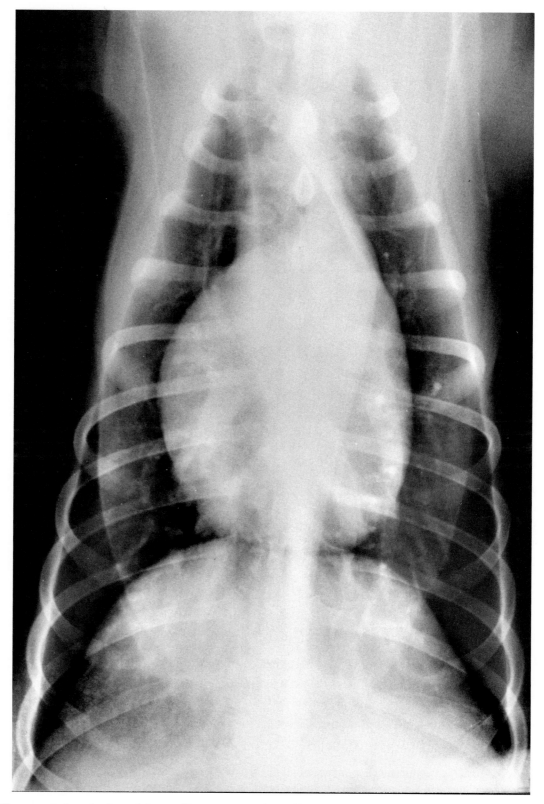

Figure 428   Dorsoventral projection of thorax. Deep, narrow chested breed of dog. Radiograph taken during general anaesthesia with full inflation of lung lobes. Doberman Pinscher dog 4 years old, entire female.

The radiograph shows the short-rounded appearance of the cardiac shadow typical in this type of chested dog. The cardiac shadow is more midline than in the normal or intermediate chested breed of dog.

Also of note are the deep costophrenic angles.

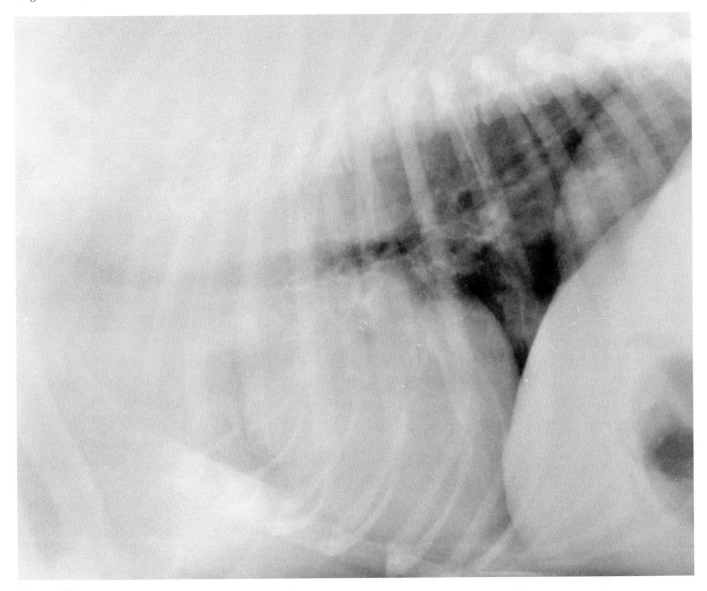

Figure 429

Figures 429 and 430   Radiographs to illustrate poor technique in thoracic radiography.

Figure 429   Right lateral recumbent projection of thorax. Radiograph taken while dog conscious using sandbag restraint.

Figure 430   Right lateral recumbent projection of thorax. Radiograph taken during general anaesthesia with full inflation of lung lobes.

Both radiographs were taken using the same radiographic equipment, exposure values and film focal distance.

Bulldog 18 months old, entire female. Same dog as in Figure 431.

In the conscious dog note the very opaque appearance of all the lung tissue, especially cranially; also the apparent narrowing of the trachea at the thoracic inlet and the 'large globular' cardiac shadow.

In the anaesthetised dog, which is now more properly positioned with full inflation of lung lobes, the lung tissue has lost its extremely opaque appearance. Also, the trachea is normal in width, and the cardiac shadow has reduced in size and is less rounded in outline.

Unfortunately, due to rotation of the chest full analysis of the cardiac shadow is not possible. However, the bulldog will have a cardiac shadow typical of a short, barrel chested breed of dog.

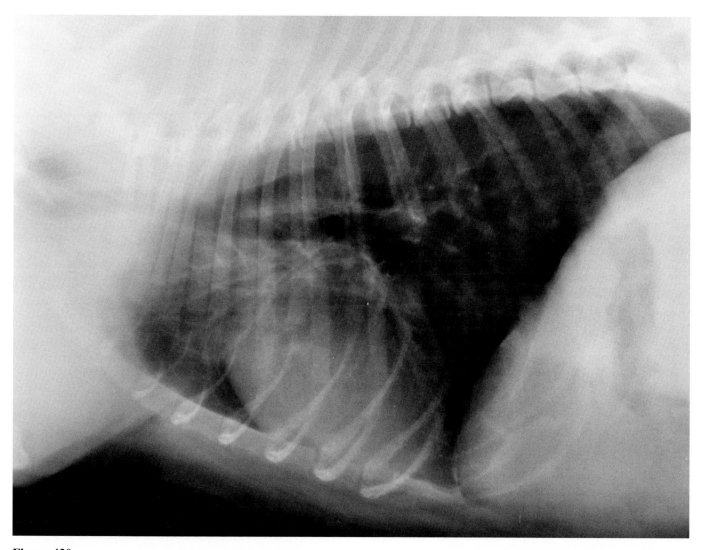

Figure 430

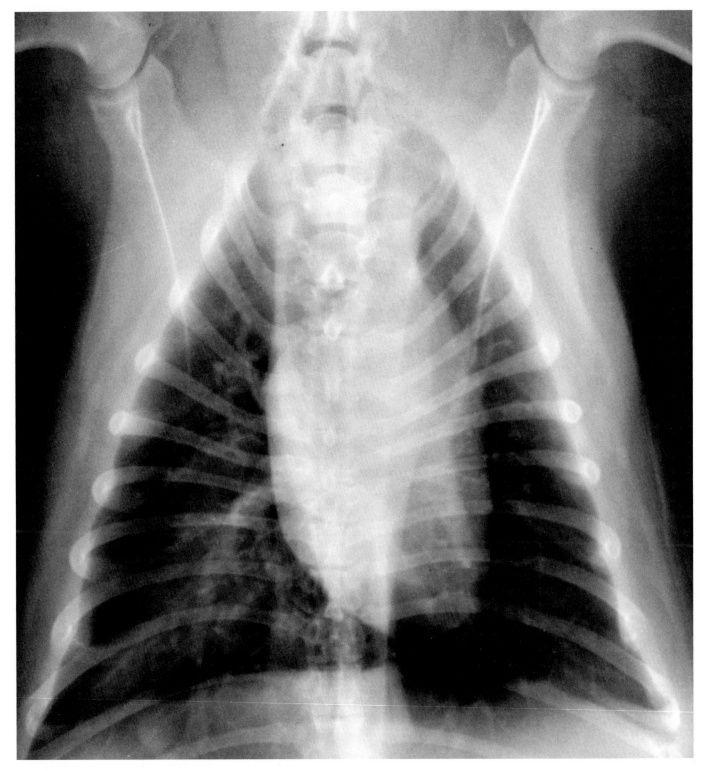

Figure 431 Ventrodorsal projection of thorax. Radiograph taken during general anaesthesia with full inflation of lung lobes. Bulldog 18 months old, entire female (same dog as in Figures 429 and 430).

The radiograph confirms that lung density is normal in both right and left lung lobes, as indicated in the right lateral recumbent projection of thorax with full inflation of lung lobes.

Note the rudimentary clavicles which are commonly seen in the ventrodorsal and dorsoventral projections of thorax. Also, at the 12th. rib level shadows of right and left nipples can be seen as distinct soft tissue shadows superimposed on lung and liver shadows. Care must be taken to ensure that nipple shadows are not misdiagnosed as neoplastic masses.

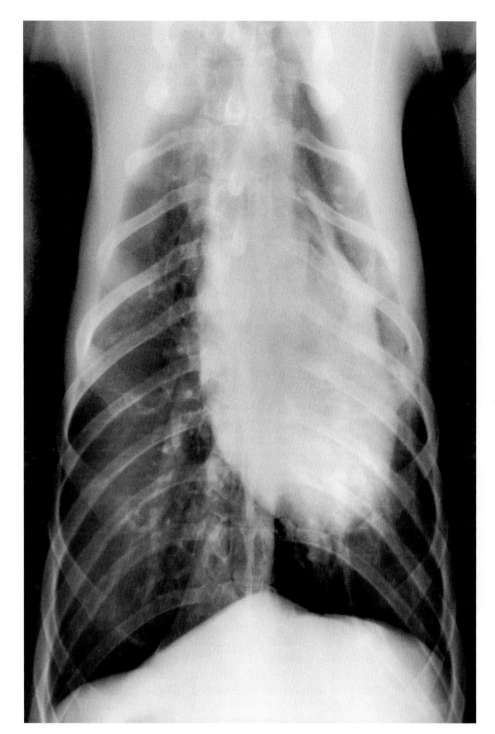

Figure 432 Ventrodorsal projection of thorax. Hypostatic congestion of lung tissue. Radiograph taken during general anaesthesia with full inflation of lung lobes. German Shepherd dog 7 years old, entire female.

The radiograph demonstrates the radiopaque appearance caused by hypostatic congestion of the left cranial lung lobe (cranial and more especially caudal parts). The congestion is collapsing of dependent lung tissue while in left lateral recumbency prior to the ventrodorsal projection being taken.

Once collapse has occurred full reinflation for a normal lung appearance is very difficult to achieve.

Although this radiograph demonstrates a normal phenomenon that will occur in any dependent lung tissue following prolonged lateral recumbency, hypostatic congestion of abnormal lung tissue can occur within minutes of lateral recumbency. Hence in radiography of clinical cases ventrodorsal or dorsoventral projections should precede lateral recumbent projections (remember that ventrodorsal projection may be contraindicated in cases of severe dyspnoea).

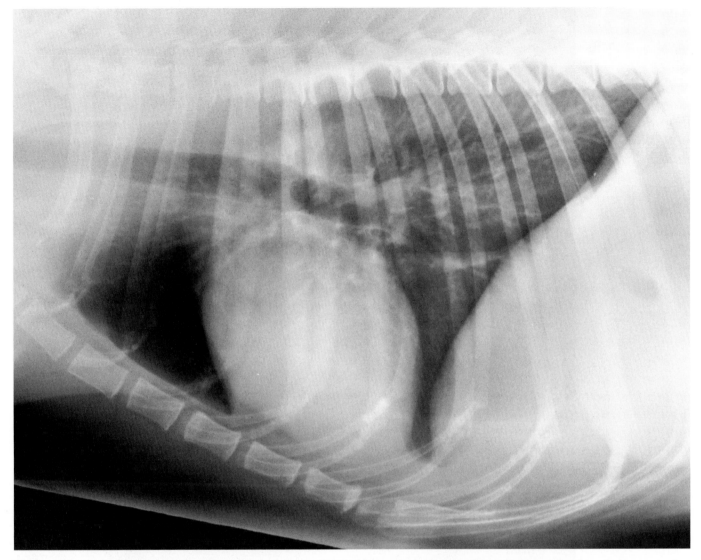

Figure 433   Right lateral recumbent projection of thorax. 'Age' changes in dog's lung tissue. Radiograph taken during general anaesthesia with full inflation of lung lobes. Golden Labrador dog 8 years old, entire female.

The radiograph shows changes within the bronchial walls and interstitial lung tissue creating an opaque mixed bronchial–interstitial pattern. The pattern is both linear and circular opacities associated with bronchial wall thickening and/or mineralisation. Interstitial involvement is also present in the form of linear and micronodular opacities. The vascular pattern is somewhat obscured by the increased interstitial radiopacity.

Such changes can commonly be seen in dogs over 4 years of age (so-called 'ageing' of lungs). 'Ageing' is progressive and in dogs over 10 years of age the radiographic appearance can be very dramatic. The latter may be difficult to differentiate from severe disease.

Urban dogs are more prone to the bronchial–interstitial changes but certain breeds appear to be more predisposed. In particular, chondrodystrophic breeds have mineralisation of their bronchial walls as they age, but changes are often seen before 4 years of age and even at 1 year old (see Figure 437, Atonic oesophagus).

Although the cat does have some 'ageing' of lung tissue, the radiographic appearance is usually a few bronchial wall thickenings scattered throughout the lung lobes. Unlike the dog the cat 'age' changes often remain limited even into geriatric years.

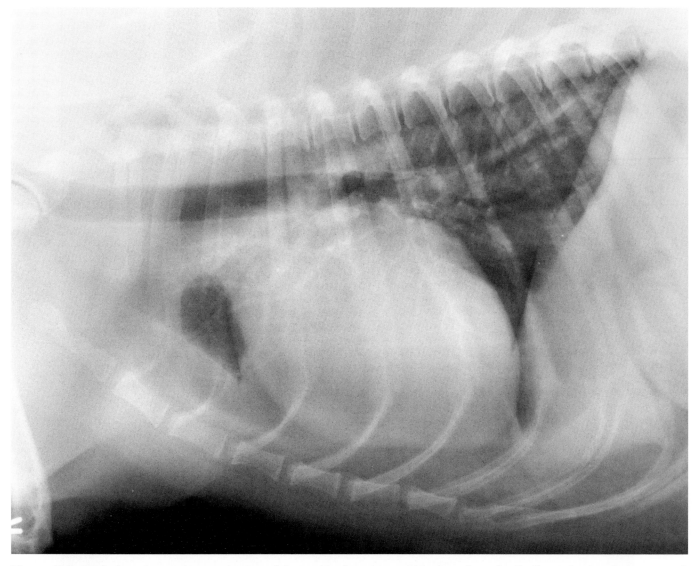

Figure 434   Right lateral recumbent projection of thorax. Fat deposition within thoracic cavity. Radiograph taken during general anaesthesia with inflation of lung lobes. Old English Sheepdog 8 years old, entire male.

The radiograph demonstrates dorsal elevation of the cardiac shadow away from the bony sternum. Ventral to the cardiac shadow the grey opacity of fat tissue can be seen.

Loss of sternal contact of the cardiac shadow caused by fat deposition must not be mistaken for a pneumothorax. In the latter case the black shadow of air will be seen ventral to the cardiac shadow.

Dorsal elevation of the cardiac shadow by fat deposition is more frequently seen in the dog than the cat.

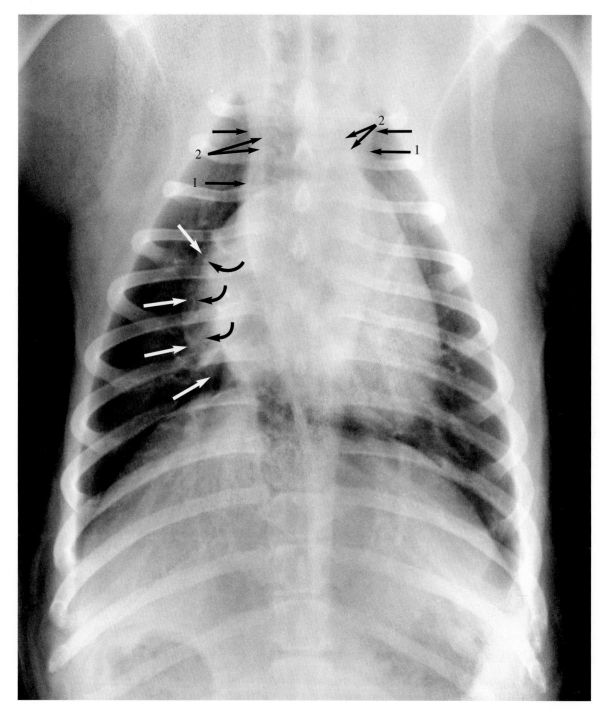

Figure 435   Dorsoventral projection of thorax. Fat deposition within thoracic cavity. Radiograph taken during general anaesthesia with inflation of lung lobes. Bulldog 1 year old, entire female.

The radiograph shows the effect of fat accumulation within the cranial mediastinum making this area appear wider than normal (closed arrows). The grey opacity of fat can be seen (1). The soft tissue opacity of the cranial mediastinum is labelled (2).

Also present is fat deposition in the ventral mediastinum and pericardial sac. This is seen to mimic cardiac 'enlargement'. The grey fat opacity outline is labelled with open arrows, while the cardiac soft tissue outline is labelled with curved arrows.

Although this fat accumulation is seen more commonly in the chondrodystrophic breed of dog, any obese dog or cat can have fat deposits in the regions described above.

Of note is the cardiac shadow which is typical of a short, barrel chested breed of dog. The left and right borders are both rounded and the rounded cardiac apex is positioned to the far left. The apex site is caused by the oblique positioning of the heart across the midline in this type of chest (see Figure 427).

An Atlas of Interpretative Radiographic Anatomy of the Dog and Cat

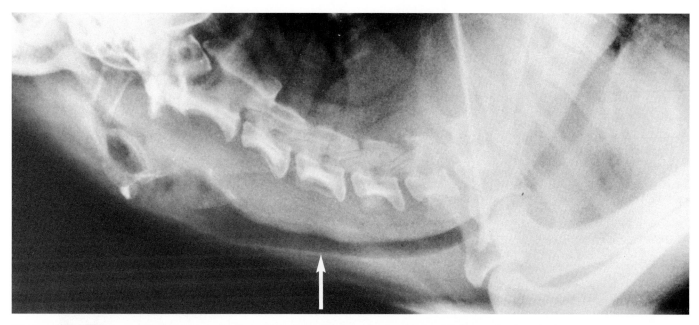

Figure 436   Hyperextended lateral projection of trachea. False tracheal collapse. Radiograph taken during general anaesthesia at full inspiration. Yorkshire Terrier dog 10 years old, neutered female.

The radiograph shows an apparent narrowing of the cervical tracheal lumen (arrow). The 'narrowing' is due to an overlying soft tissue shadow of the oesophagus and ventral neck muscles.

This soft tissue shadow at the dorsal aspect of the trachea commonly creates a 'false' tracheal collapse, especially with hyperextension of the neck. Differentiation from abnormality is aided by studying the pharyngeal spaces and thoracic trachea. Pharyngeal air spaces and the thoracic trachea are of a normal size, i.e. are not enlarged, in this dog.

If there is doubt in interpretation of tracheal collapse further radiography must be undertaken. This includes lateral projections of the cervical and thoracic trachea, with the neck in a normal extended position, at both full inspiration and full expiration. In cases of tracheal collapse, collapse of cervical trachea will be seen at inspiration while thoracic trachea collapses at expiration.

Alternatively, or additionally, a cross section of the lower cervical tracheal shadow can be obtained by special tracheal positioning. While the dog is in sternal recumbency the neck is hyperflexed. The vertical primary beam is then directed tangentially to the trachea.

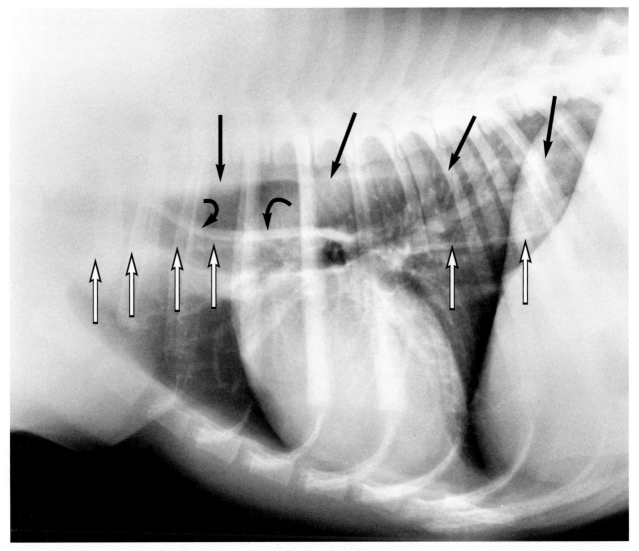

Figure 437   Left lateral recumbent projection of thorax. Atonic oesophagus caused by general anaesthesia. Radiograph taken during general anaesthesia with full inflation of lung lobes. Bull Terrier dog 18 months old, entire male.

The radiograph highlights the atonic effect of general anaesthesia on the oesophagus. This type of atony must not be misdiagnosed as an abnormality of the muscle, or even as an enlargement, i.e. megaoesophagus. The oesophagus will return to its normal size, and function, following recovery from the general anaesthetic.

Closed arrows = Dorsal wall of oesophagus

Open arrows = Ventral wall of oesophagus

Note the linear radiolucent area between the two types of arrow

Curved arrows = Tracheoesophageal stripe sign. This occurs normally when the oesophagus is distended with gas. It is not a thickening of the tracheal or oesophageal wall. The appearance is due to oesophageal lumenal gas contrast allowing the soft tissue of the dorsal tracheal wall and the contacting oesophageal wall to be seen as a single shadow.

Also of note is the obvious bronchial pattern even though the dog is only 18 months old. This is due to calcification of the bronchial walls in a chondrodystrophic breed of dog. Micronodular calcified plaques are also present throughout the interstitial tissue.

Although cardiac shadow analysis should be made from the right lateral recumbent projection, the cardiac shadow here is typical of a short, barrel chested breed of dog (see Figure 425).

Cardiac shadow appears more horizontal in thoracic position with increase in sternal contact. This effect gives rounding of cardiac borders and the craniocaudal measurement of the heart is larger than compared with the normal or intermediate chested breeds of dog.

Most terrier breeds of dog have this type of cardiac shadow.

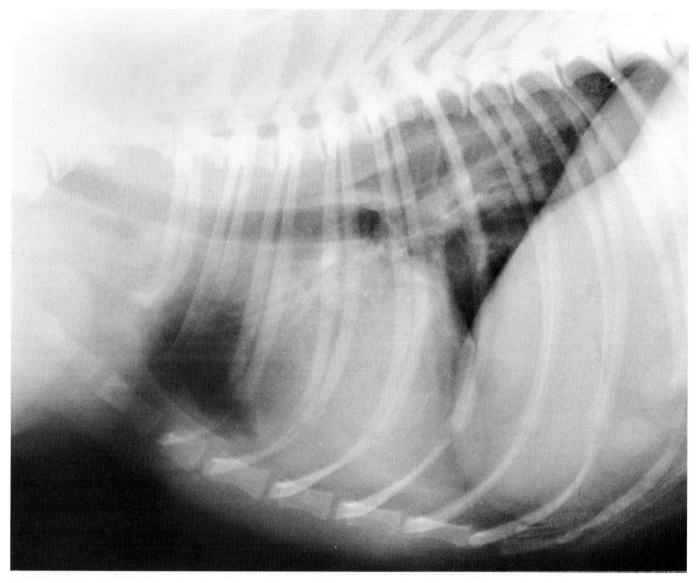

Figure 438   Left lateral recumbent projection of thorax. Congenital oesophageal diverticulum. Radiograph taken during general anaesthesia with no inflation of lung lobes. Boston Terrier dog 20 months old, entire female.

The radiograph shows a gas pocket depicting a congenital oesophageal diverticulum at the thoracic inlet. Diverticula in this region of the oesophagus are not uncommon especially in the brachycephalic breed of dog. Usually they are of no clinical significance.

The presence of gas in the oesophagus is normal for an animal under a general anaesthetic. However, any evidence of oesophageal gas in the conscious animal must be treated with suspicion as it indicates abnormal oesophageal function.

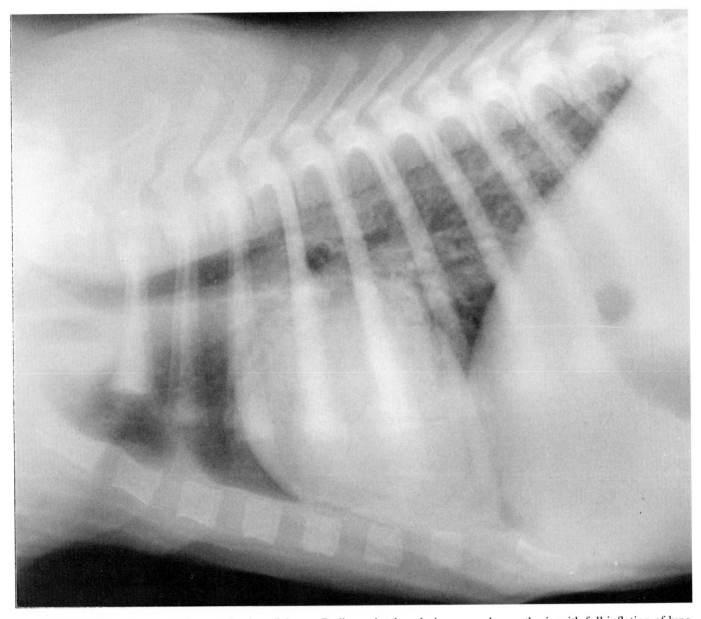

Figure 439   Right lateral recumbent projection of thorax. Radiograph taken during general anaesthesia with full inflation of lung lobes. Weimaraner dog 7 weeks old, entire female.

The radiograph shows the opaque appearance of lung tissue in the very young animal. This opacity is thought to be due to fluid within the interstitial tissue not present in the adult. It must not be misdiagnosed as disease.

Also of note is the large cardiac shadow. Young dogs of every breed, that is all type chested breeds, have comparatively large cardiac shadows with rounded borders and increase in sternal contact. Again the shadow must not be confused with an abnormality.

When adult, the Weimaraner cardiac shadow would be the normal or intermediate chested breed of dog (see Figure 396).

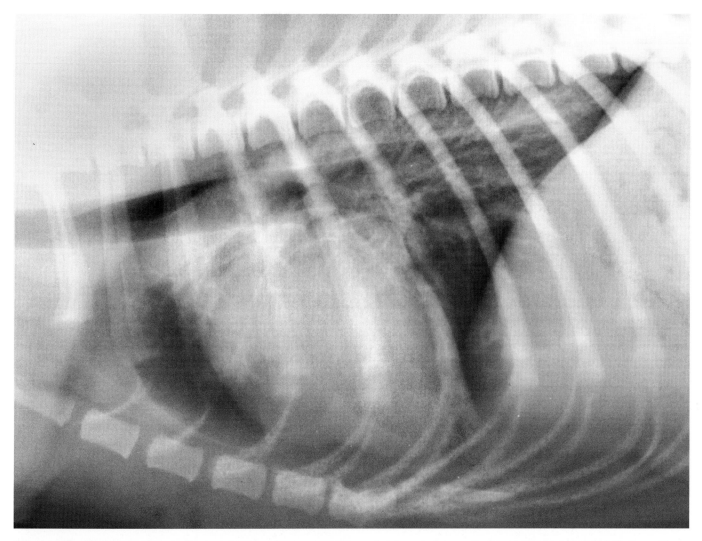

Figure 440   Right lateral recumbent projection of thorax. Radiograph taken during general anaesthesia with full inflation of lung lobes. Golden Labrador dog 20 weeks old, entire female.

The radiograph demonstrates a linear radiopaque interstitial pattern which is normal for a dog of this age. Some bronchial markings are also present where the interstitial fluid has involved the peribronchial tissue.

The cardiac shadow appears to have enlargement, especially of the cranial border or right ventricle. A ventral indentation can be seen at the junction of the right and left ventricle. These signs must not be mistaken for cardiac abnormality as a dog of 20 weeks of age normally has a large cardiac shadow compared to the adult.

The Labrador dog is a normal or intermediate chested breed of dog and when mature this dog will lose its apparent right-sided cardiac enlargement.

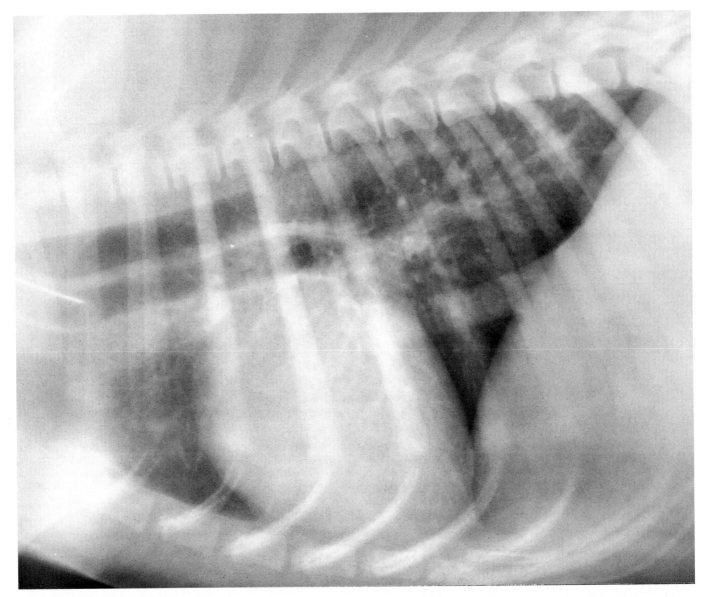

Figure 441 Right lateral recumbent projection of thorax. Radiograph taken during general anaesthesia with full inflation of lung lobes. Samoyed crossbred dog 25 weeks old, entire male (same dog as in Figure 442).

Although the radiograph shows the radiopaque appearance of the lung lobes, which is usually seen in the immature animal, the long woolly coat of this dog has caused an additional mottled soft tissue opacity over the entire thorax. However, the linear and circular lung opacity of the interstitial and bronchial tissue can still be identified.

The cardiac shadow appears abnormally rounded, especially the cranial border. This is normal for a short, barrel chested breed of dog at 25 weeks of age.

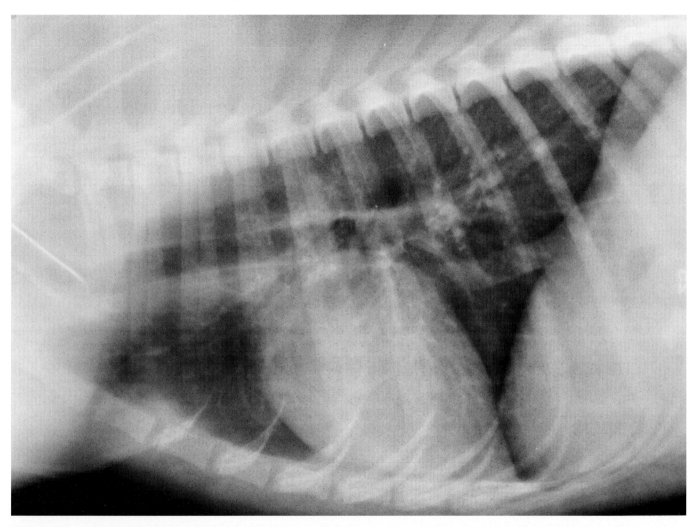

Figure 442   Right lateral recumbent projection of thorax. Radiograph taken during general anaesthesia with full inflation of lung lobes. Samoyed crossbred dog 38 weeks old, entire male (same dog as in Figure 441).

The radiograph now shows that the cardiac shadow has become typical for a short, barrel chested breed of dog. The extreme rounding of the borders, especially the cranial border or right ventricle, has disappeared.

The lung tissue still appears opaque at this age, but repeat radiography of the same dog at 52 weeks old, showed overall reduction of both interstitial and bronchial patterns. Cardiac shadow at 52 weeks of age was similar in size and shape to this 38 week film.

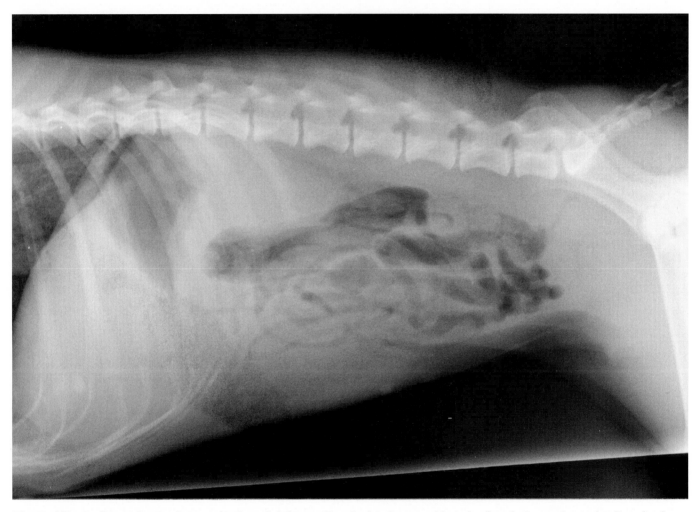

Figure 443   Left lateral recumbent projection of abdomen. Beagle dog 2 years old, entire female (same dog as in all projections of the abdomen of the female).

An Atlas of Interpretative Radiographic Anatomy of the Dog and Cat

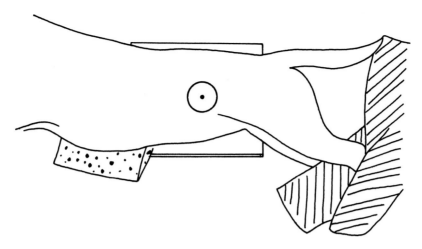

Figure 444 Line drawing of photograph representing radiographic positioning for Figure 443.

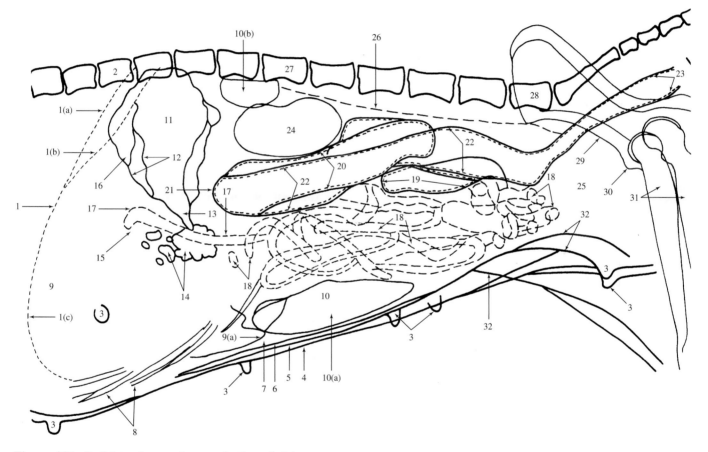

Figure 445 Left lateral recumbent projection of abdomen.

1	Diaphragmatic shadow	4	Skin margin
	1(a) Left 'crus'	5	Subcutaneous fat
	1(b) Right 'crus'	6	M.rectus abdominis
	1(c) Cupola	7	Intraperitoneal fat
2	11th. thoracic vertebra	8	Calcified costal cartilages
3	Soft tissue shadows of nipples		

9 Soft tissue shadow of liver
   9(a) Caudoventral margin of liver. Normally seen just beyond costal arch forming an acute angle of 30 degrees or less.

Note that in aged and obese animals this shadow often projects beyond the costal arch due to stretching of the ligaments supporting the liver. A right lateral recumbent projection shows the dorsal extent of the liver to be less in these cases than in younger, non-obesed dogs.

The liver shadow is slightly more caudally positioned during inspiration but most abdominal radiography is performed during expiration.

10 Spleen
   10(a) Ventral extremity. Normally seen at this position but varies depending on gastric distention.
   10(b) Dorsal extremity

11 Gas in gastric fundus. (In this radiograph there is an abnormally large volume of gas seen for left lateral recumbency.)

The fundus is dependent in this projection and is usually fluid filled. Normally most of the gastric gas will be found in the pyloric part, as this is uppermost in left lateral recumbency.

12 Gastric mucosa

13 Gastric body

14 Pyloric part, antrum and canal, of gastric shadow. (Some gas is present due to left lateral recumbency, see number 11.)

15 Position of pylorus (pylorus not seen in this film)

The term pylorus is often incorrectly used to mean pyloric antrum and canal.

16 Position of gastric cardia (cardia not seen in this film)

Contrast media normally required to demonstrate numbers 15 and 16.

17 Duodenal shadow (seen due to the presence of lumenal gas contrast)

18 Jejunum and ileum (seen due to the presence of lumenal gas contrast)

Loops of bowel are normally visible, their lumens filled with gas or fluid, or a mixture of both. The mixture of luminal gas and fluid can mimic wall 'thickening' when lateral recumbent projections are taken. This is caused by the fluid lining the lumen being in contact with the wall while gas is in the centre of the lumen. Fluid and soft tissue have the same radiographic opacity and hence cannot be differentiated in plain radiographs. A bowel fluid line, i.e. a gas and fluid interface, will only be seen in lateral standing projections of the abdomen.

In the dog radiographed for this film, very little abdominal intraperitoneal fat was present. This resulted in poor soft tissue contrast and has made the gas-filled gastrointestinal shadows most obvious.

The long jejunum is indistinguishable from the short ileum and generally the diameter of all the bowel is equal; the rule of thumb is, maximum width normally equal to the height of the lumbar vertebra's body.

It has been noted that the terminal ileum can be greater in diameter as it approaches the caecum. The terminal ileum is usually located in the central abdomen, just to the right of the midline.

19 Caecal shadow (elongated comma shape is not clearly seen in this film)

20 Ascending colon

21 Transverse colon

22 Descending colon

23 Rectum

24 Left kidney

The left kidney is more mobile than the right. In obese dogs the craniocaudal axis often becomes more vertical than horizontal and fat opacity is present dorsally.

Kidney shape varies from bean to elliptical but the outline is always smooth. Size is 2.5 to 3.5 times the length of the 2nd. lumbar vertebral body.

Kidneys and ureters, not visible in the normal dog in plain films, are retroperitoneal.

25 Region of urinary bladder

Although not seen in this film, the urine-filled bladder is usually clearly identifiable. It extends cranially in a ventral position.

The genital system of the non-pregnant normal female dog is not usually seen without contrast material.

26 Sublumbar muscles; m.psoas minor, m.iliopsoas and m.quadratus lumborum

Also included in this shadow are ureters, lymph nodes plus aorta, caudal vena cava and other vessels.

The shadow gradually decreases in opacity caudal to the 4th. lumbar vertebra as the m.iliopsoas diverge to insert on the proximal femora. The m.quadratus lumborum inserts on the wing of the ilium. The caudal vena cava forms from the iliac veins and the aorta divides to form the left and right internal and external arteries.

27 2nd. lumbar vertebra

28 7th. lumbar vertebra

29 Body of ilium

30 Iliopubic or iliopectineal eminence

31 Femoral bodies

32 Skin folds

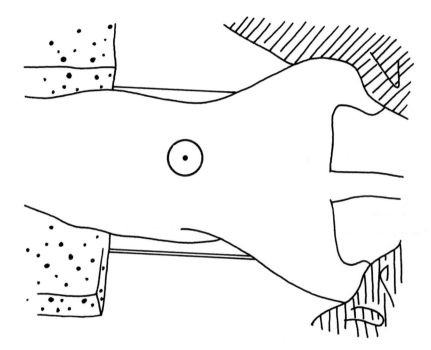

Figure 446   Line drawing of photograph representing radiographic positioning for Figure 447.

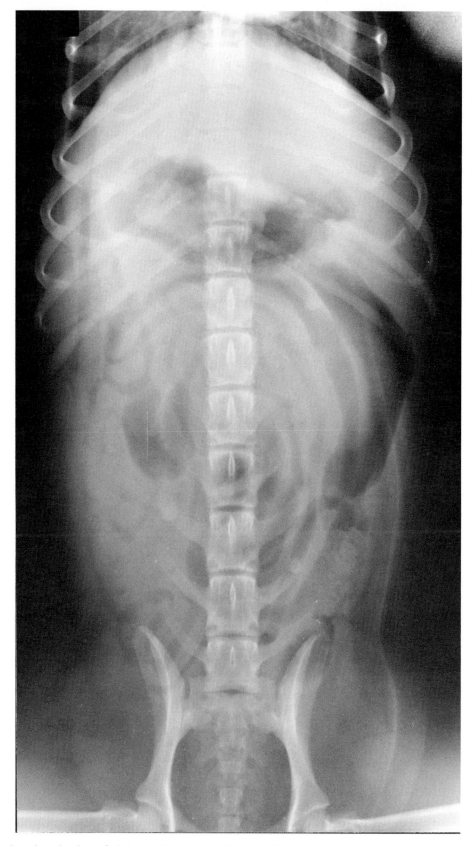

Figure 447 Ventrodorsal projection of abdomen. Beagle dog 2 years old, entire female (same dog as in all projections of abdomen of the female).

An Atlas of Interpretative Radiographic Anatomy of the Dog and Cat

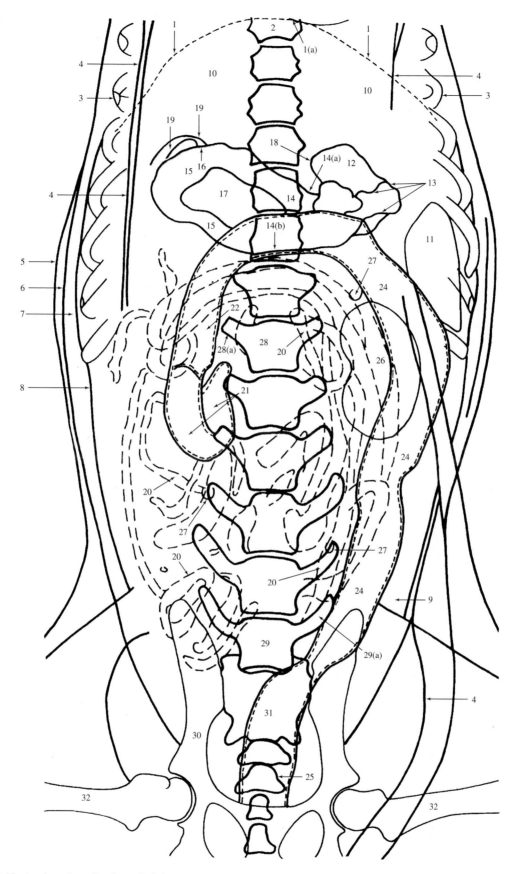

Figure 448   Ventrodorsal projection of abdomen.

(448 continued.)

1 Diaphragmatic shadow
  1(a) Cupola

2 8th. thoracic vertebra

3 8th. rib

4 Skin folds

5 Skin margin

6 Subcutaneous fat. (Only just visible in this dog as a thin grey line between the outer skin and the first superficial muscle layer of the lateral abdominal wall.)

7 M.obliquus externus abdominis

8 Very thin layer of fat overlying the superficial surface of the caudal ribs.

This layer usually serves to separate the m.obliquus externus abdominis from the m.obliquus internus abdominis and m.transversus abdominis. Unfortunately the fat layer is too thin to distinguish clearly between the two muscle layers in this female dog.

9 Intraperitoneal fat

10 Soft tissue shadow of liver

11 Dorsal extremity of spleen

12 Gastric fundus

13 Gastric mucosa

14 Gastric body. (Contains most of gas within the gastric structures due to the ventrodorsal positioning allowing gas to collect in the uppermost part of gastric shadow.)
  14(a) Lesser curvature
  14(b) Greater curvature

15 Pyloric part of gastric shadow; Pyloric antrum and canal.

16 Pylorus; pyloric sphincter muscle. The term pylorus is often misused to mean pyloric antrum and canal.

17 Ingesta within gastric lumen

18 Position of gastric cardia (cardia not visible in this film)

19 Duodenal shadow (seen due to the presence of gas in the lumen)

20 Jejunum and ileum (seen due to the presence of gas in the lumen)

See (18) in left lateral recumbent projection of abdomen of female, Figure 445, for additional information.

21 Caecal shadow. (Comma shape more obvious in this film than in the corresponding dorsoventral projection line drawing, Figure 451.)

22 Ascending colon

23 Transverse colon (superimposed in part by gastric shadow)

24 Descending colon

25 Rectum

26 Left kidney (only just visible)

See (24) in left lateral recumbent projection of abdomen of female, Figure 445, for more information.

The right kidney is not visible in this film due to the small amount of perirenal fat contrast.

27 Soft tissue shadows representing nipples

28 2nd. lumbar vertebra
  28(a) Transverse process

29 7th. lumbar vertebra
  29(a) Transverse process

30 Body of ilium

31 Sacrum

32 Femoral bodies

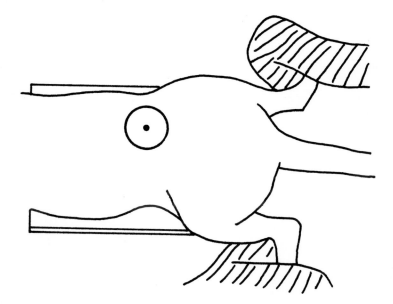

Figure 449   Line drawing of photograph representing radiographic positioning for Figure 450

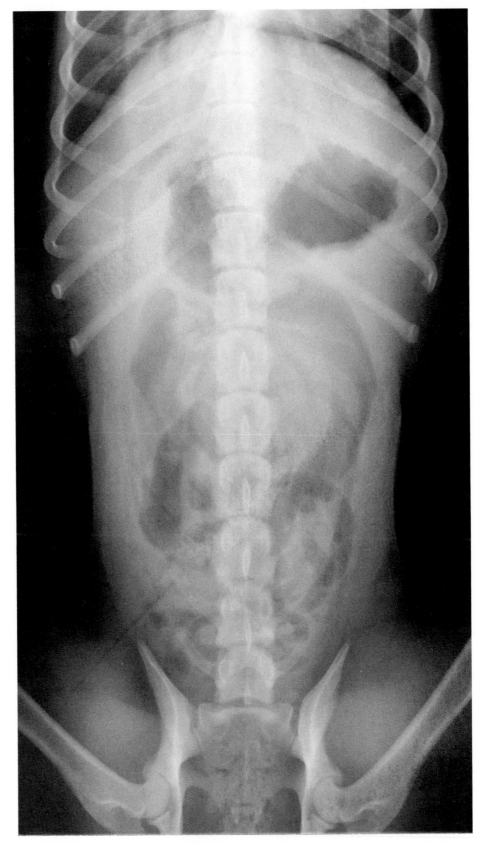

Figure 450   Dorsoventral projection of abdomen. Beagle dog 2 years old, entire female (same dog as in all projections of abdomen of the female).

An Atlas of Interpretative Radiographic Anatomy of the Dog and Cat

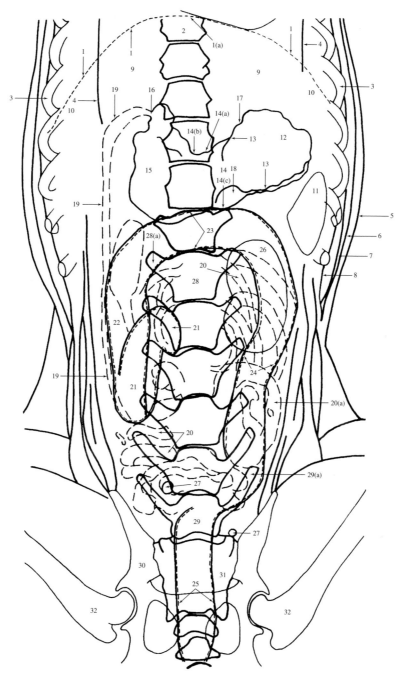

Figure 451 Dorsoventral projection of abdomen.

Although the dorsoventral projection is not routinely used as a standard abdominal projection, comparison of the ventrodorsal and dorsoventral projections, in the same female dog, highlights how free gas within the gastrointestinal tract changes position. In addition, structures further away from the filmed cassette, e.g. kidneys (in the dorsoventral projection), are less well defined. Also note the shape of the pelvis in the dorsoventral projection, as opposed to the usual appearance in the ventrodorsal projection.

1 Diaphragmatic shadow
  1(a) Cupola

2 9th. thoracic vertebra

3 9th. rib

4 Skin folds

5 Skin margin

6 Subcutaneous fat

(451 continued.)

7 M.obliquus externus abdominis

8 Very thin fat layer

See (8) in ventrodorsal projection of abdomen of female, Figure 448, for additional details.

9 Soft tissue shadow of liver

10 Lucent gas shadows of caudal lung lobes superimposed over soft tissue shadow of liver

11 Dorsal extremity of spleen (most of the triangular shadow lines are only just visible)

12 Gastric fundus. (Contains most of the gas in the stomach due to positioning causing gas to rise to the uppermost part of the stomach, i.e. fundus in dorsoventral projection.)

13 Gastric mucosa

14 Gastric body
    14(a) Lesser curvature
    14(b) Angular notch
    14(c) Greater curvature

15 Pyloric part of gastric shadow; Pyloric antrum and canal.

16 Pylorus; pyloric part of the stomach containing the pyloric sphincter muscle. The term pylorus is often misused to mean pyloric antrum and canal.

17 Position of gastric cardia (cardia not visible in this film)

18 Ingesta within gastric lumen

19 Duodenum. (Shadow seen due to the presence of gas in lumen and can be seen more extensively than in the corresponding ventrodorsal projection, Figure 448.)

20 Jejunum and ileum. See (18) in left lateral recumbent abdominal projection of female, Figure 445, for additional information.

    20(a) Terminal portion of ileum. Apart from this bowel shadow jejunum and ileum can not be differentiated between in plain radiographs.

21 Caecal shadow

22 Ascending colon

23 Transverse colon. (Superimposition less in this film than the corresponding ventrodorsal projection in Figure 448.)

24 Descending colon

25 Rectum

26 Left kidney (only the craniolateral pole is visible with the aid of colonic gas contrast)

See (24) in left lateral recumbent projection of abdomen of female, Figure 445, for additional information.

The right kidney is not visible in this film due to insufficient perirenal fat contrast and radiographic projection.

27 Soft tissue shadows representing nipples

28 2nd. lumbar vertebra
    28(a) Ttransverse process

29 7th. lumbar vertebra
    29(a) Transverse process

30 Body of ilium

31 Sacrum

32 Femoral bodies

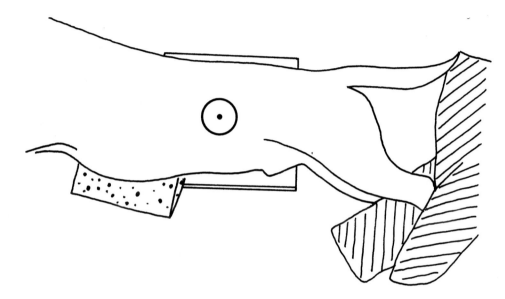

Figure 452   Line drawing of photograph representing radiographic positioning for Figure 453.

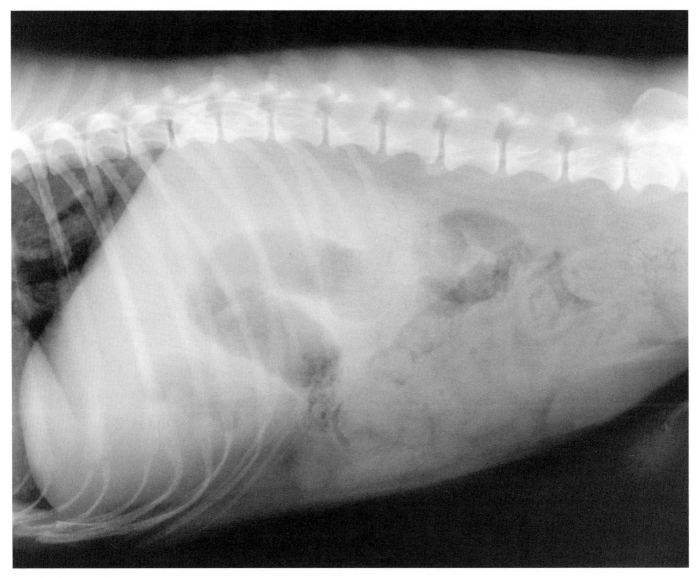

Figure 453 Left lateral recumbent projection of abdomen. Cranially centred. Beagle dog 7 years old, entire male (same dog as in all projections of abdomen of the male).

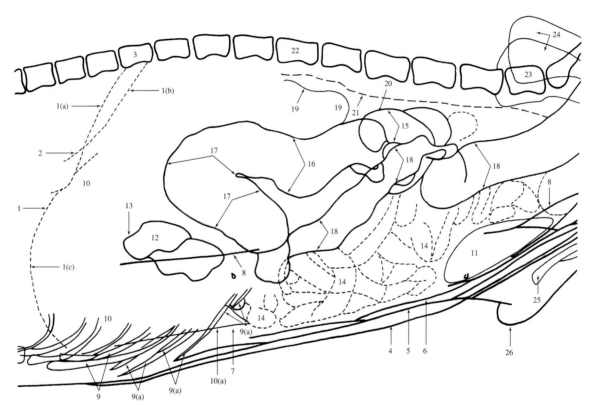

Figure 454   Left lateral recumbent projection of abdomen. Cranially centred.

1   Diaphragmatic shadow
   1(a)   Left 'crus'
   1(b)   Right 'crus'
   1(c)   Cupola

2   Caudal vena cava entering the central tendon just right of the midline

3   11th. thoracic vertebra

4   Skin margin

5   Subcutaneous fat

6   M.rectus abdominis

7   Fat in falciform ligament of the liver

8   Skin folds

9   Calcified costal cartilages
   9(a)   Costal arch. (Formed by costal cartilages 10, 11 and 12.)

(*454 continued.*)

10   Soft tissue shadow of liver. See (9) in left lateral recumbent projection abdomen of female, Figure 445, for more details.

  10(a) Caudoventral margin. (Acute angle not clearly seen due to superimposition of fluid-filled intestinal shadow.)

11   Ventral extremity of spleen

12   Pyloric part, antrum and canal, of gastric shadow. (Large volume of gas present due to left lateral recumbency resulting in gas entering the uppermost part of the gastric shadow. No other part of the gastric shadow is seen in this film.)

13   Position of pylorus; sphincter at entrance of duodenum.

   The term pylorus is often incorrectly used to mean the pyloric antrum and canal. (Not seen as a separate structure in this film.)

14   Jejunum and ileum. (Seen as fluid filled viscera with a few gas pockets in lumens.)

   See (18) in left lateral recumbent projection abdomen of female, Figure 445, for more details.

15   Caecal shadow. (Contrast of gas in the lumen makes the comma shape of the caecum distinguishable from the surrounding intestinal shadows.)

16   Ascending colon

17   Transverse colon

18   Descending colon

19   Right kidney. See (24) in left lateral recumbent projection of abdomen of female, Figure 445, for additional kidney information.

20   Position of left kidney. (Shadow cannot be seen as it is obscured by caecal and colonic shadows.)

   See ventrodorsal and dorsoventral projections line drawing, Figures 464–469 and 471–475, for left kidney in this dog.

21   Sublumbar muscles. For more details see (26) in left lateral recumbent projection of abdomen of female, Figure 445.

22   2nd. lumbar vertebra

23   7th. lumbar vertebra. (A degenerative bony change, spondylosis, is present on the ventral aspect of cranial endplate. See 'normality' in the Introduction.)

24   Ilia

25   Os penis

26   Preputial shadow

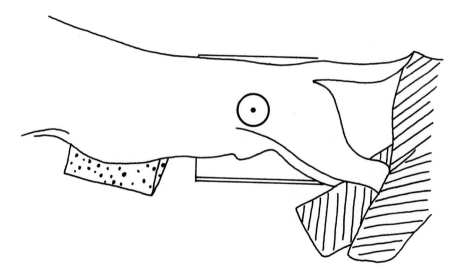

Figure 455   Line drawing of photograph representing radiographic positioning for Figure 456.

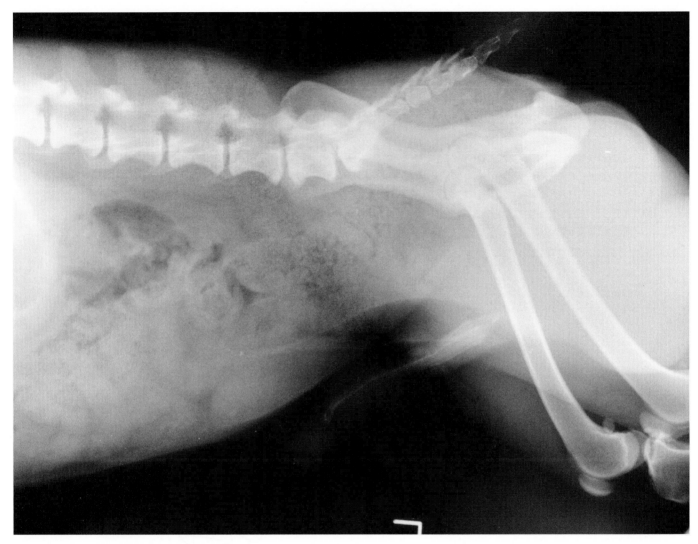

Figure 456   Left lateral recumbent projection of abdomen. Caudally centred. Beagle dog 7 years old, entire male (same dog as in all projections of abdomen of the male).

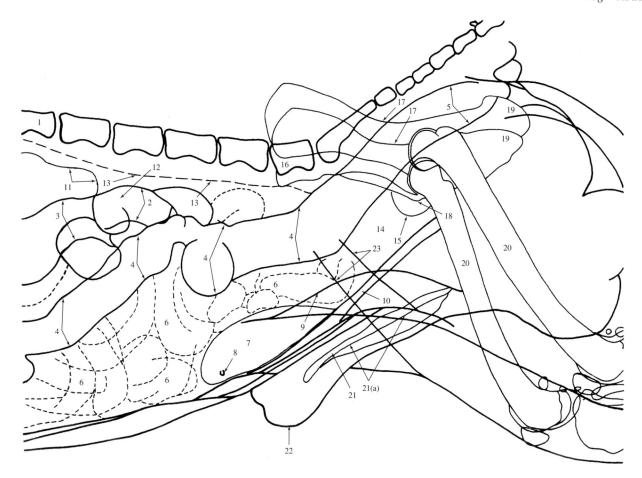

Figure 457 Left lateral recumbent projection of abdomen. Caudally centred.

1 2nd. lumbar vertebra

2 Caecal shadow

3 Ascending colon

4 Descending colon

5 Rectum

6 Jejunum and ileum. See (18) in left lateral recumbent projection of abdomen of female, Figure 445, for more details.

7 Ventral extremity of spleen

8 Soft tissue shadow of nipple

9 Skin fold

10 M.rectus abdominis

11 Right kidney. See (24) in left lateral recumbent projection of abdomen of female, Figure 445, for more kidney details.

12 Position of left kidney. (Shadow cannot be seen as it is obscured by caecal and colonic shadows.)

See ventrodorsal and dorsoventral projections line drawings, Figures 464–469 and 471–475, for left kidney in this dog.

13 Sublumbar muscles. For more details see (26) in left lateral recumbent projection of abdomen of female, Figure 445.

14 Region of urinary bladder. When distended with urine a distinct soft tissue shadow can be seen but when empty the urinary bladder lies almost entirely within the pelvis.

15 Soft tissue shadow of prostatic gland

16 7th. lumbar vertebra. (A degenerative bony change, spondylosis, is present on the ventral aspect of the cranial endplate. See 'normality' in the Introduction.)

17 Body of ilium

18 Iliopubic or iliopectineal eminence

19 Ischiatic tuberosity

20 Femoral bodies

21 Os penis
    21(a) Roof of urethral sulcus

22 Preputial shadow

23 Soft tissue shadows of hind limb muscles

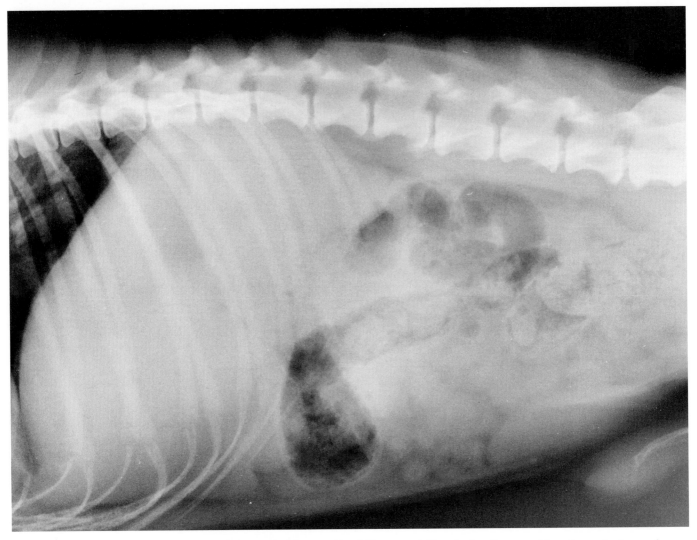

Figure 458   Right lateral recumbent projection of abdomen. Cranially centred. Beagle dog 7 years old, entire male (same dog as in all projections of abdomen of the male).

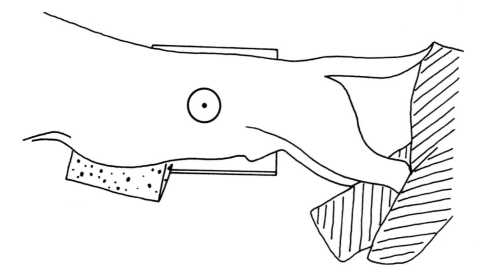

Figure 459   Line drawing of photograph representing radiographic positioning for Figure 458.

An Atlas of Interpretative Radiographic Anatomy of the Dog and Cat

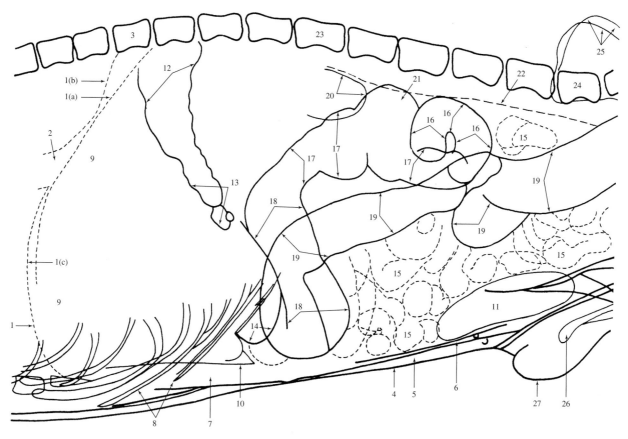

Figure 460   Right lateral recumbent projection of abdomen. Cranially centred.

For a routine survey radiograph of the abdomen, a right lateral recumbency is often preferred by many radiographers/radiologists. The most important factor is being consistent with one's radiographic approach and hence radiographic appraisal and interpretation.

1 Diaphragmatic shadow
   1(a) Left 'crus'
   1(b) Right 'crus'
   1(c) Cupola

2 Caudal vena cava entering the central tendon just right of the midline

3 11th. thoracic vertebra

4 Skin margin

5 Subcutaneous fat

6 M.rectus abdominis

7 Fat within the falciform ligament of the liver

8 Calcified costal cartilages

9 Soft tissue shadow of liver

10 Caudoventral margin of liver. (Acute angle just visible.)

See (9) in left lateral recumbent projection of abdomen of female, Figure 445, for aditional information.

11 Ventral extremity of spleen

12 Gas in gastric fundus. (Large volume is present due to right lateral recumbency resulting in gas rising into uppermost part of gastric structure.)

13 Gas in gastric body

14 Pyloric part, antrum and canal, of gastric shadow. (Seen as a rounded soft tissue shadow due to the presence of fluid gravitating to this part in right lateral recumbency. The most ventral aspect of the shadow is the antrum.)

The pyloric part shadow in right lateral recumbency can be mistaken for a ball within the gastric lumen. However, the 'ball' appearance will disappear in left lateral recumbency as fluid shifts to the dependent gastric fundus.

Radiography of both lateral recumbencies is very important for all gastric region analysis.

15 Jejunum and ileum. (Seen as fluid-filled viscera with a few lumenal gas shadows.)

(*460 continued.*)

See (18) in left lateral recumbent projection of abdomen of female, Figure 445, for more details.

16 Caecal shadow. (Lumenal gas contrast showing its shape.)

17 Ascending colon

18 Transverse colon

19 Descending colon

Numbers 17 to 19 should be compared with the same shadows seen in left lateral recumbency line drawing, Figures 454 and 457. The different appearances are due to the shifting lumenal gas contrast. Identification of intestinal shadows may require both lateral recumbencies.

20 Right kidney. See (24) in left lateral recumbent projection of abdomen of female, Figure 445, for more kidney details.

21 Position of left kidney in this dog. (Shadow cannot be seen as it is obscured by caecal and colonic shadows.) See ventrodorsal and dorsoventral projections line drawing, Figures 464–469 and 471–475, for the left kidney shadow in this dog.

22 Sublumbar muscles. See (26), left lateral recumbent projection of abdomen of female, Figure 445, for more details.

23 2nd. lumbar vertebra

24 7th. lumbar vertebra. (A degenerative bony change, spondylosis, is present on the ventral aspect of the cranial endplate. See 'normality' in the Introduction.)

25 Ilia

26 Os penis

27 Preputial shadow

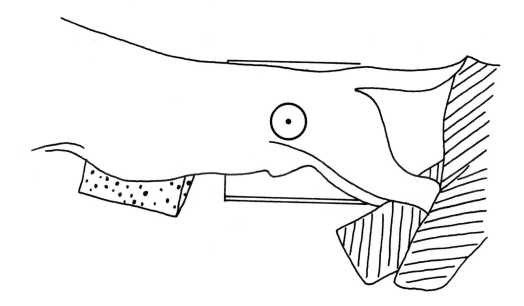

Figure 461 Line drawing of photograph representing radiographic positioning for Figure 462.

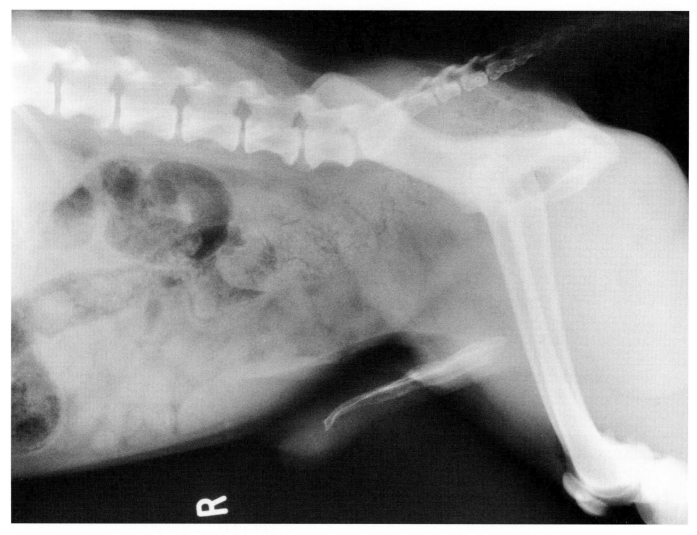

Figure 462   Right lateral recumbent projection of abdomen. Caudally centred. Beagle dog 7 years old, entire male (same dog as in all projections of abdomen of the male).

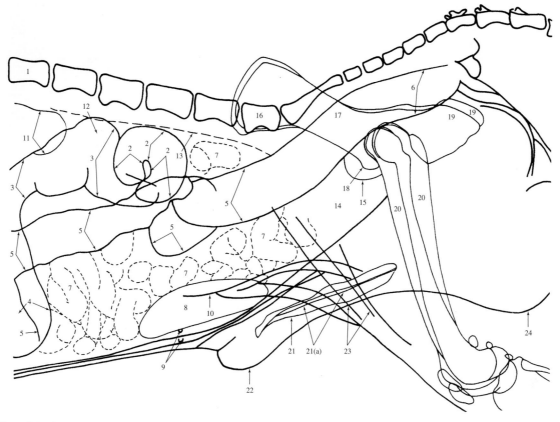

Figure 463 Right lateral recumbent projection of abdomen. Caudally centred.

For a routine survey radiograph of the abdomen, a right lateral recumbency is often preferred by many radiographers/radiologists. The most important factor is being consistent with one's radiographic approach and hence radiographic appraisal and interpretation.

1 2nd. lumbar vertebra

2 Caecal shadow

3 Ascending colon

4 Transverse colon

5 Descending colon

6 Rectum

7 Jejunum and ileum. See (18) in left lateral recumbent projection of abdomen of female, Figure 445, for more details.

8 Ventral extremity of spleen

9 Soft tissue shadows of nipples

10 Skin fold

11 Right kidney. See (24) in left lateral recumbent projection of abdomen of female, Figure 445, for additional kidney information.

12 Position of left kidney. (Shadow cannot be seen as it is obscured by caecal and colonic shadows.)

See ventrodorsal and dorsoventral projections line drawing, Figures 464–469 and 471–475, for the left kidney shadow in this dog.

13 Sublumbar muscles. For more details see (26) in left lateral recumbent abdomen projection of female, Figure 445.

14 Region of distended urinary bladder. (Distinct soft tissue shadow not seen in this film.)

15 Soft tissue shadow of the prostatic gland

16 7th. lumbar vertebra. (A degenerative bony change, spondylosis, is present on the ventral aspect of the cranial endplate. See 'normality' in the Introduction.)

17 Body of ilium

18 Iliopubic or iliopectineal eminence

19 Ischiatic tuberosity

20 Femoral body

21 Os penis
   21(a) Roof of urethral sulcus

22 Preputial shadow

23 Soft tissue shadows of hind limb muscles

24 Scrotal shadow

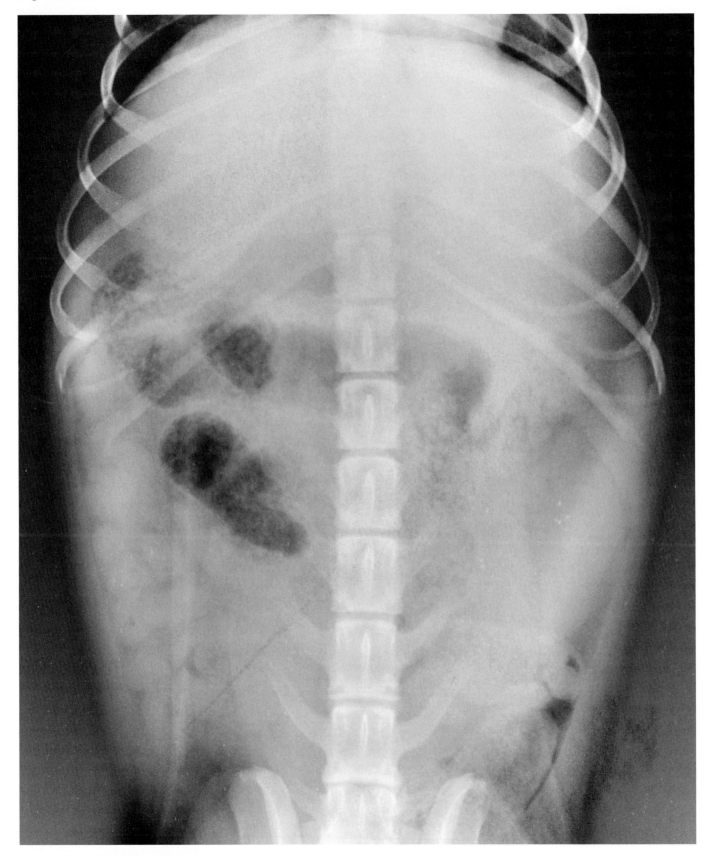

Figure 464   Ventrodorsal projection of abdomen. Cranially centred. Beagle dog 7 years old, entire male (same dog as in all projections of abdomen of the male).

An Atlas of Interpretative Radiographic Anatomy of the Dog and Cat

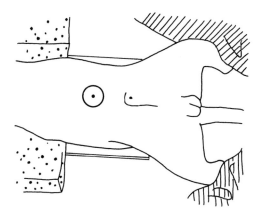

Figure 465 Line drawing of photograph representing radiographic positioning for Figure 464.

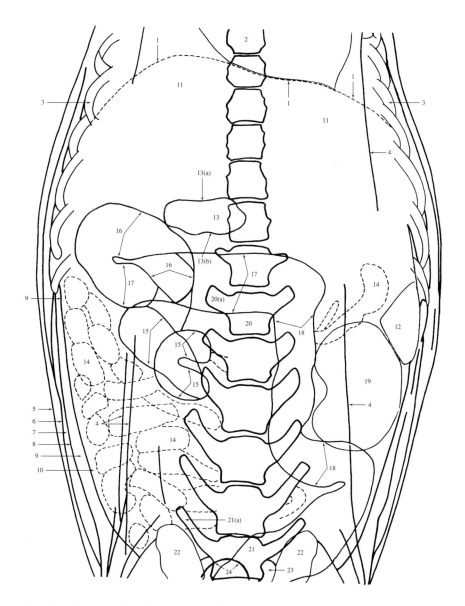

Figure 466 Ventrodorsal projection of abdomen. Cranially centred.

(466 continued.)

1 Diaphragmatic shadow

2 8th. thoracic vertebra

3 8th. rib

4 Skin folds

5 Skin margin

6 Subcutaneous fat. (Only just visible in this dog as a grey line between the outer skin and first muscle layer of the lateral wall of the middle abdomen.)

7 M.obliquus externus abdominis

8 Very thin layer of fat originating from superficial surface of caudal ribs. This layer usually serves to separate the m.obliquus externus abdominis from the m.obliquus internus abdominis and m.transversus abdominis. (The fat layer which differentiates these muscle layers of the lateral wall is only just visible in this dog.)

9 M.obliquus internus abdominis and m.transversus abdominis. Seen as a single soft tissue linear shadow extending from the caudal margin of the rib cage. These muscles attach to the last two ribs and the medial aspect of the last four or five ribs and costal cartilage, respectively.

10 Fat layer of peritoneal cavity

11 Soft tissue shadow of liver

12 Dorsal extremity of spleen

13 Pyloric antrum. (Contains most of the gas within the gastric lumen due to ventrodorsal projection resulting in gas rising to the uppermost part. No other gastric part is clearly visible.)
    13(a) Lesser curvature
    13(b) Greater curvature

14 Jejunum and ileum. (Seen as fluid-filled viscera with a few small gas shadows within the lumens.)

For more details on these structures see (18) Left lateral recumbent projection of abdomen of female Figure 445.

15 Caecal shadow

16 Ascending colon

17 Transverse colon

18 Descending colon

19 Left kidney. (Medial surface cannot be seen and in both lateral recumbencies, line drawings Figures 454/457 and 460/463, this kidney was not visible. Note that in this dog its position is relatively caudal, extending from mid 2nd. lumbar vertebra to cranial 5th. lumbar vertebral levels.)

See (24) in left lateral recumbent projection of abdomen of female, Figure 445, for more kidney information.

The right kidney is not visible in this film due to insufficient perirenal fat contrast. The caudal pole of this kidney was visible in both lateral recumbencies, line drawings Figures 454/457 and 460/463, extending to cranial 3rd. lumbar vertebral level.

20 2nd. lumbar vertebra
    20(a) Transverse process

21 7th. lumbar vertebra (A degenerative bony change, spondylosis, is present left lateral aspect of cranial endplate. See 'normality' in the Introduction.)
    21(a) Transverse process

22 Ilium

23 Sacrum

24 Preputial shadow. (This shadow is only just visible but it can be seen clearly in the caudally centred projection, (13) in Figure 469. In this latter film the shadow may be mistaken as an abnormal vertebral bony opacity rather than a superimposed soft tissue opacity.)

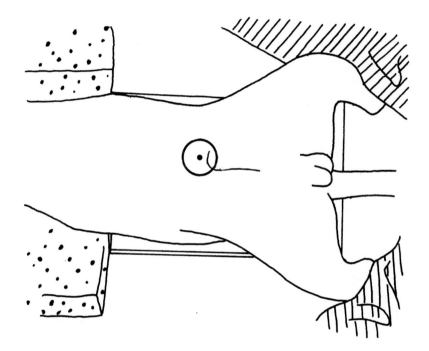

Figure 467   Line drawing of photograph representing radiographic positioning for Figure 468.

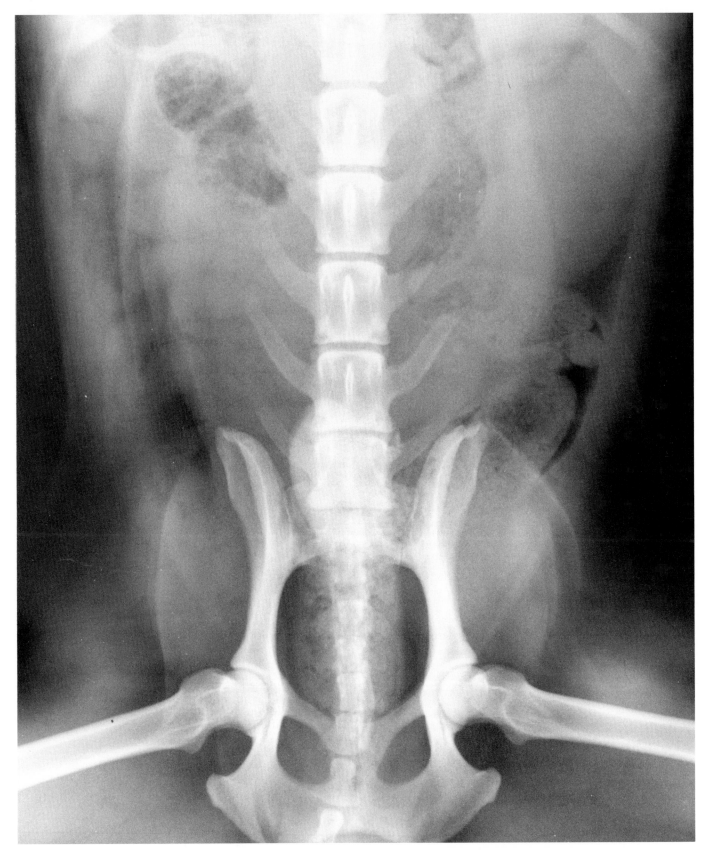

Figure 468 Ventrodorsal projection of abdomen caudally centred. Beagle dog 7 years old, entire male (same dog as in all projections of abdomen of the male).

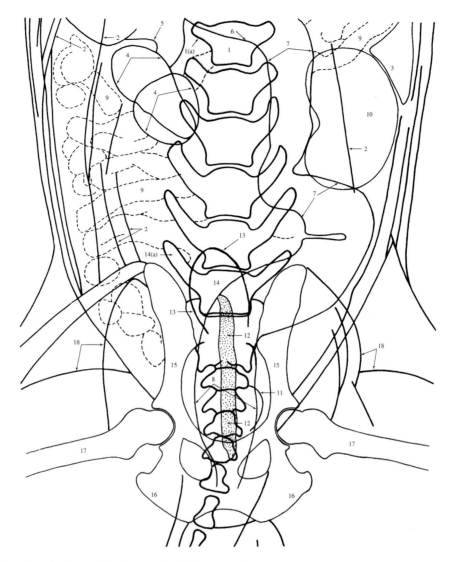

Figure 469   Ventrodorsal projection of abdomen. Caudally centred.

1 2nd. lumbar vertebra
   1(a) Transverse process

2 Skin folds

3 Dorsal extremity of spleen

4 Caecal shadow

5 Ascending colon

6 Transverse colon

7 Descending colon

8 Rectum

9 Jejunum and ileum. (Seen as fluid-filled viscera with a few small gas shadows within the lumens.)

See (18) in left lateral recumbent projection of abdomen of female, Figure 445, for more details.

10 Left kidney. (Medial surface can not be seen in this film and left kidney was not visible in either lateral recumbency line drawing Figures 454/457 and 460/463. Note the relatively caudal position of the kidney in this dog extending from mid 2nd. lumbar vertebra to cranial 5th. lumbar vertebral levels.)

See (24) in left lateral recumbent projection of abdomen of female, Figure 445, for more kidney information.
The right kidney is not visible in this film due to insufficient perirenal fat contrast. The caudal pole of this kidney is seen in both lateral recumbencies, line drawings Figures 454/457 and 460/463, extending to cranial 3rd. lumbar vertebral level.

(469 continued.)

11 Prostatic shadow

12 Os penis (shaded in drawing)

13 Preputial shadow

14 7th. lumbar vertebra. (A degenerative bony change, spondylosis, is present in the left lateral aspect of the cranial endplate. See 'normality' in the Introduction.) 14(a)Transverse process

15 Body of ilium

16 Ischial tuberosity

17 Femoral body

18 Soft tissue shadows of hindlimb muscles

The individual lateral abdominal wall layers are not clearly seen with this caudally centred film. Please refer to the cranially centred film line drawing, Figure 466.

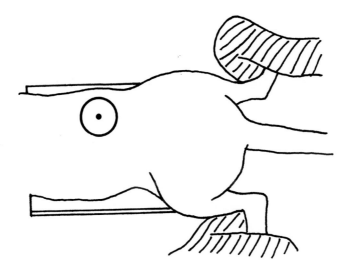

Figure 470   Line drawing of photograph representing radiographic positioning for Figure 471.

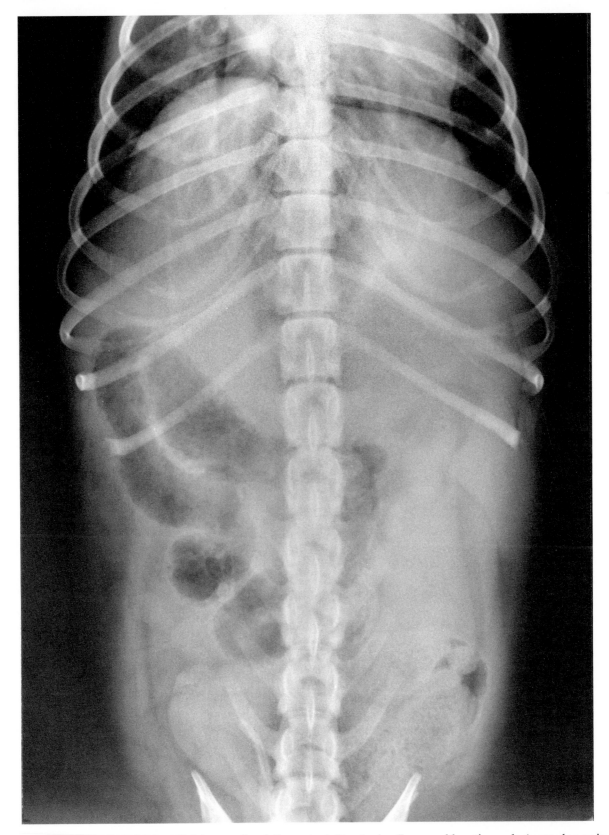

Figure 471   Dorsoventral projection of abdomen. Cranially centred. Beagle dog 7 years old, entire male (same dog as in all projections of abdomen of the male).

An Atlas of Interpretative Radiographic Anatomy of the Dog and Cat

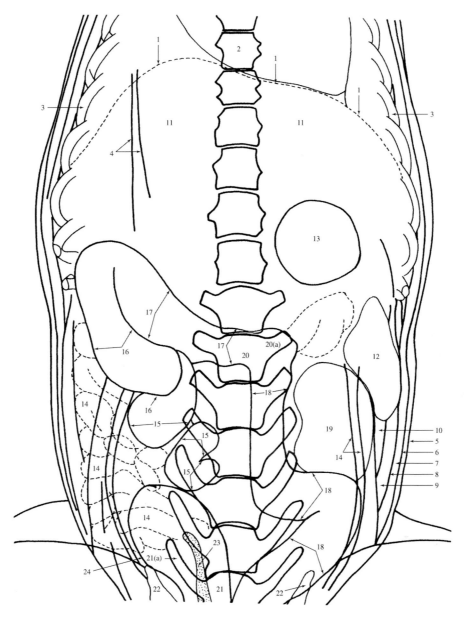

Figure 472 Dorsoventral projection of abdomen. Cranially centred.

1 Diaphragmatic shadow

2 8th. thoracic vertebra

3 8th. rib

4 Skin folds

5 Skin margin

6 Subcutaneous fat

7 M.obliquus externus abdominis

8 Very thin layer of fat originating from superficial surface of caudal ribs

9 M.obliquus internus abdominis and m.transversus abdominis

Note that numbers (6) to (9) are seen more clearly in the ventrodorsal projection of abdomen, Figure 466. Please refer to the latter if numbers (6) to (9) in this film are confusing.

10 Fat layer of the peritoneal cavity

11 Soft tissue shadow of liver

12 Dorsal extremity of spleen

13 Gastric fundus. (Contains most of the gas within gastric lumen due to dorsoventral projection resulting in gas rising to the uppermost part. No other gastric part is clearly seen.)

14 Jejunum and ileum (seen as fluid-filled viscera).

See (18) in left lateral recumbent projection of abdomen of female, Figure 445, for more details.

(472 continued.)

15 Caecal shadow

16 Ascending colon

17 Transverse colon

18 Descending colon

19 Left kidney. (Medial surface just visible in film but caudal pole obscured by colonic shadow. This kidney is not seen in either lateral recumbency line drawing, Figures 454/457 and 460/463, of this dog and does appear to be slightly more caudal in position than normal.)

See (24) in left lateral recumbent projection of abdomen of female, Figure 445, for additional kidney information.

The right kidney is not visible due to insufficient perirenal fat contrast. The caudal pole is seen in both lateral recumbencies line drawings Figures 454/457 and 460/463, extending to cranial 3rd. lumbar vertebral level.

20 2nd. lumbar vertebra
   20(a) Transverse process

21 7th. lumbar vertebra. (A degenerative bony change, spondylosis, is present in the left lateral aspect of the cranial endplate. See 'normality' in the Introduction.)
   21(a) Transverse process

22 Ilium

23 Os penis (shaded in drawing)

24 Preputial shadow

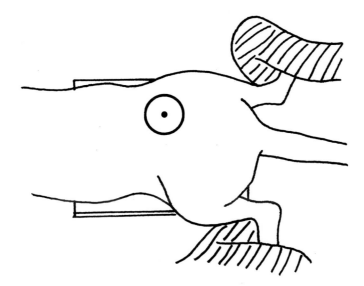

Figure 473   Line drawing of photograph representing radiographic positioning for Figure 474.

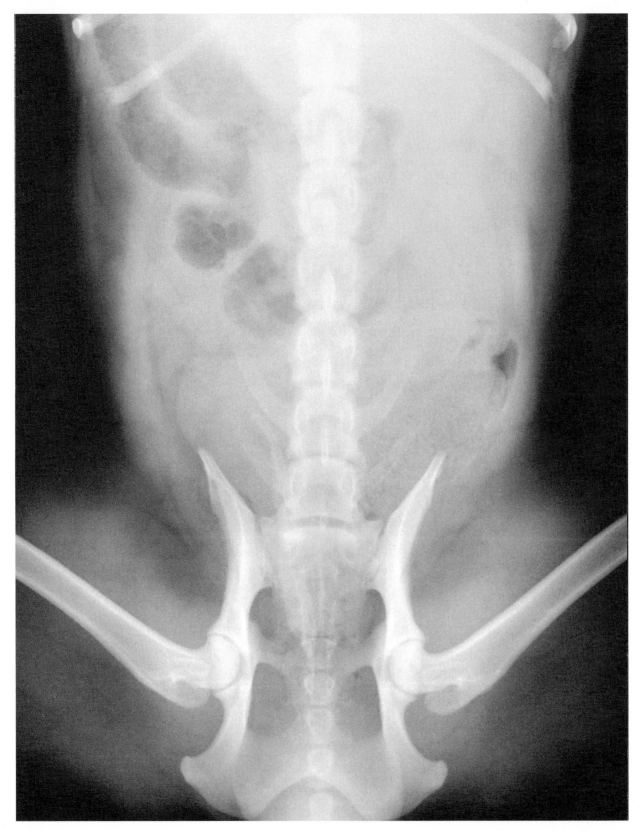

Figure 474 Dorsoventral projection of abdomen. Caudally centred. Beagle dog 7 years old, entire male (same dog as in all projections of abdomen of the male).

An Atlas of Interpretative Radiographic Anatomy of the Dog and Cat

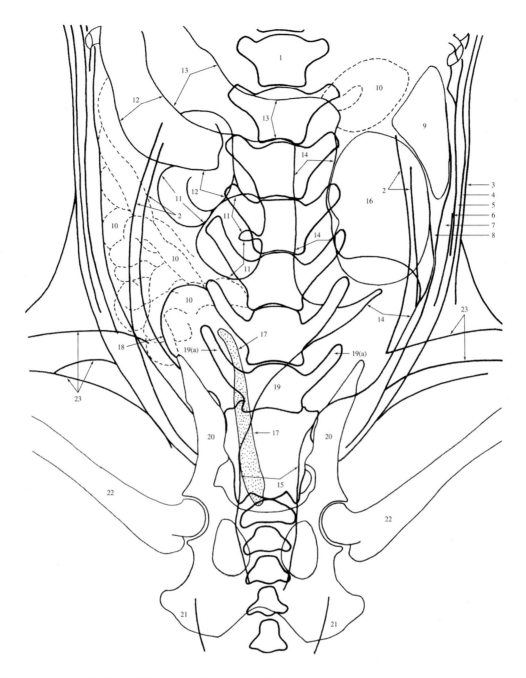

Figure 475   Dorsoventral projection of abdomen. Caudally centred.

1 1st. lumbar vertebra

2 Skin folds

3 Skin margin

4 Subcutaneous fat

5 M.obliquus externus abdominis

6 Very thin layer of fat

7 M.obliquus internus abdominis and m.transversus
   abdominis

8 Fat layer of peritoneal cavity

9 Dorsal extremity of spleen

10 Jejunum and ileum. (Seen as fluid-filled viscera with a
    few gas shadows within the lumens.)

See (18) in left lateral recumbent projection of abdomen of
female, Figure 445, for more details.

11 Caecal shadow

12 Ascending colon

13 Transverse colon

14 Descending colon

15 Rectum

16 Left kidney. (Caudal pole just visible superimposed on colonic shadow. This kidney is not seen in either lateral recumbency line drawing, Figures 454/457 and 460/463, in this dog. In addition it does appear to be slightly more caudal than normal.)

Please see (24) Left lateral recumbent projection of abdomen of female Figure 445 for more kidney information.

The right kidney is not visible due to insufficient perirenal fat contrast. The caudal pole is seen in both lateral recumben- cies, line drawings Figures 454/457 and 460/463, extending to cranial 3rd. lumbar vertebral level.

17 Os penis (shaded in drawing)

18 Preputial shadow

19 7th. lumbar vertebra. (A degenerative bony change, spondylosis, is present in the left lateral aspect of the cranial endplate. See 'normality' in the Introduction.)
19(a) Transverse process

20 Body of ilium

21 Ischial tuberosity

22 Femoral body

23 Soft tissue shadows of hindlimb muscles

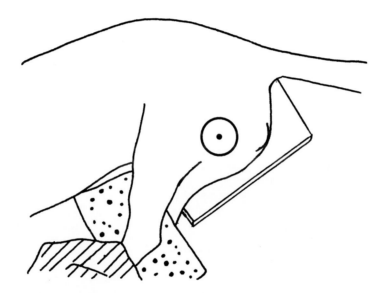

Figure 476   Line drawing of photograph representing radiographic positioning for Figure 477.

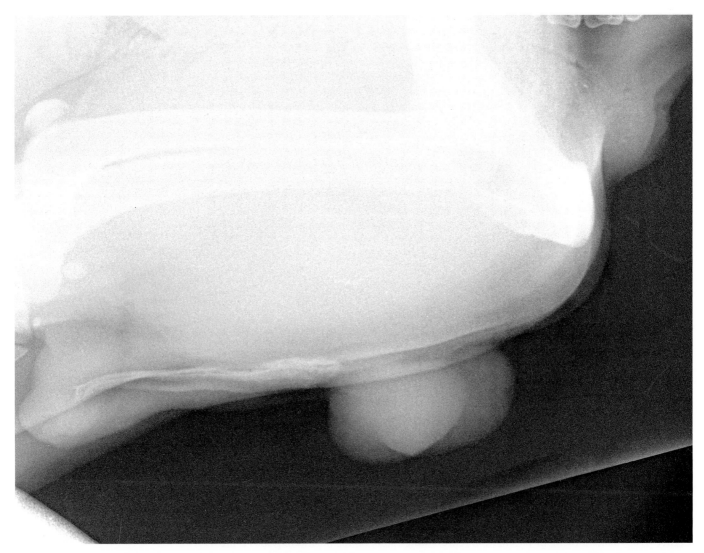

Figure 477   Lateral recumbent projection of urethra with hyperflexion of hindlegs. Beagle dog 7 years old, entire male.

An Atlas of Interpretative Radiographic Anatomy of the Dog and Cat

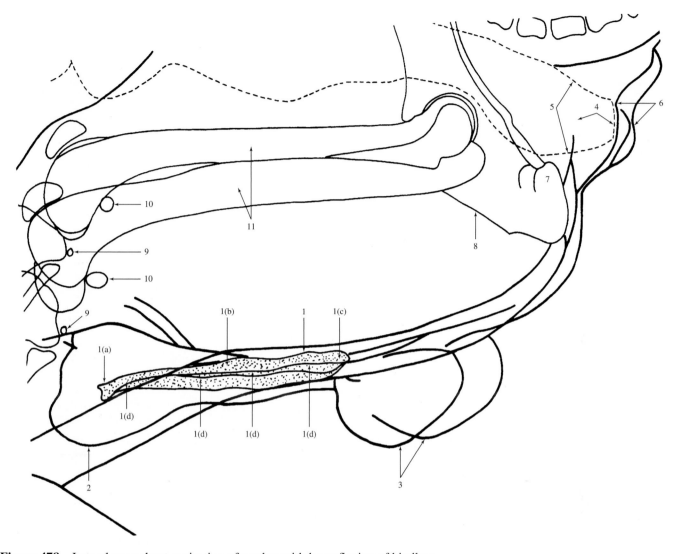

Figure 478   Lateral recumbent projection of urethra with hyperflexion of hindlegs.

1 Os penis (shaded in drawing). Ossification of the distal extremity of the corpora cavernosa penis. It is surrounded by the bulbus glandis and pars longa glandis.

  1(a)   Apex. Ends in cartilaginous tip attached by a ligament to the corona of the glans penis.

  1(b)   Body. Ventrally contains the urethral groove. The urethra, surrounded by corpus spongiosum penis, runs in this groove.

  1(c)   Base. Attaches to the fibrous tissues of the corpora cavernosa penis.

  1(d)   Roof of urethral sulcus

2 Prepuce

3 Scrotum

4 Extent of the external anal sphincter muscle

5 Rectum

6 Folds of skin encircling the anus

7 Ischiatic tuberosity

8 Pelvic symphysis

9 Popliteal fabella

10 Gastrocneumius fabella

11 Femoral bodies

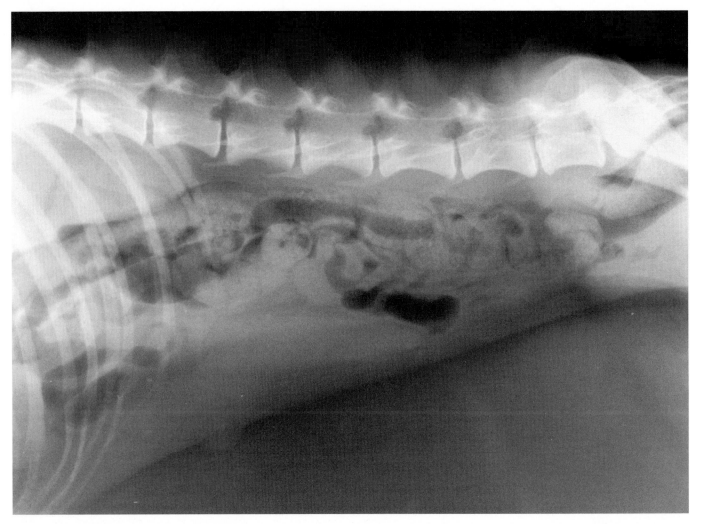

Figure 479 Right lateral recumbent projection of abdomen. Breed of dog with deep, narrow chest and long, shallow abdomen. Afghan Hound dog 2 years old, entire female.

The radiograph shows the economical use of space for the gut viscera in this type of abdomen. This dog was also very lean, emphasising the narrow appearance of the abdomen.

The lack of fat contrast makes differentiation of soft tissue structures more difficult but in this type of abdomen left kidney shadow can sometimes be seen to cause 'ventral displacement' of the descending colon, e.g. in Great Danes. When seen in this type of breed, the colonic position is due to the long, shallow abdomen and not to disease.

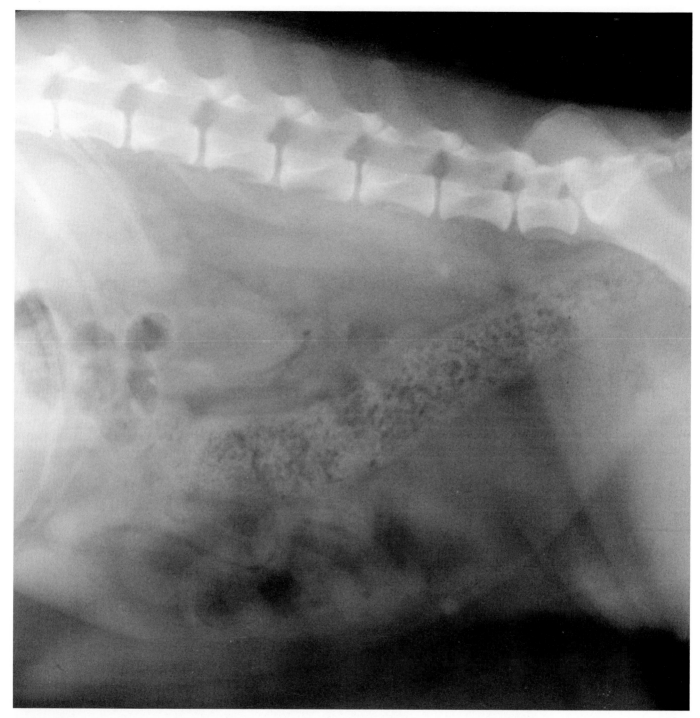

Figure 480   Right lateral recumbent projection of abdomen. Colon variant. Samoyed dog 6 years old, entire female.

The radiograph shows extreme ventral positioning of the descending colon. Such a ventral deviation may be linked to displacement by an abnormal organ, especially a neoplastic left kidney. In this case the shadows dorsal to the colon are within normal radiographic limits and both kidneys are visible.

The large amount of abdominal fat in this dog has enhanced contrast making identification of soft tissue shadows easier.

The ventrodorsal projection of this dog has not been included but the descending colon was in the normal left abdominal position.

The descending colon commonly has another positional variation. This is to be found on the ventrodorsal or dorsoventral projections where the descending colon is curved towards the midline and not running parallel to the abdominal wall. Again, careful evaluation of radiographic shadows is necessary to ensure that a disease process is not the cause of the unusual colonic position.

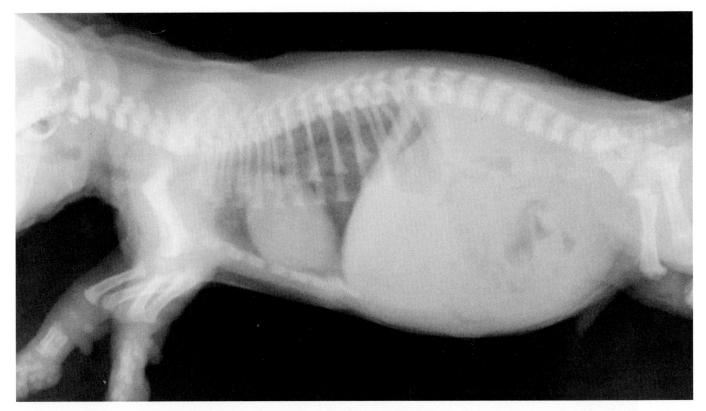

Figure 481   Right lateral recumbent projection of whole body of puppy. Shih Tzu dog 4 weeks old, entire male.

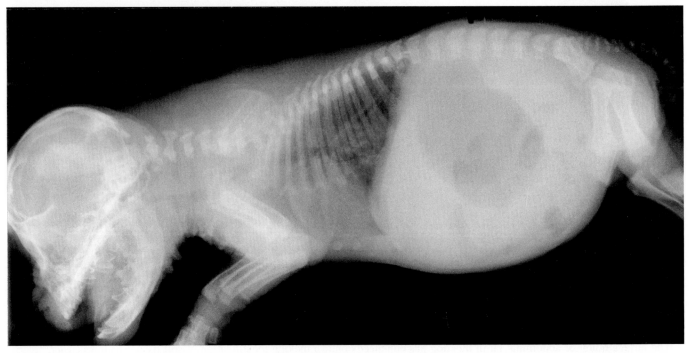

Figure 482   Right lateral recumbent projection of whole body of puppy. Bulldog 12 days old, entire male (same dog as in Figure 483).

In the juvenile section of the Samoyed crossbred dog radiography of the axial skeleton was not performed until 13 weeks of age. Note the appearance of the atlas and axis in this dog, especially the separate ossification centres for the atlas body and the axis dens. These must not be confused as fractures. Compare this figure with the 4-week whole body of puppy (Figure 481).

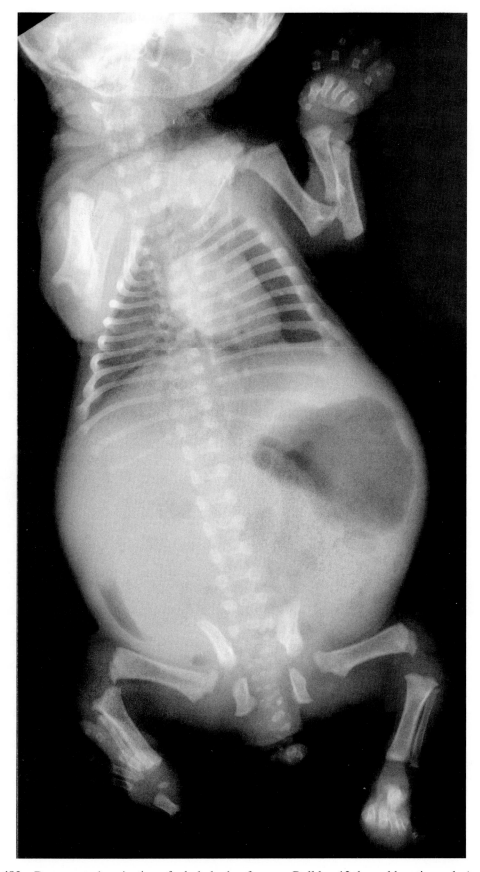

Figure 483   Dorsoventral projection of whole body of puppy. Bulldog 12 days old, entire male (same dog as in Figure 482).

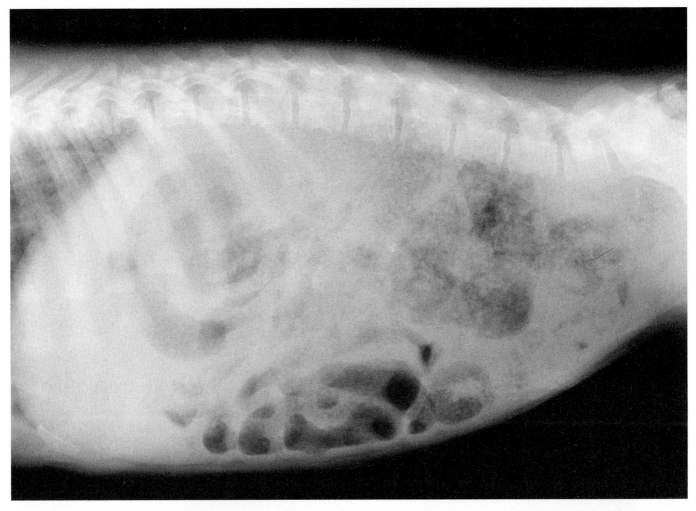

Figure 484   Right lateral recumbent projection of abdomen. Absence of abdominal fat tissue in the young animal. Weimaraner dog 7 weeks old, entire female.

The radiograph shows the effect of lack of abdominal fat which results in a marked reduction of contrast within the abdominal cavity. Most of the distinct inner surface of the abdominal wall and serosal surface of bowel are lost.

Differentiation of viscera is only possible in this radiograph by the presence of gas, ingesta and faecal material. A very small amount of grey opacity, fat, is seen outlining the caudoventral lobe of the liver separating it from the soft tissue opacity of the ventral abdominal wall.

This abdominal radiograph is typical of the young animal and must not be confused with disease. In this case the somewhat mottled appearance of the opaque abdomen may be misdiagnosed as peritonitis (also see Figure 735 of the mature animal with extreme loss of abdominal fat contrast).

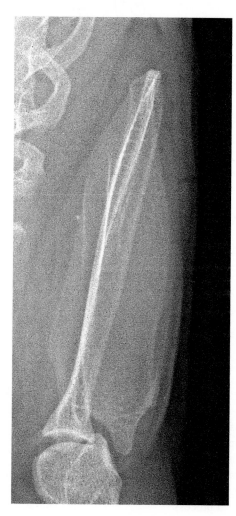

Figure 485 Caudocranial projection of scapula. British domestic short haired cat 2 years old, neutered female.

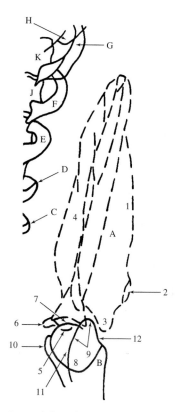

Figure 486 Caudocranial projection of scapula.

A Scapula
  1 Spine
  2 Metacromion
  3 Acromion
  4 Subscapular fossa
  5 Supraglenoid tubercle
  6 Coracoid process
  7 Glenoid cavity

B Humerus
  8 Head
  9 Greater tubercle
  10 Lesser tubercle
  11 Intertubercular groove
  12 Fossa for m.infraspinatus
     insertion

C 1st. rib

D 2nd. rib

E 3rd. rib

F 4th. rib

G 5th. rib

H 6th. rib

I 3rd. thoracic vertebra

J 4th. thoracic vertebra

K 5th. thoracic vertebra

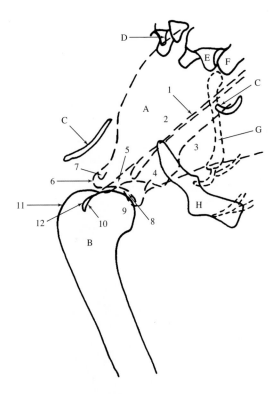

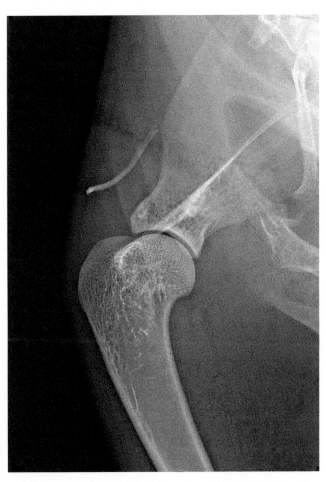

Figure 487   Mediolateral projection of shoulder joint.
Siamese cat 3 years old, neutered male.

Figure 488   Mediolateral projection of shoulder joint.

A Scapula
  1 Spine
  2 Supraspinous fossa
  3 Infraspinous fossa
  4 Metacromion
  5 Acromion
  6 Supraglenoid tubercle
  7 Coracoid process
  8 Glenoid cavity

B Humerus
  9 Head
  10 Lesser tubercle

  11 Greater tubercle
  12 Intertubercular
      groove

C Clavicle

D 6th. cervical vertebra

E 7th. cervical vertebra

F 1st. thoracic vertebra

G 1st. rib

H Manubrium of sternum

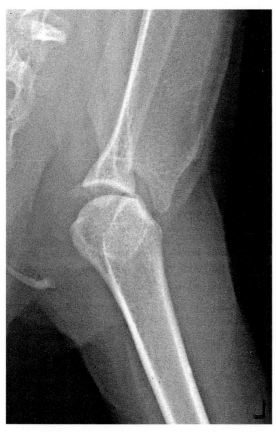

Figure 489 Caudocranial projection of shoulder joint. British domestic short haired cat 2 years old, neutered female.

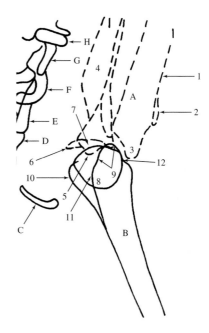

Figure 490 Caudocranial projection of shoulder joint

A Scapula
  1 Spine
  2 Metacromion
  3 Acromion
  4 Subscapular fossa
  5 Supraglenoid tubercle
  6 Coracoid process
  7 Glenoid cavity

B Humerus
  8 Head
  9 Greater tubercle
 10 Lesser tubercle

 11 Intertubercular groove
 12 Fossa for m.infra-
      spinatus insertion

C Clavicle

D 4th. cervical vertebra

E 5th. cervical vertebra

F 6th. cervical vertebra

G 7th. cervical vertebra

H 1st. rib

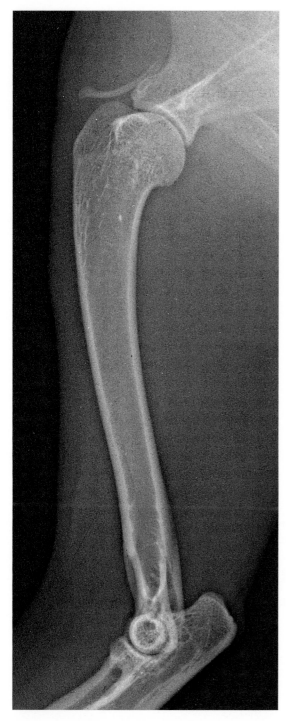

Figure 491　Mediolateral projection of humerus. British domestic short haired cat 2 years old, neutered female.

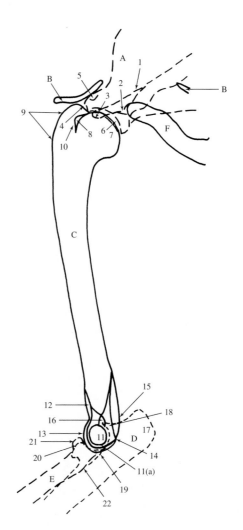

Figure 492　Mediolateral projection of humerus

A　Scapula
　　1　Spine
　　2　Metacromion
　　3　Acromion
　　4　Supraglenoid tubercle
　　5　Coracoid process
　　6　Glenoid cavity

B　Clavicle

C　Humerus
　　7　Head
　　8　Lesser tubercle
　　9　Greater tubercle
　　10　Intertubercular groove
　　11　Condyle
　　　　11(a)　Radiodense circular shadow formed by condylar groove
　　12　Supracondyloid foramen
　　13　Trochlea of condyle. Trochlea is on the medial

aspect of the condyle while the capitulum is lateral. The capitulum is not clearly defined in this radiograph.
　　14　Medial epicondyle
　　15　Lateral epicondyle
　　16　Olecranon fossa

D　Ulna
　　17　Olecranon
　　18　Anconeal process
　　19　Position of lateral coronoid process
　　20　Medial coronoid process

E　Radius
　　21　Head
　　22　Tuberosity

F　Manubrium of sternum

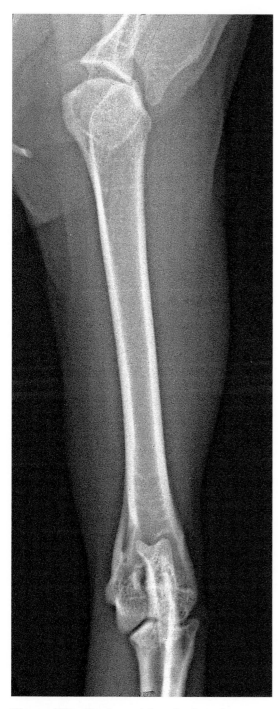

Figure 493 Caudocranial projection of humerus. British domestic short haired cat 2 years old, neutered female.

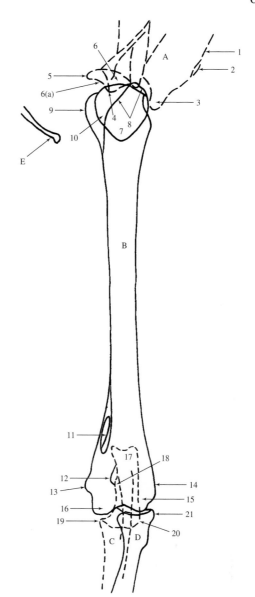

Figure 494 Caudocranial projection of humerus.

A Scapula
  1 Spine
  2 Metacromion
  3 Acromion
  4 Supraglenoid tubercle
  5 Coracoid process
  6 Glenoid cavity
    6(a) Medial aspect of glenoid cavity

B Humerus
  7 Head
  8 Greater tubercle
  9 Lesser tubercle
  10 Intertubercular groove
  11 Supracondyloid foramen

12 Olecranon fossa
13 Medial epicondyle
14 Lateral epicondyle
15 Capitulum of condyle
16 Trochlea of condyle

C Ulna
  17 Olecranon
  18 Anconeal process
  19 Medial coronoid process
  20 Lateral coronoid process

D Radius
  21 Head

E Clavicle

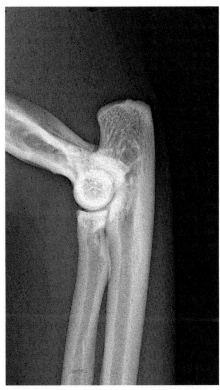

Figure 495 Extended mediolateral projection of elbow joint. British domestic short haired cat 6 years old, neutered female.

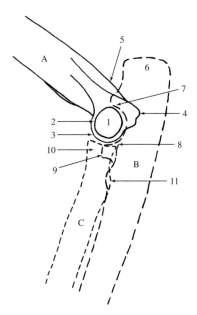

Figure 496 Extended mediolateral projection of elbow joint.

A Humerus
   1 Condyle
   2 Groove of condyle
   3 Trochlea of condyle.
      Trochlea is on the medial
      aspect of the condyle while
      the capitulum is lateral. The
      capitulum cannot be seen in
      this radiograph.
   4 Medial epicondyle
   5 Lateral epicondyle

B Ulna
   6 Olecranon
   7 Anconeal process
   8 Lateral coronoid process
   9 Medial coronoid process

C Radius
   10 Head
   11 Tuberosity

         An Atlas of Interpretative Radiographic Anatomy of the Dog and Cat

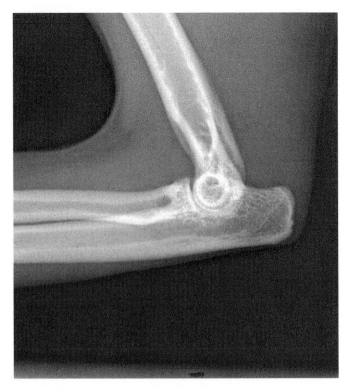

Figure 497   Flexed mediolateral projection of elbow joint.
British domestic short haired cat 2 years old, neutered
female.

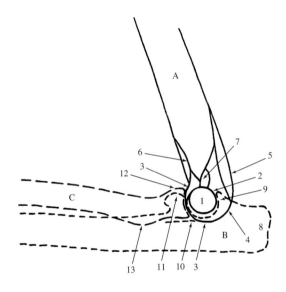

Figure 498   Flexed mediolateral projection of elbow joint.

A   Humerus
   1   Condyle
   2   Groove of condyle
   3   Trochlea of condyle. The
      trochlea is on the medial aspect
      of the condyle while the capitu-
      lum is lateral. The capitulum
      cannot be seen in this radio-
      graph. There is only one humer-
      al condyle although the terms
      medial and lateral condyle are
      often incorrectly used.
   4   Medial epicondyle

   5   Lateral epicondyle
   6   Supracondyloid foramen
   7   Olecranon fossa

B   Ulna
   8   Olecranon
   9   Anconeal process
  10   Position of lateral coronoid
      process
  11   Medial coronoid process

C   Radius
  12   Head
  13   Tuberosity

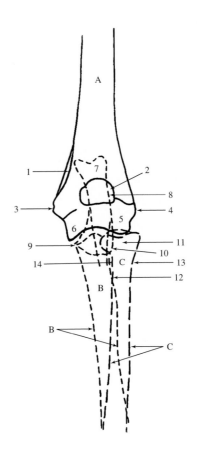

Figure 500 Caudocranial projection of elbow joint.

A Humerus
1 Supracondyloid foramen
2 Olecranon fossa
3 Medial epicondyle
4 Lateral epicondyle
5 Capitulum of condyle
6 Trochlea of condyle

B Ulna
7 Olecranon
8 Position of anconeal process
9 Medial coronoid process
10 Lateral coronoid process

C Radius
11 Head
12 Tuberosity
13 Neck
14 Interosseous space

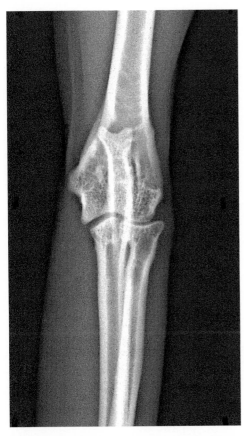

Figure 499 Caudocranial projection of elbow joint. British domestic short haired cat 2 years old, neutered female.

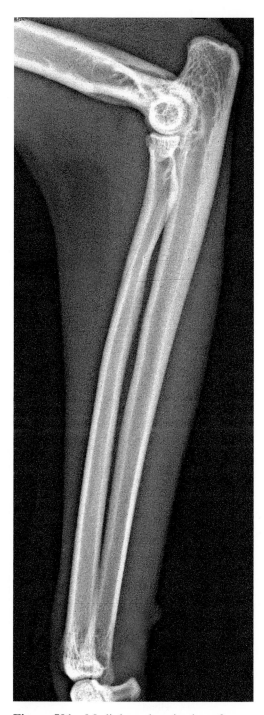

Figure 501 Mediolateral projection of radius and ulna. British domestic short haired cat 2 years old, neutered female.

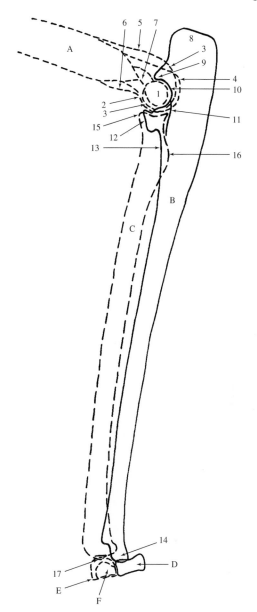

Figure 502 Mediolateral projection of radius and ulna.

A Humerus
  1 Condyle
  2 Trochlea of condyle.Medial aspect of condyle.
  3 Capitulum of condyle. Lateral aspect of condyle.
  4 Medial epicondyle
  5 Lateral epicondyle
  6 Supracondyloid foramen
  7 Olecranon fossa

B Ulna
  8 Olecranon
  9 Anconeal process

10 Trochlear notch
11 Lateral coronoid process
12 Medial coronoid process
13 Cranial cortical margin
14 Lateral styloid process

C Radius
  15 Head
  16 Tuberosity
  17 Medial styloid process

D Accessory carpal bone

E Radial carpal bone

F Ulnar carpal bone

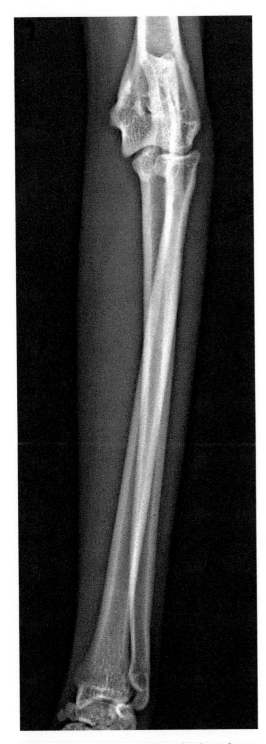

Figure 503 Craniocaudal projection of radius and ulna. British domestic short haired cat 2 years old, neutered female.

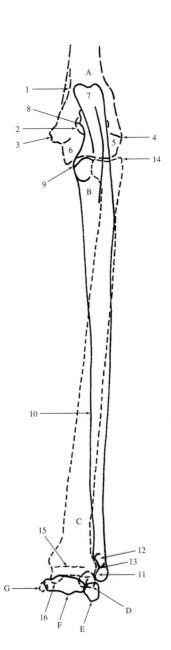

Figure 504 Craniocaudal projection of radius and ulna.

A Humerus
 1 Supracondyloid foramen
 2 Olecranon fossa
 3 Medial epicondyle
 4 Lateral epicondyle
 5 Capitulum of condyle
 6 Trochlea of condyle

B Ulna
 7 Olecranon
 8 Anconeal process
 9 Medial coronoid process
 10 Medial cortical margin
 11 Lateral styloid process

 12 Circular lucency often present
    in region of growth plate scar
 13 Growth plate scar

C Radius
 14 Head
 15 Growth plate scar
 16 Medial styloid process

D Accessory carpal bone

E Ulnar carpal bone

F Radial carpal bone

G Sesamoid bone of the tendon of
  the m.abductor pollicis longus

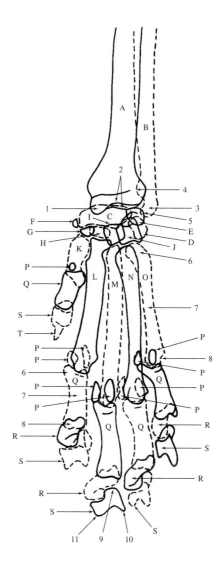

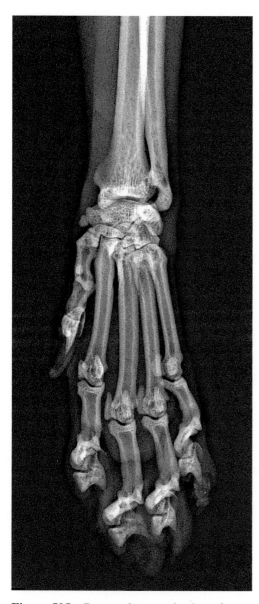

Figure 505 Dorsopalmar projection of manus. British domestic short haired cat 6 years old, neutered female.

Figure 506 Dorsopalmar projection of manus.

A Radius
  1 Medial styloid process
  2 Radiocarpal articulation

B Ulna
  3 Lateral styloid process
  4 Radioulnar articulation
  5 Ulnarcarpal articulation

C Radial carpal bone

D Ulnar carpal bone

E Accessory carpal bone

F Sesamoid bone in the tendon of the m.abductor pollicis longus

G Carpal bone 1

H Carpal bone 2

I Carpal bone 3

J Carpal bone 4

K Metacarpal bone 1

L Metacarpal bone 2

M Metacarpal bone 3

N Metacarpal bone 4

O Metacarpal bone 5

P Proximal sesamoid bones

Q Proximal phalanges

R Middle phalanges
  6 Base
  7 Body
  8 Head

S Distal phalanges
  9 Ungual crest
  10 Ungual process
  11 Flexor tubercle

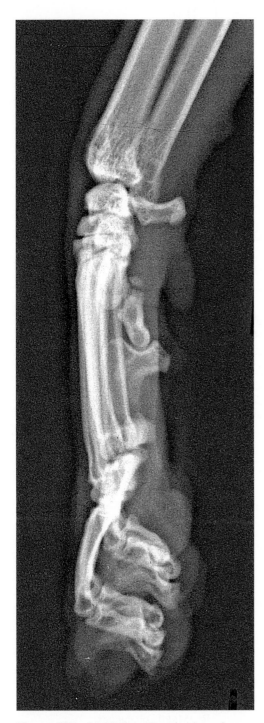

Figure 507 Mediolateral projection of manus. British domestic short haired cat 2 years old, neutered female.

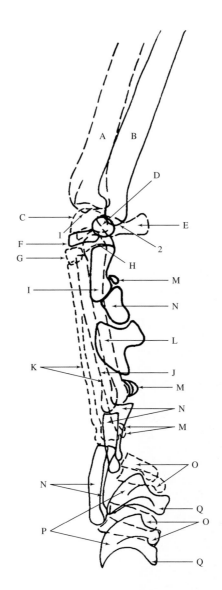

Figure 508 Mediolateral projection of manus.

A Radius
   1 Medial styloid process

B Ulna
   2 Lateral styloid process

C Radial carpal bone

D Ulnar carpal bone

E Accessory carpal bone

F Carpal bone 2

G Carpal bone 3

H Carpal bone 4 (Carpal bone 1 is superimposed but cannot be seen as a separate shadow)

I Metacarpal bone 1

J Metacarpal bone 2

K Metacarpal bones 3 and 4 (superimposed shadows)

L Metacarpal bone 5

M Proximal sesamoid bones

N Proximal phalanges

O Middle phalanges

P Distal phalanges

Q Ungual process

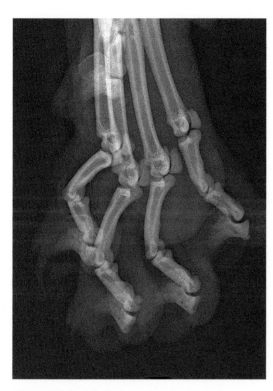

Figure 509 Mediolateral projection of phalanges. Digits stressed. British domestic short haired cat 6 years old, neutered male.

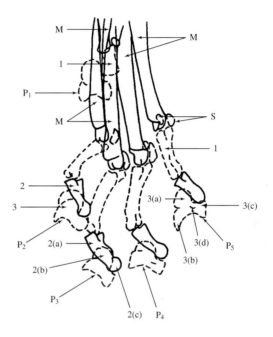

Figure 510 Mediolateral projection of phalanges. Digits stressed.

M   Metacarpal bones

P1 1st. digit

P2 2nd. digit

P3 3rd. digit

P4 4th. digit

P5 5th. digit
    1   Proximal phalanx
    2   Middle phalanx

2(a) Base
2(b) Body
2(c) Head
3   Distal phalanx
    3(a) Ungual crest
    3(b) Ungual process
    3(c) Flexor tuberosity
    3(d) Solar foramen

S   Proximal sesamoid bones

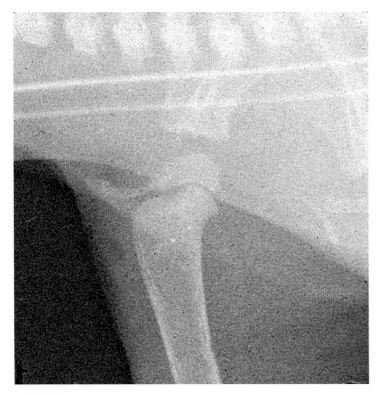

Figure 511   Age 4 weeks male   **Figure 511**

Figures 511, 512, 513, 514, 515, 516, 517, 518, 519, 520   Mediolateral projection of shoulder joint.

British domestic short haired cats at 4 weeks entire male, 8 weeks entire male, 12 weeks entire male, 16 weeks entire female, 20 weeks entire male, 24 weeks entire male, 46 weeks entire female, 68 weeks entire male, 80 weeks entire female, and 96 weeks entire female.

Correlating line drawings for all ages except 96 weeks.

A Scapula
  1 Epiphysis of supraglenoid tubercle
  2 Growth plate
    2(a) Open
  3 Coracoid process

B Humerus
  4 Proximal epiphysis
  5 Proximal growth plate
    5(a) Open
    5(b) Closing

C Clavicle

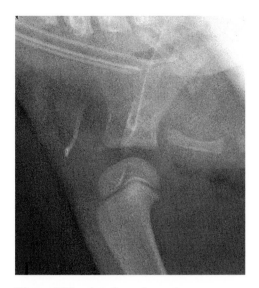

Figure 512 Age 8 weeks male

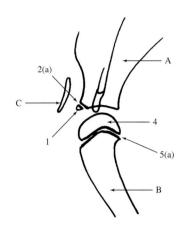

Figure 512

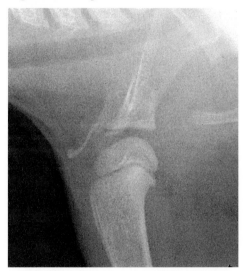

Figure 513 Age 12 weeks male

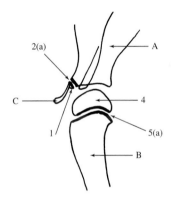

Figure 513

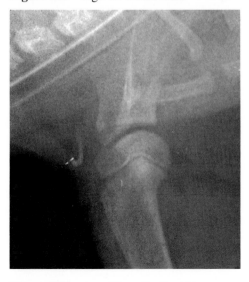

Figure 514 Age 16 weeks female

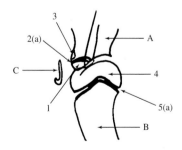

Figure 514

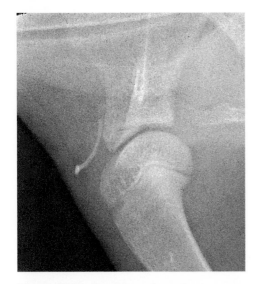

Figure 515   Age 20 weeks male

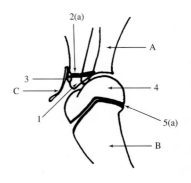

Figure 515

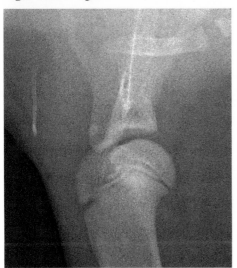

Figure 516   Age 24 weeks male

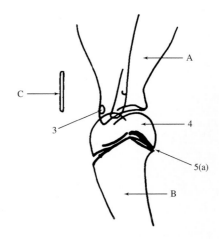

Figure 516

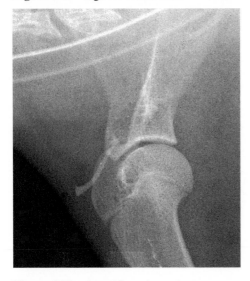

Figure 517   Age 46 weeks male

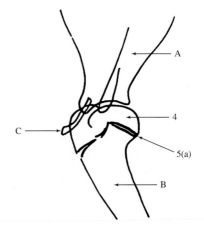

Figure 517

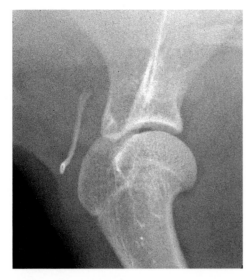

Figure 518   Age 68 weeks male

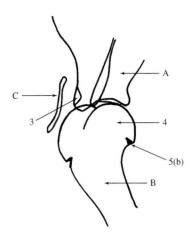

Figure 518

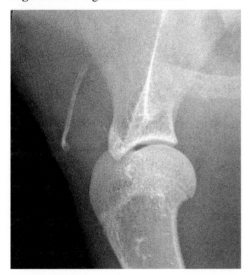

Figure 519   Age 80 weeks female

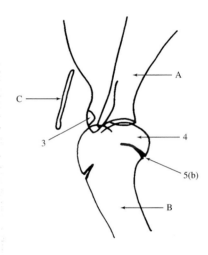

Figure 519

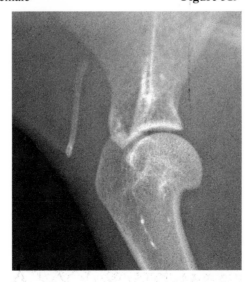

Figure 520   Age 96 weeks female

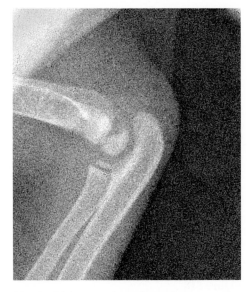

Figure 521   Age 4 weeks male

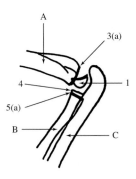

Figure 521

Figures 521, 522, 523, 524, 525, 526, 527, 528, 529, 530   Mediolateral projection of elbow joint.

British domestic short haired cats at 4 weeks entire male, 8 weeks entire male, 12 weeks entire male, 16 weeks entire female, 20 weeks entire male, 24 weeks entire male, 28 weeks entire female, 36 weeks entire female, 40 weeks entire female, and 46 weeks entire female.

Correlating line drawings for all ages except 46 weeks.

A Humerus
   1 Distal epiphysis.
     Initially two separate ossification centres for medial and lateral condylar centres.
   2 Medial epicondyle
   3 Distal growth plates
     3(a) Open
     3(b) Closing

B Radius
   4 Proximal epiphysis
   5 Proximal growth plate
     5(a) Open
     5(b) Closing

C Ulna
   6 Proximal epiphysis
   7 Proximal growth plate
     7(a) Open
     7(b) Closing
     7(c) Remnant

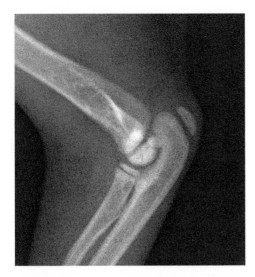

Figure 522 Age 8 weeks male

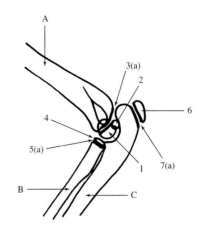

Figure 522

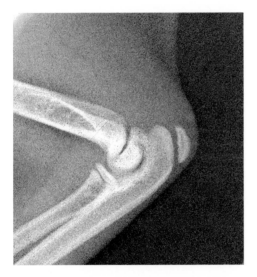

Figure 523 Age 12 weeks male

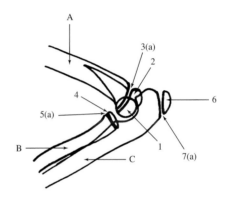

Figure 523

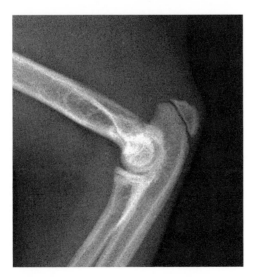

Figure 524 Age 16 weeks female

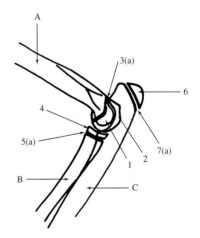

Figure 524

An Atlas of Interpretative Radiographic Anatomy of the Dog and Cat

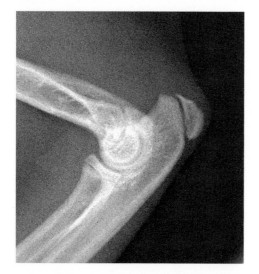

Figure 525   Age 20 weeks male

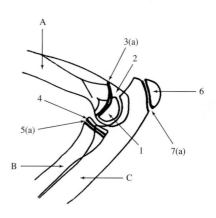

Figure 525

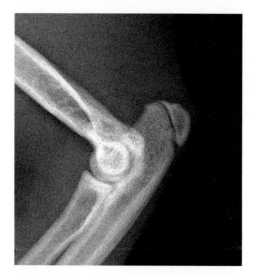

Figure 526   Age 24 weeks male

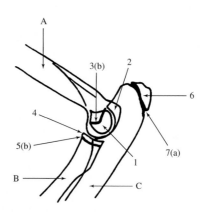

Figure 526

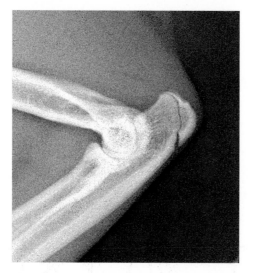

Figure 527   Age 28 weeks female

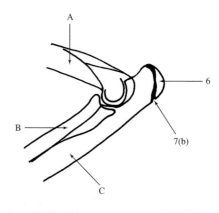

Figure 527

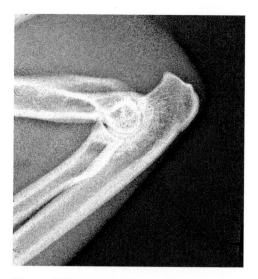

Figure 528   Age 36 weeks female

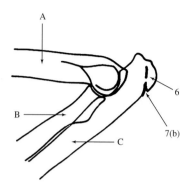

Figure 528

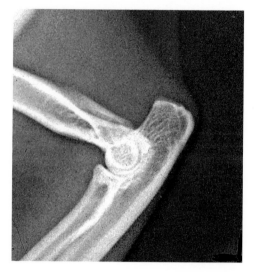

Figure 529   Age 40 weeks female

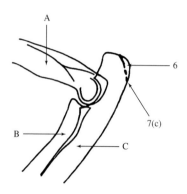

Figure 529

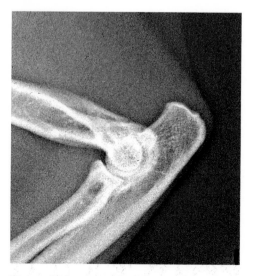

Figure 530   Age 46 weeks female

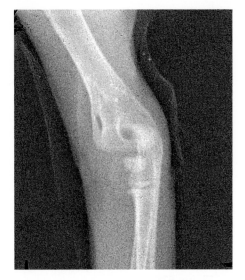

Figure 531   Age 4 weeks male

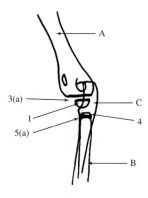

Figure 531

Figures 531, 532, 533, 534, 535, 536, 537, 538, 539   Craniocaudal projection of elbow joint.

British domestic short haired cats at 4 weeks entire male, 8 weeks entire male, 12 weeks entire male, 16 weeks entire female, 20 weeks entire male, 24 weeks entire male, 28 weeks entire female, 36 weeks entire female, and 46 weeks entire female.

Correlating line drawings for all ages except 46 weeks.

A   Humerus
  1   Distal epiphysis.
      Initially two separate ossification centres for medial and lateral condylar centres.
  2   Medial epicondyle
  3   Distal growth plate
      3(a)   Open
      3(b)   Closing

B   Radius
  4   Proximal epiphysis
  5   Proximal growth plate
      5(a)   Open
      5(b)   Closing

C   Ulna
  6   Proximal epiphysis
  7   Proximal growth plate
      7(a)   Open
      7(b)   Closing

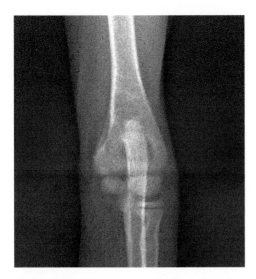

Figure 532 Age 8 weeks male

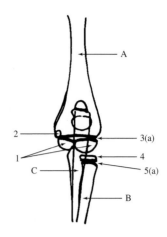

Figure 532

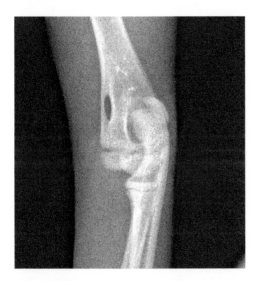

Figure 533 Age 12 weeks male

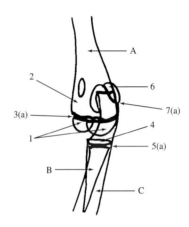

Figure 533

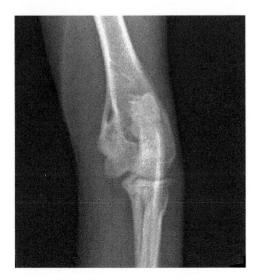

Figure 534 Age 16 weeks female

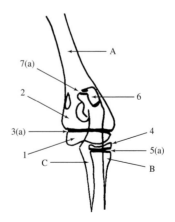

Figure 534

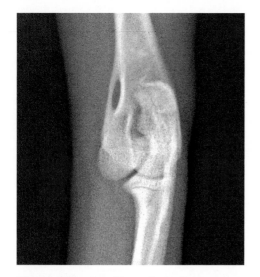

Figure 535 Age 20 weeks male

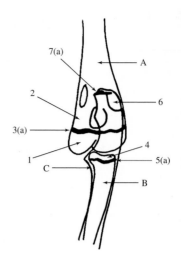

Figure 535

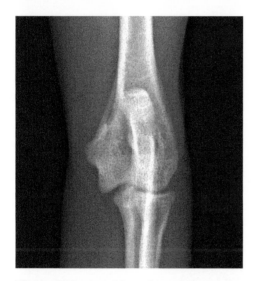

Figure 536 Age 24 weeks male

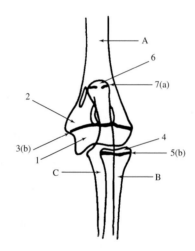

Figure 536

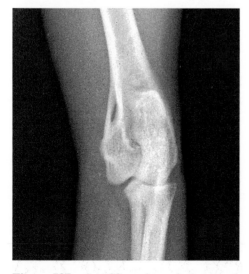

Figure 537 Age 28 weeks male

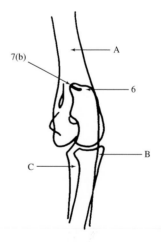

Figure 537

An Atlas of Interpretative Radiographic Anatomy of the Dog and Cat

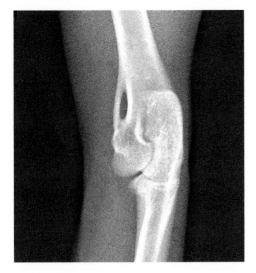

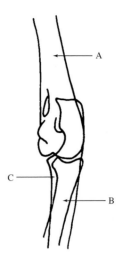

Figure 538   Age 36 weeks female   **Figure 538**

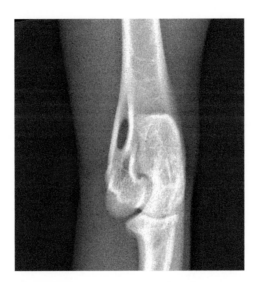

Figure 539   Age 46 weeks female

Figures 540, 541, 542, 543, 544, 545, 546, 547, 548, 549   Dorsopalmar projection of carpus, metacarpal bones and phalanges.

British domestic short haired cats at 4 weeks entire male, 8 weeks entire male, 12 weeks entire male, 16 weeks entire female, 24 weeks entire male, 32 weeks entire male, 46 weeks entire female, 54 weeks entire female, 68 weeks entire male, and 96 weeks entire female.

Correlating line drawings for all ages except 96 weeks.

A Radius
   1 Distal epiphysis
   2 Distal growth plate
     2(a) Open
     2(b) Closing
     2(c) Remnant

B Ulna
   3 Distal epiphysis
   4 Distal growth plate
     4(a) Open
     4(b) Closing
     4(c) Remnant

C Carpus

D Metacarpal bone 5 (2, 3 and 4 similar)
   5 Epiphysis.
     Note that there is only a distal epiphysis in these metacarpal bones.
   6 Growth plate
     6(a) Open
     6(b) Closing
   7 Proximal sesamoid bone (lateral)

E Proximal phalanx of digit 2 (3, 4 and 5 similar)
   8 Epiphysis.
     Note that there is only a proximal epiphysis in the proximal phalanx.
   9 Growth plate
     9(a) Open
     9(b) Closing
     9(c) Remnant

F Middle phalanx of digit 2 (3, 4 and 5 similar)
  Epiphysis and growth plate similar to proximal phalanx

G Distal phalanx of digit 2 (3, 4 and 5 similar)

H Metacarpal 1
  10 Epiphysis.
  Note that there is only a proximal epiphysis in this bone.
  11 Growth plate
     11(a) Open
     11(b) Closing

I Proximal phalanx of digit 1
  Epiphysis and growth plate similar to proximal phalanx of digit 2

J Distal phalanx of digit 1

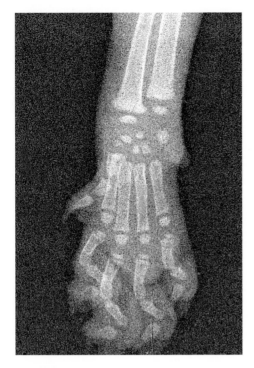

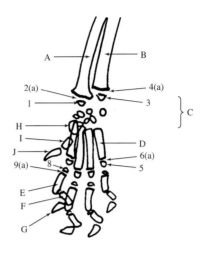

Figure 540   Age 4 weeks male

Figure 540

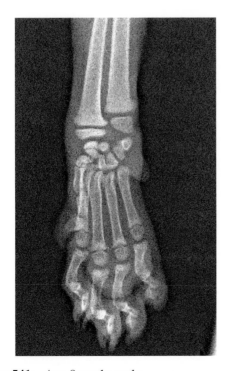

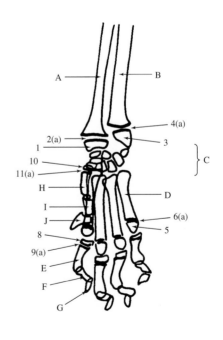

Figure 541   Age 8 weeks male

Figure 541

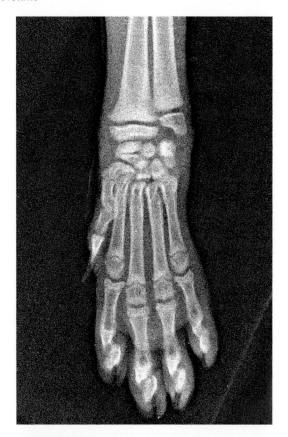

Figure 542   Age 12 weeks male

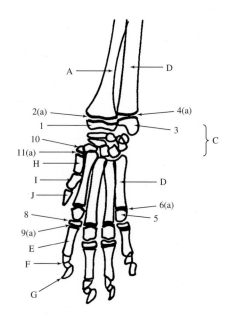

Figure 542

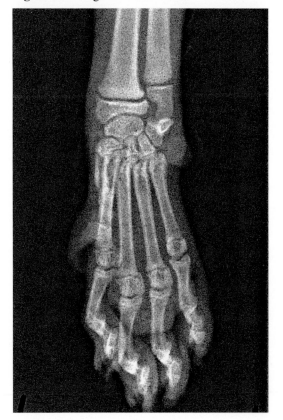

Figure 543   Age 16 weeks female

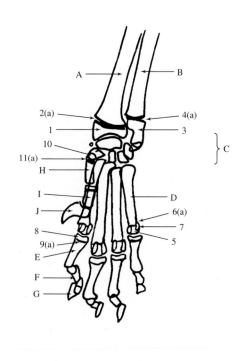

Figure 543

An Atlas of Interpretative Radiographic Anatomy of the Dog and Cat

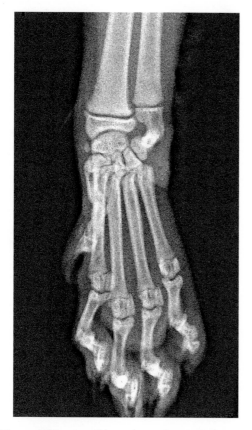

Figure 544   Age 24 weeks male

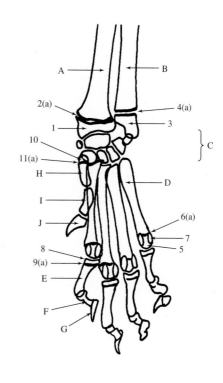

Figure 544

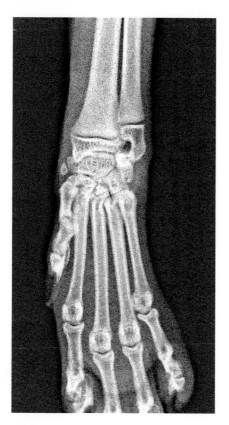

Figure 545   Age 32 weeks male

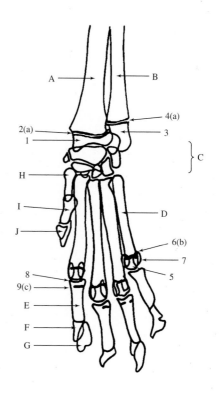

Figure 545

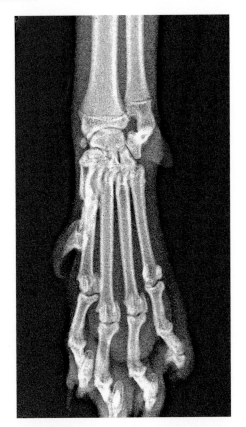

Figure 546   Age 46 weeks female

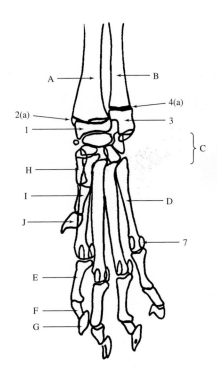

Figure 546

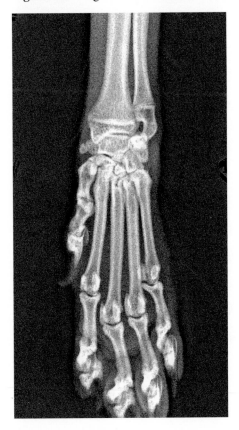

Figure 547   Age 54 weeks female

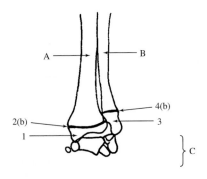

Figure 547

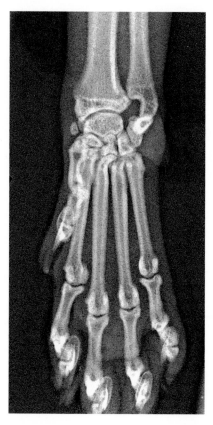

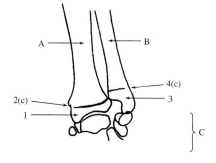

Figure 548   Age 68 weeks male   **Figure 548**

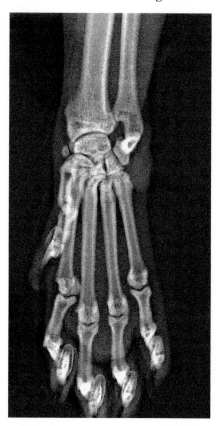

Figure 549   Age 96 weeks female

Figures 550, 551, 552, 553, 554, 555, 556, 557, 558, 559   Mediolateral projection of carpus, metacarpal bones and phalanges.

British domestic short haired cats at 4 weeks entire male, 8 weeks entire male, 12 weeks entire male, 16 weeks entire female, 24 weeks entire male, 32 weeks entire male, 46 weeks entire female, 54 weeks entire female, 68 weeks entire female, and 96 weeks entire female.

Correlating line drawings for all ages except 96 weeks.

A Radius
   1 Distal epiphysis
   2 Distal growth plate
     2(a) Open
     2(b) Closing
     2(c) Remnant

B Ulna
   3 Distal epiphysis
   4 Distal growth plate
     4(a) Open
     4(b) Closing
     4(c) Remnant

C Carpus
   5 Epiphysis of accessory carpal bone
   6 Accessory carpal bone growth plate
     6(a) Open

D Metacarpal bone 3 or 4 (2 and 5 similar but shorter)
   7 Epiphysis.
     Note that there is only a distal epiphysis in these metacarpal bones.
   8 Growth plate
     8(a) Open
     8(b) Closing
   9 Proximal sesamoids

E Proximal phalanx of digits 3 or 4 (2 and 5 similar)
  10 Epiphysis.
     Note that there is only a proximal epiphysis in the proximal phalanges.

  11 Growth plate
     11(a) Open
     11(b) Closing

F Middle phalanx of digits 3 or 4 (2 and 5 similar)
   Epiphysis and growth plate are similar to proximal phalanx.

G Distal phalanx of digits 3 or 4 (2 and 5 similar)

H Metacarpal bone 1
   Epiphysis and growth plate are proximal

I Proximal phalanx of digit 1

J Distal phalanx of digit 1

An Atlas of Interpretative Radiographic Anatomy of the Dog and Cat

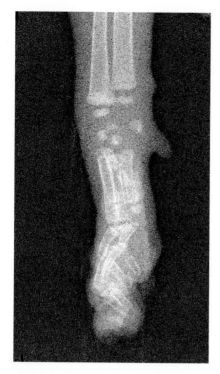

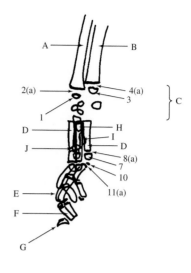

Figure 550   Age 4 weeks male

Figure 550

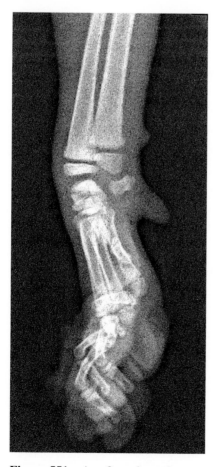

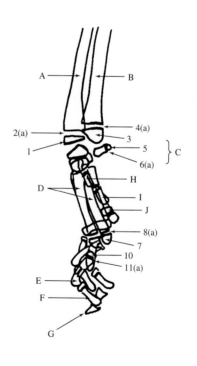

Figure 551   Age 8 weeks male

Figure 551

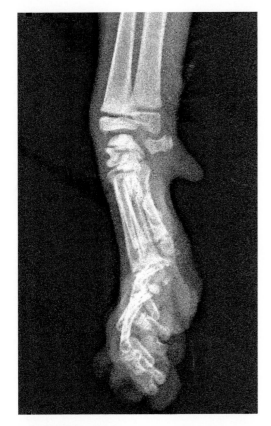

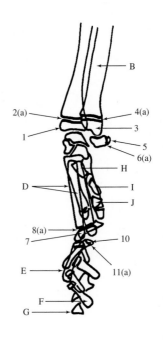

Figure 552   Age 12 weeks male

Figure 552

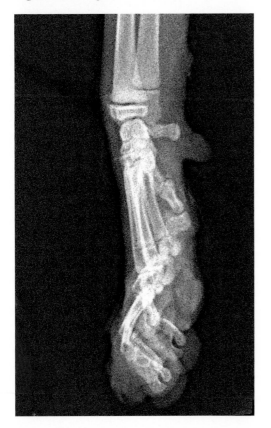

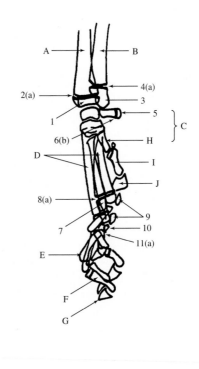

Figure 553   Age 16 weeks female

Figure 553

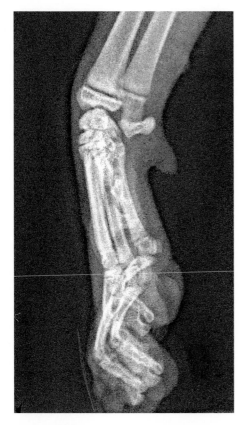

Figure 554   Age 24 weeks male

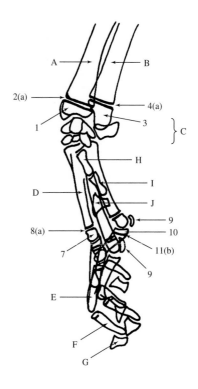

Figure 554

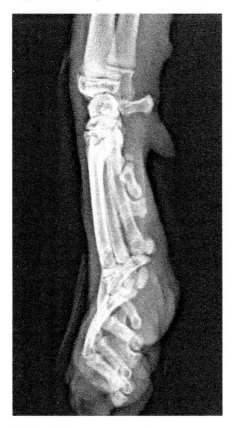

Figure 555   Age 32 weeks male

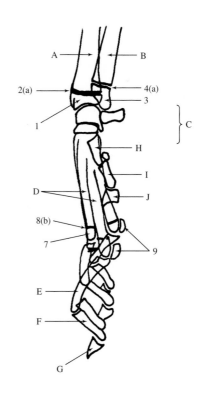

Figure 555

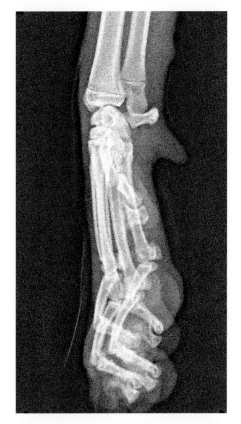

Figure 556   Age 46 weeks female

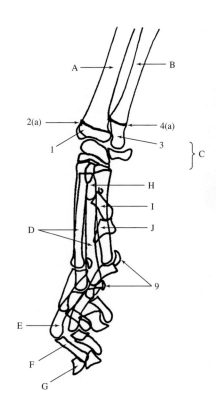

Figure 556

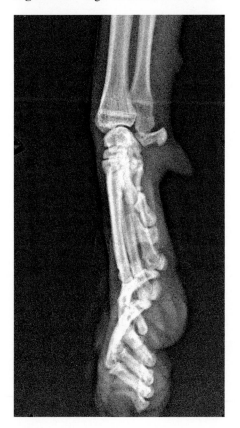

Figure 557   Age 54 weeks female

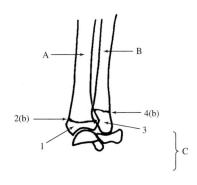

Figure 557

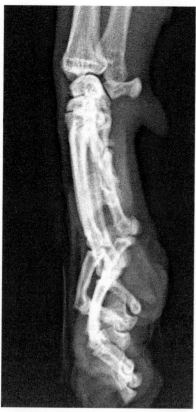

Figure 558   Age 68 weeks female

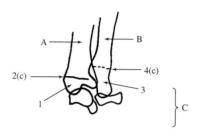

Figure 558

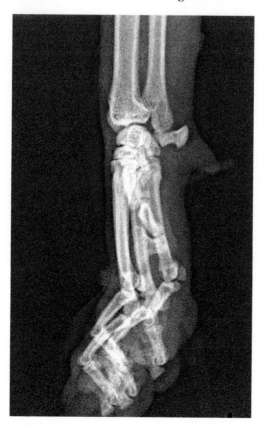

Figure 559   Age 96 weeks female

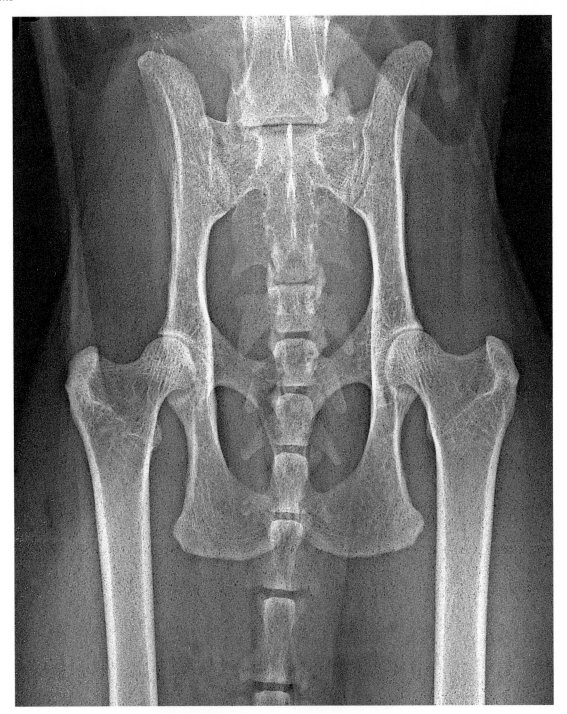

Figure 560   Ventrodorsal projection of hip joints and pelvis. British domestic short haired cat 6 years old, neutered male.

An Atlas of Interpretative Radiographic Anatomy of the Dog and Cat

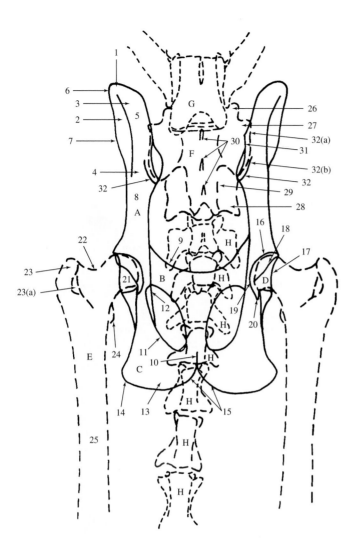

Figure 561   Ventrodorsal projection of hip joints and pelvis.

To simplify the labelling each structure has been numbered on one side or the other but not on both sides. Also the vertebral column has not been fully labelled.

A Ilium
  1 Crest
  2 Gluteal surface
  3 Cranial dorsal iliac spine
  4 Caudal dorsal iliac spine

Numbers 3 and 4 form the tuber sacrale or dorsal iliac spine

  5 Wing
  6 Cranial ventral iliac spine
  7 Caudal ventral iliac spine

Numbers 6 and 7 form the tuber coxae or ventral iliac spine

  8 Body

B Pubis
  9 Pecten

Pubic symphysis, part of the symphysis of the pelvis, is not recognisable due to superimposition of coccygeal or caudal vertebrae.

C Ischium
  10 Ischiatic symphysis, part of the symphysis of the pelvis
  11 Obturator foramen

  12 Ischiatic spine
  13 Ischiatic table
  14 Ischiatic tuberosity
  15 Ischiatic arch

D Acetabulum
  16 Cranial acetabular edge
  17 Dorsal acetabular edge
  18 Ventral acetabular edge
  19 Acetabular fossa
  20 Acetabular notch

E Femur
  21 Head
  22 Neck
  23 Greater trochanter
    23(a) Trochanteric fossa
  24 Lesser trochanter
  25 Body

F Sacrum
  26 Cranial articular process
  27 Wing
  28 Lateral sacral crest
  29 Intermediate sacral crest
  30 Median sacral crest
  31 Articular surface with ilium wing
  32 Sacroiliac joint
    32(a) Region of synchrondrosis
    32(b) Region of synovial joint

G 7th. lumbar vertebra

H Coccygeal or caudal vertebra

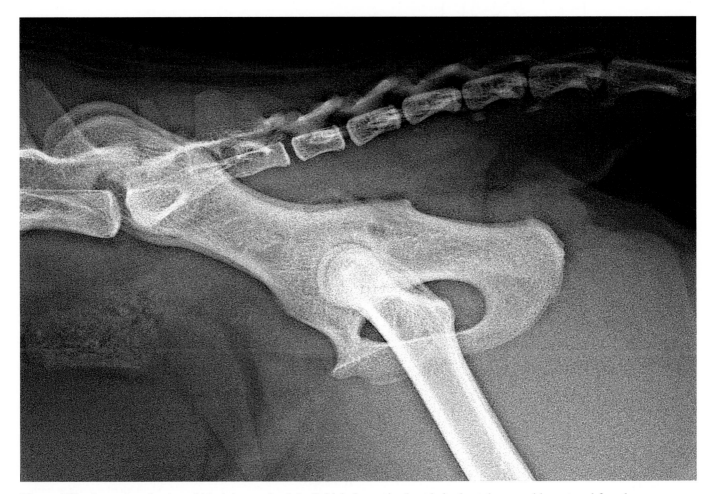

Figure 562   Lateral projection of hip joints and pelvis. British domestic short haired cat 4 years old, neutered female.

An Atlas of Interpretative Radiographic Anatomy of the Dog and Cat

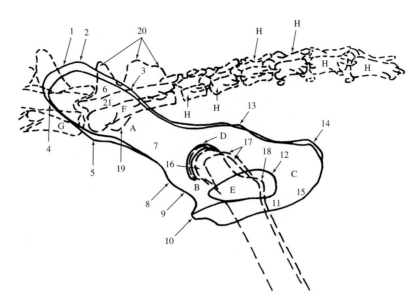

Figure 563   Lateral projection of hip joints and pelvis.

A Ilium
   1 Crest
   2 Cranial dorsal iliac spine
   3 Caudal dorsal iliac spine

Numbers 2 and 3 form the tuber sacrale or dorsal iliac spine

   4 Cranial ventral iliac spine
   5 Caudal ventral iliac spine

Numbers 4 and 5 form the tuber coxae or ventral iliac spine

   6 Wing
   7 Body

B Pubis
   8 Iliopubic eminence
   9 Pecten
  10 Pubic tubercle. Cranial limit of the pubic part of the pelvic symphysis.

C Ischium
  11 Pelvic symphysis
  12 Obturator foramen
  13 Ischiatic spine
  14 Ischiatic tuberosity
  15 Ischiatic table

D Acetabulum

E Femur
  16 Head
  17 Greater trochanter
  18 Lesser trochanter

F Sacrum
  19 Sacroiliac articulation
  20 Spinal processes
  21 Vertebral canal

G 7th. lumbar vertebra

H Coccygeal or caudal vertebra

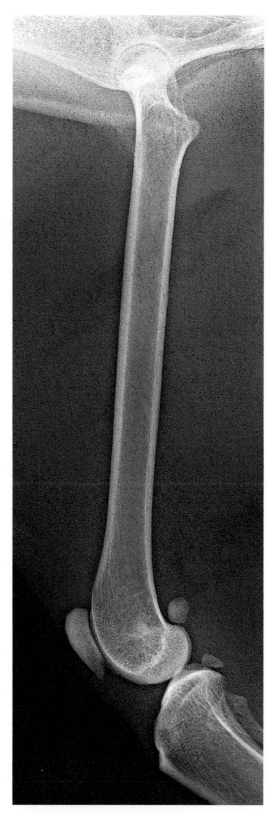

Figure 564   Mediolateral projection of femur. British domestic short haired cat 6 years old, neutered male.

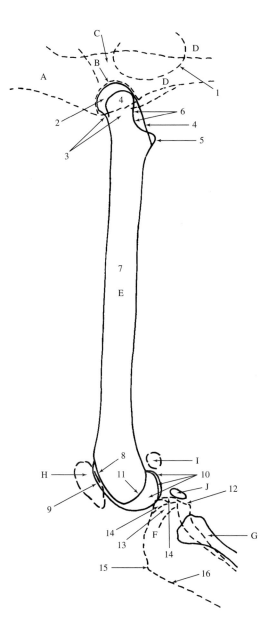

Figure 565   Mediolateral projection of femur.

A Ilium

B Acetabulum

C Pubis

D Ischium
   1   Obturator foramen

E Femur
   2   Head
   3   Neck
   4   Greater trochanter
   5   Lesser trochanter
   6   Trochanteric fossa
   7   Body
   8   Trochlear groove
   9   Trochlear ridge
   10   Superimposed lateral and
       medial condyles
   11   Base of intercondyloid fossa

F Tibia
   12   Lateral condyle

13   Medial condyle
14   Intercondyloid eminence
    (more caudal shadow is that
    of the lateral intercondyloid
    tubercle)
15   Tibial tuberosity
16   Cranial border or 'tibial crest'
    as formerly known

G Fibula

H Patella

I Fabella of lateral head of
  m.gastrocnemius. (No ossified
  fabella visible on the medial side
  in this cat. This is a common
  finding in the cat. Figures 564
  and 566 of the femur are of the
  same cat.)

J Fabella of m.popliteus

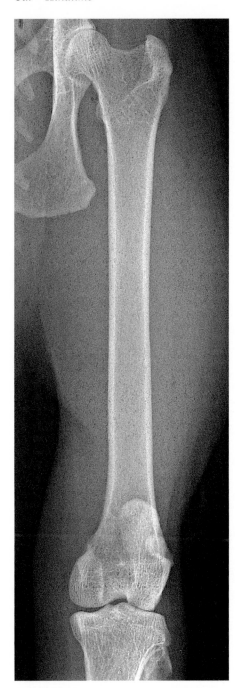

Figure 566 Craniocaudal projection of femur. British domestic short haired cat 6 years old, neutered male

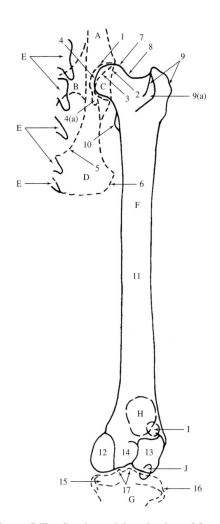

Figure 567 Craniocaudal projection of femur.

A Ilium

B Pubis

C Acetabulum
  1 Cranial acetabular edge
  2 Dorsal acetabular edge
  3 Ventral acetabular edge
  4 Acetabular fossa
    4(a) Acetabular fissure

D Ischium
  5 Obturator foramen
  6 Ischiatic tuberosity

E Coccygeal or caudal vertebrae

F Femur
  7 Head
  8 Neck
  9 Greater trochanter
    9(a) Trochanteric fossa

10 Lesser trochanter
11 Body
12 Medial condyle
13 Lateral condyle
14 Intercondyloid fossa

G Tibia
  15 Medial condyle
  16 Lateral condyle
  17 Intercondyloid eminence (medial and lateral intercondyloid tubercles are clearly seen)

H Patella

I Lateral fabella of m.gastrocnemius. (No ossified medial fabella is visible in this cat. This is a common finding in the cat. Figures 564 and 566 of the femur are of the same cat.)

J Fabella of m.popliteus

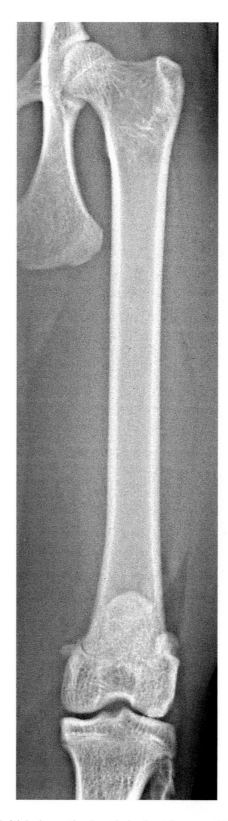

Figure 568 Craniocaudal projection of femur. British domestic short haired cat 2 years old, neutered female.

The radiograph has been included to demonstrate the ossified medial fabella in the tendon of the m.gastrocnemius. The medial fabella is commonly not seen in radiographs. This is usually due to non-mineralisation of the sesamoid fibrocartilage rather than agenesis.

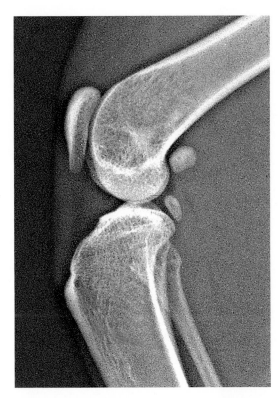

Figure 569 Mediolateral projection of stifle joint. British domestic short haired cat 2 years old, neutered female.

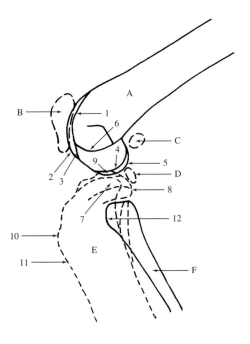

Figure 570 Mediolateral projection of stifle joint.

A Femur
   1 Trochlear groove
   2 Medial trochlear ridge
   3 Lateral trochlear ridge
   4 Medial condyle
   5 Lateral condyle
   6 Intercondyloid fossa

B Patella

C Lateral fabella of m.gastrocnemius
   (No ossified medial fabella is
   visible in this cat. Also not seen in
   radiograph and line drawing,
   Figures 571 and 572, of the 6-year-
   old cat.)

D Fabella of m.popliteus

E Tibia
   7 Medial condyle
   8 Lateral condyle
   9 Intercondyloid
     eminence
  10 Tibial tuberosity
  11 Cranial border or 'tibial crest'
     as formerly known.

F Fibula
  12 Head

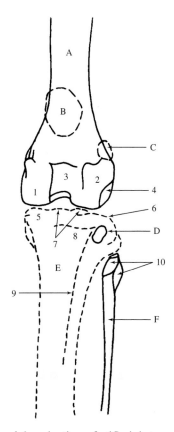

Figure 572 Caudocranial projection of stifle joint.

A Femur
  1 Medial condyle
  2 Lateral condyle
  3 Intercondyloid fossa
  4 Popliteal fossa

B Patella

C Lateral fabella of m.gastrocnemius
(No ossified medial fabella is
visible in this cat. Also not seen
in radiograph and line drawing,
Figures 569 and 570, of the 2-
year-old cat.)

D Fabella of m.popliteus

E Tibia
  5 Medial condyle
  6 Lateral condyle
  7 Intercondyloid eminence
(Medial and lateral intercondyloid tubercles)
  8 Tibial tuberosity
  9 Cranial border or 'tibial crest'
as formerly known.

F Fibula
10 Head

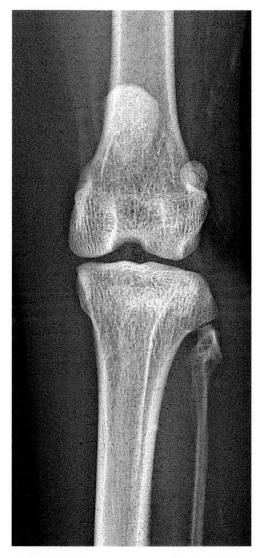

Figure 571 Caudocranial projection of
stifle joint. British domestic short haired cat 6
years old, neutered male.

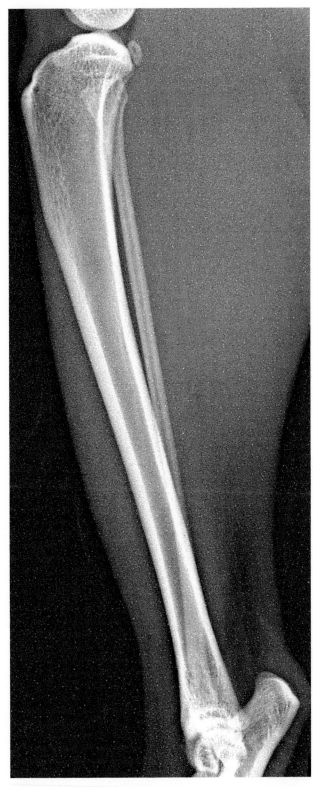

Figure 573 Mediolateral projection of tibia and fibula. British domestic short haired cat 2 years old, neutered female.

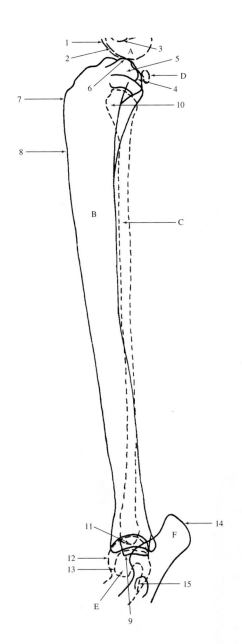

Figure 574 Mediolateral projection of tibia and fibula.

A Femur
  1 Lateral condyle
  2 Medial condyle
  3 Base of intercondyloid fossa

B Tibia
  4 Lateral condyle
  5 Medial condyle
  6 Intercondyloid eminence
  7 Tibial tuberosity
  8 Cranial border or 'tibial crest' as formerly known
  9 Medial malleolus

C Fibula
  10 Head
  11 Lateral malleolus

D Fabella of m.popliteus

E Tibial tarsal bone or talus
  12 Medial trochlear ridge
  13 Lateral trochlear ridge

F Fibular tarsal bone or calcaneus
  14 Calcaneal tuber
  15 Sustentaculum tali

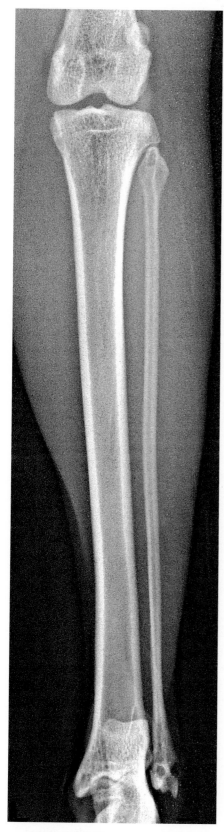

Figure 575 Caudocranial projection of tibia and fibula. British domestic short haired cat 2 years old, neutered female.

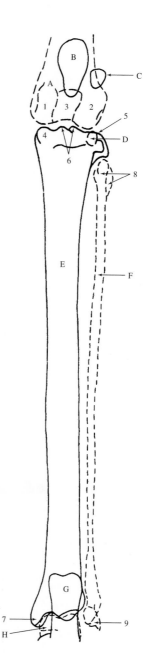

Figure 576 Caudocranial projection of tibia and fibula.

A Femur
  1 Medial condyle
  2 Lateral condyle
  3 Intercondyloid fossa

B Patella

C Lateral fabella of m.gastrocnemius. (No ossified medial fabella is visible in this cat.)

D Fabella of m.popliteus

E Tibia
  4 Medial condyle

  5 Lateral condyle
  6 Intercondyloid eminence (lateral and medial intercondyloid tubercles)
  7 Medial malleolus

F Fibula
  8 Head
  9 Lateral malleolus

G Fibular tarsal bone or calcaneus

H Tibial tarsal bone or talus

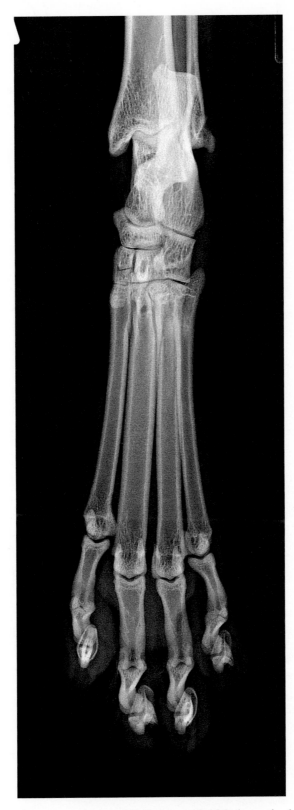

Figure 577   Plantarodorsal projection of tarsus, metatarsus and phalanges. British domestic short haired cat 3 years old, neutered male.

An Atlas of Interpretative Radiographic Anatomy of the Dog and Cat

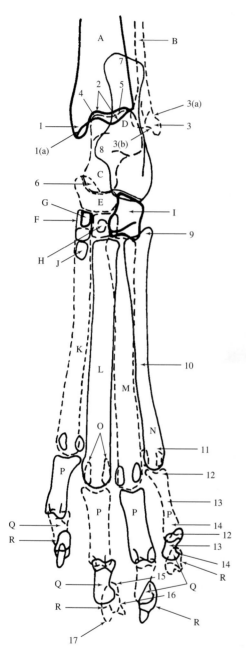

Figure 578 Plantarodorsal projection of tarsus, metatarsus and phalanges.

A Tibia
  1 Medial malleolus
    1(a) Groove for tendon of
        m.flexor digitorum
        longus
  2 Distal articular borders

B Fibula
  3 Lateral malleolus
    3(a) Groove for tendon of
        m.fibularis longus
    3(b) Groove for tendon of
        m.fibularis brevis and
        m.extensor digitorum later-
        alis

C Tibial tarsal bone or talus
  4 Medial trochlear ridge
  5 Lateral trochlear ridge
  6 Head

D Fibular tarsal bone or calcaneus
  7 Calcaneal tuber
  8 Sustentaculum tali

E Central tarsal bone

F Tarsal bone 1

G Tarsal bone 2

H Tarsal bone 3

I Tarsal bone 4

J Metatarsal bone 1

K Metatarsal bone 2

L Metatarsal bone 3

M Metatarsal bone 4

N Metatarsal bone 5
  9 Base
  10 Body
  11 Head

O Proximal sesamoids. Present on the
  plantar aspect.

P Proximal phalanges

Q Middle phalanges
  12 Base
  13 Body
  14 Head

R Distal phalanges
  15 Ungual crest
  16 Ungual process
  17 Flexor tuberosity

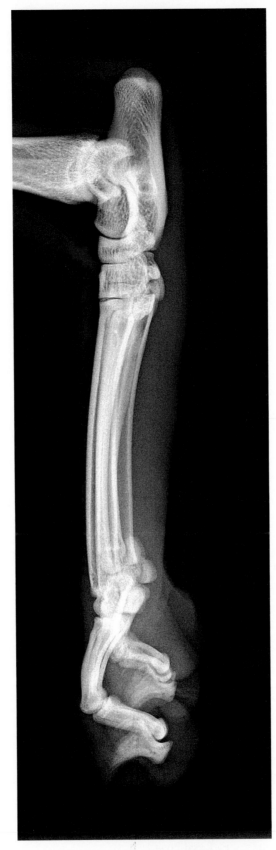

Figure 579 Mediolateral projection of tarsus, metatarsus and phalanges. British domestic short haired cat 3 years old, neutered male.

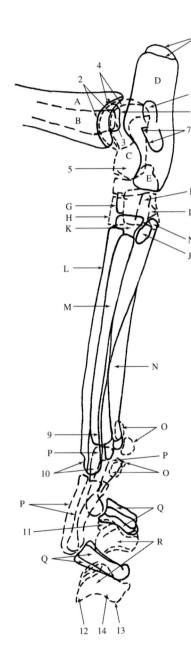

Figure 580 Mediolateral projection of tarsus, metatarsus and phalanges.

A Tibia
  1 Medial malleolus
  2 Distal articular borders (lateral border is proximal to the medial)

B Fibula
  3 Lateral malleolus

C Tibial tarsal bone or talus
  4 Trochlear ridges (lateral ridge is proximal to the medial)
  5 Head

D Fibular tarsal bone or calcaneus
  6 Calcaneal tuber
  7 Sustentaculum tali
  8 Depression for attachment of the short part of the lateral collateral ligament

E Central tarsal bone

F Tarsal bone 1

G Tarsal bone 2

H Tarsal bone 3

I Tarsal bone 4

J Metatarsal bone 1

K Metatarsal bone 2

L Metatarsal bone 3

M Metatarsal bone 4

N Metatarsal bone 5
  9 Superimposed heads of metatarsal bones 2 and 5
  10 Superimposed heads of metatarsal bones 3 and 4

O Proximal sesamoids

P Proximal phalanges

Q Middle phalanges

R Distal phalanges
  11 Ungual crest
  12 Ungual process
  13 Flexor tuberosity
  14 Solar foramen

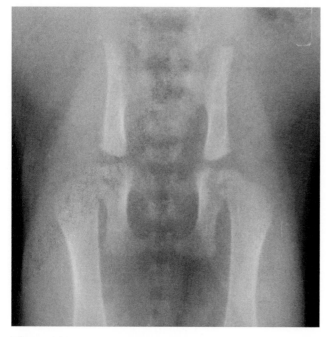

Figure 581   Age 4 weeks male

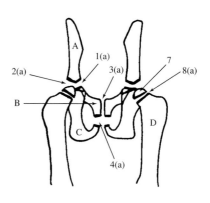

Figure 581

Figures 581, 582, 583, 584, 585, 586, 587, 588, 589, 590   Ventrodorsal projection of pelvis and craniocaudal proximal femur. British domestic short haired cats at 4 weeks entire male, 8 weeks entire male, 12 weeks entire male, 16 weeks entire female, 20 weeks entire male, 24 weeks entire male, 32 weeks entire male, 36 weeks entire female, 40 weeks entire female, and 54 weeks entire female.

Correlating line drawings for all ages except 54 weeks.

A Ilium
   1 Iliopubic growth plate
      1(a) Open
      1(b) Closing
      1(c) Remnant
   2 Ilioischial growth plate
      2(a) Open
      2(b) Closing

B Pubis

C Ischium
   3 Symphysis of pelvis
      3(a) Open
   4 Ischiopubic growth plate
      4(a) Open
      4(b) Closing

   5 Ischiatic tuberosity
   6 Ischiatic tuberosity growth plate
      6(a) Open

D Femur
   7 Femoral head
   8 Proximal growth plate
      8(a) Open
      8(b) Closing
      8(c) Remnant
   9 Greater trochanter
   10 Greater trochanter growth plate
      10(a) Open
      10(b) Closing
   11 Lesser trochanter

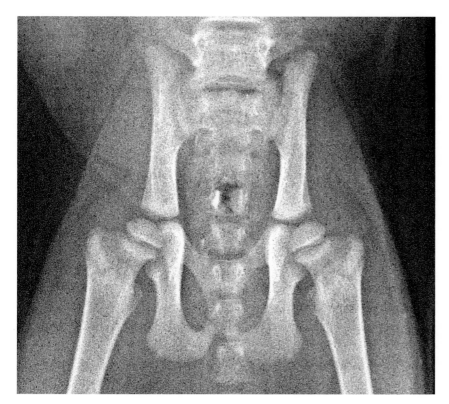
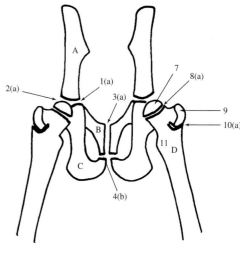

Figure 582   Age 8 weeks male

Figure 582

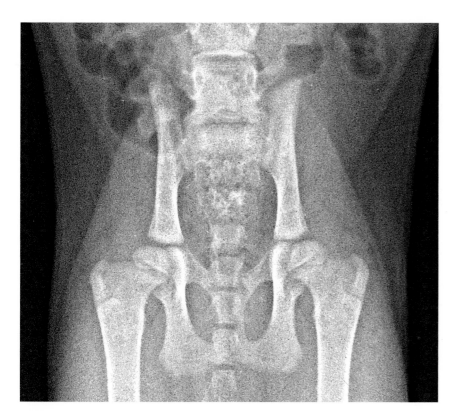
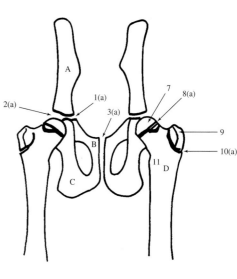

Figure 583   Age 12 weeks male

Figure 583

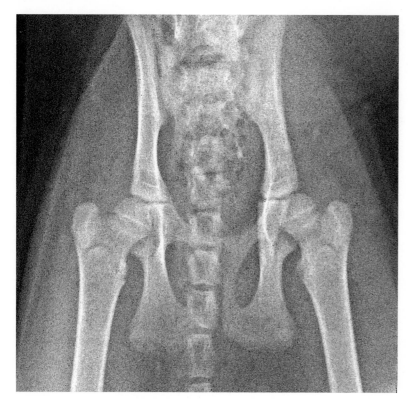

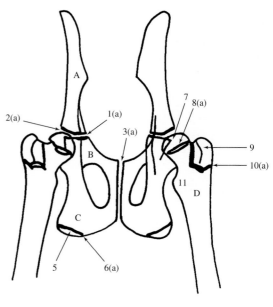

Figure 584   Age 16 weeks female

Figure 584

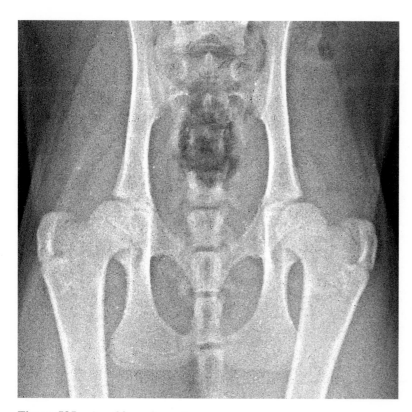

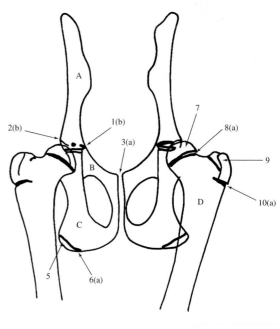

Figure 585   Age 20 weeks male

Figure 585

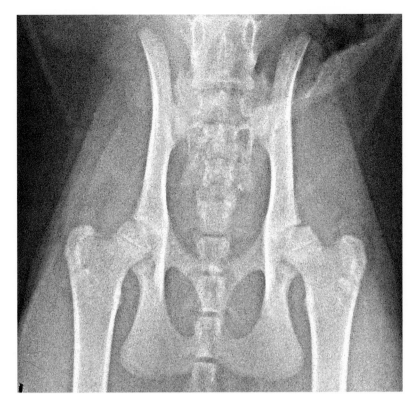

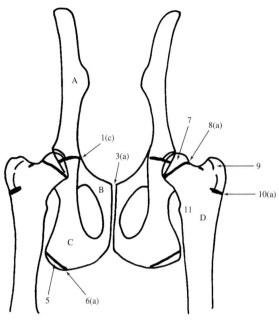

Figure 586   Age 24 weeks male

Figure 586

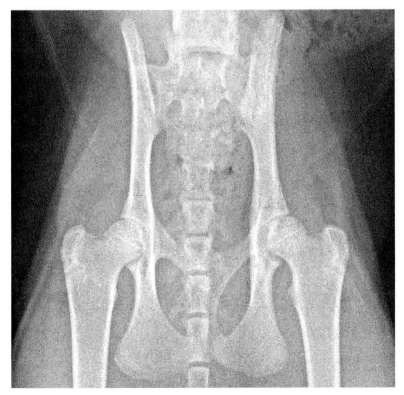

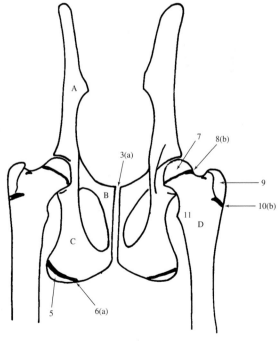

Figure 587   Age 32 weeks male

Figure 587

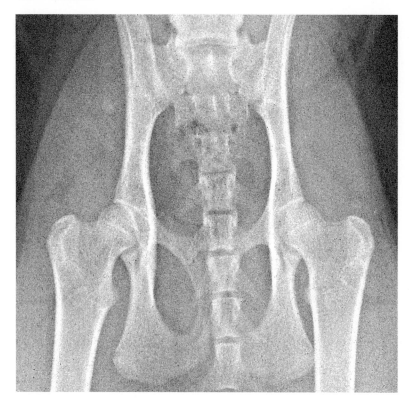

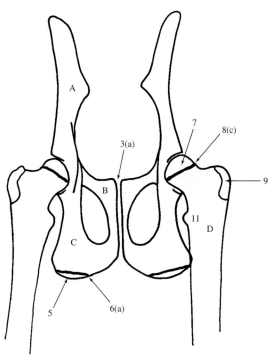

Figure 588 Age 36 weeks female

Figure 588

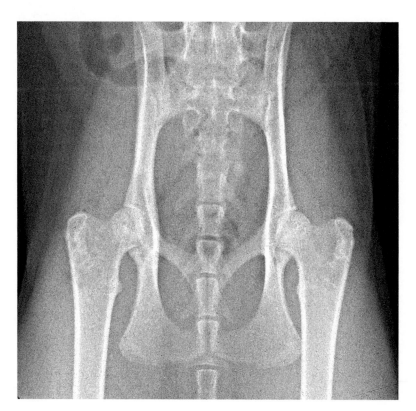

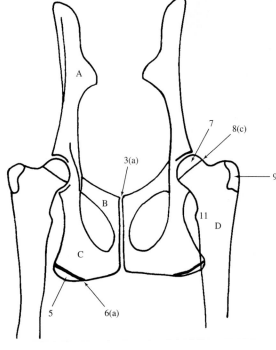

Figure 589 Age 40 weeks female

Figure 589

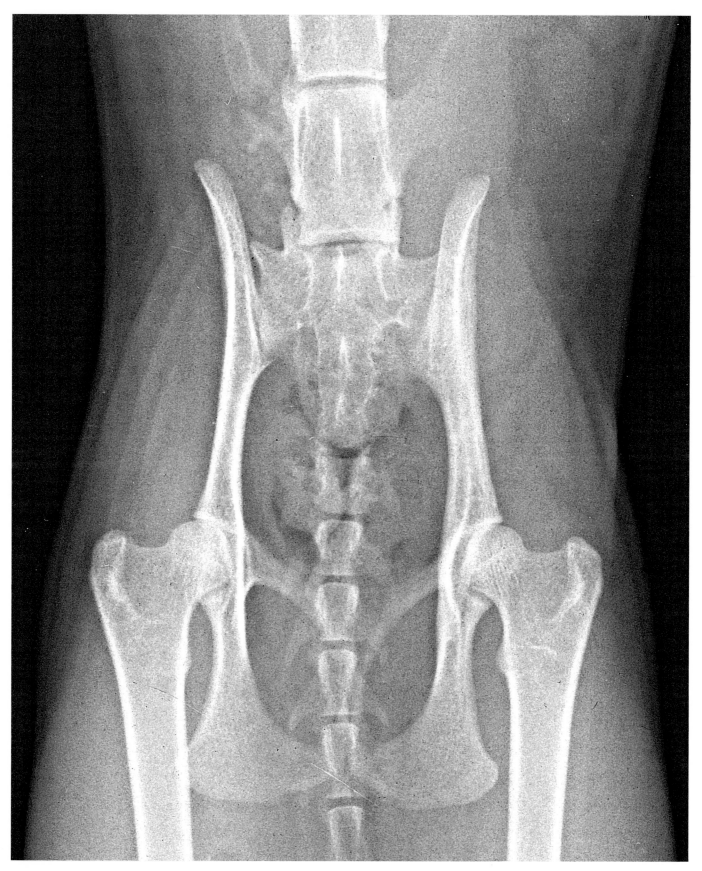

Figure 590   Age 54 weeks female

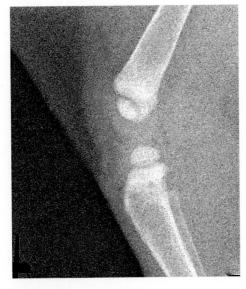

Figure 591   Age 4 weeks male

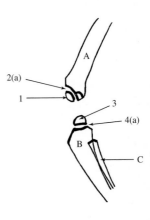

Figure 591

Figures 591, 592, 593, 594, 595, 596, 597, 598, 599, 600, 601   Mediolateral projection of stifle joint.

British domestic short haired cats at 4 weeks entire male, 8 weeks entire male, 12 weeks entire male, 16 weeks entire female, 20 weeks entire male, 24 weeks entire male, 32 weeks entire male, 36 weeks entire female, 46 weeks entire female, 54 weeks entire female, and 80 weeks entire female.

Correlating line drawings for all ages except 80 weeks

A Femur
  1   Distal epiphysis
  2   Distal growth plate
    2(a)   Open
    2(b)   Closing
    2(c)   Remnant

B Tibia
  3   Proximal epiphysis
  4   Proximal growth plate
    4(a)   Open
    4(b)   Closing
    4(c)   Remnant
  5   Tibial tuberosity
  6   Tibial tuberosity growth plate to diaphysis
    6(a)   Open
    6(b)   Closing
    6(c)   Remnant

  7   Tibial tuberosity growth plate to proximal epiphysis
    7(a)   Open
    7(b)   Closing

C Fibula
  8   Proximal epiphysis
  9   Proximal growth plate
    9(a)   Open
    9(b)   Closing
    9(c)   Remnant

D Patella

E Lateral fabella of m.gastrocnemius
  Note the apparent absence of the medial fabella. The fibro-cartilage of this sesamoid bone often remains in a non-mineralised state (see adult section).

F Fabella of m.popliteal

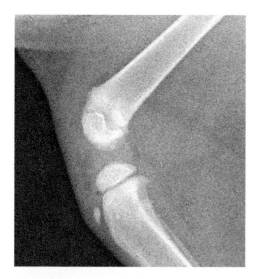

Figure 592   Age 8 weeks male

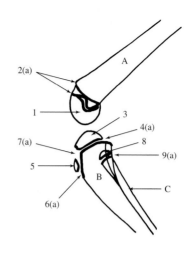

Figure 592

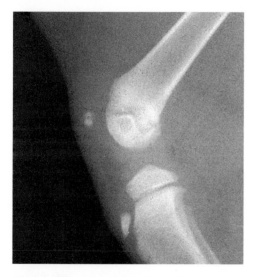

Figure 593   Age 12 weeks male

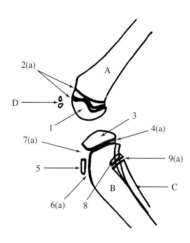

Figure 593

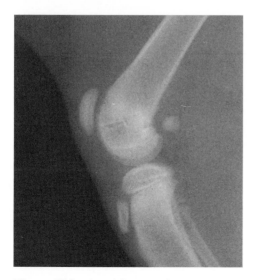

Figure 594   Age 16 weeks female

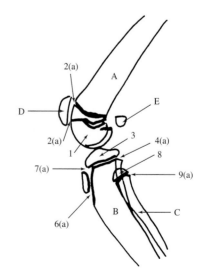

Figure 594

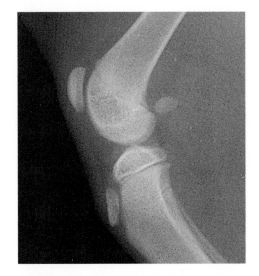

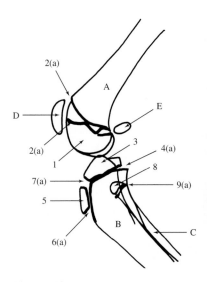

Figure 595   Age 20 weeks male

Figure 595

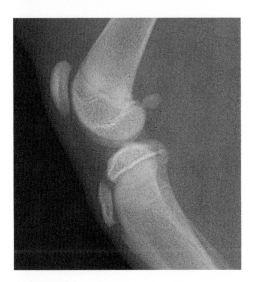

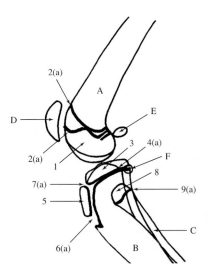

Figure 596   Age 24 weeks male

Figure 596

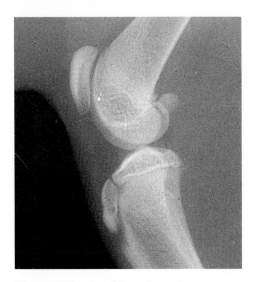

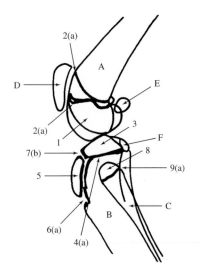

Figure 597   Age 32 weeks male

Figure 597

An Atlas of Interpretative Radiographic Anatomy of the Dog and Cat

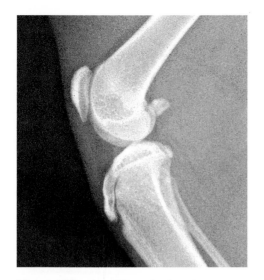

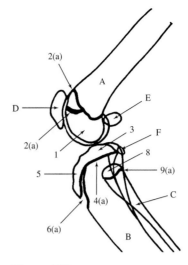

Figure 598 Age 36 weeks female

Figure 598

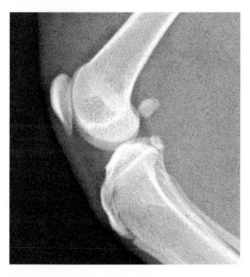

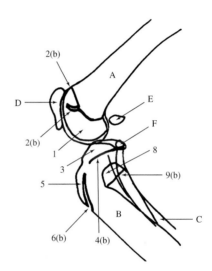

Figure 599 Age 46 weeks female

Figure 599

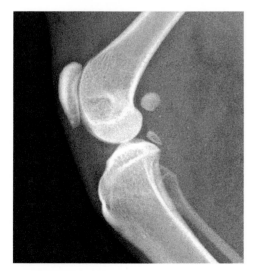

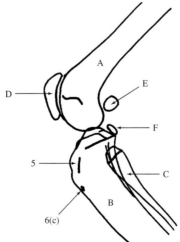

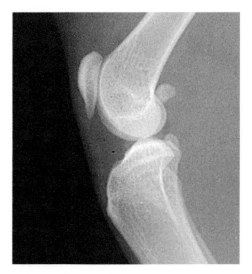

Figure 600 Age 54 weeks female

Figure 600

Figure 601 Age 80 weeks female

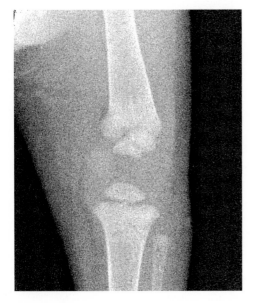

Figure 602   Age 4 weeks male

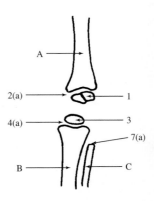

Figure 602

Figures 602, 603, 604, 605, 606, 607, 608, 609, 610, 611   Craniocaudal projection of stifle joint.

British domestic short haired cats at 4 weeks entire male, 8 weeks entire male, 12 weeks entire male, 16 weeks entire male, 20 weeks entire male, 28 weeks entire female, 36 weeks entire female, 46 weeks entire female, 54 weeks entire female, and 80 weeks entire female.

Correlating line drawings for all ages except 80 weeks.

A Femur
  1   Distal epiphysis
  2   Distal growth plate
      2(a) Open
      2(b) Closing
      2(c) Remnant

B Tibia
  3   Proximal epiphysis
  4   Proximal growth plate
      4(a) Open
      4(b) Closing
      4(c) Remnant
  5   Tibial tuberosity

C Fibula
  6 Proximal epiphysis
  7   Proximal growth plate
      7(a) Open
      7(b) Closing
      7(c) Remnant

D Patella

E Lateral fabella of m.gastrocnemius
  Note the apparent absence of the medial fabella. The fibro-cartilage of this sesamoid bone often remains in a non-mineralised state (see adult section).

F Fabella of m.popliteal

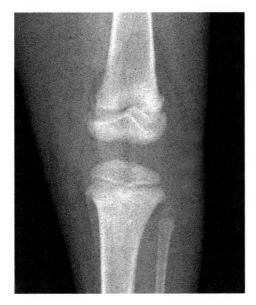

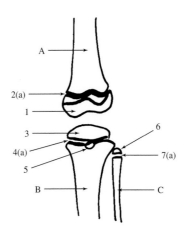

Figure 603   Age 8 weeks male

Figure 603

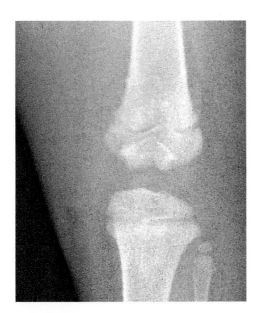

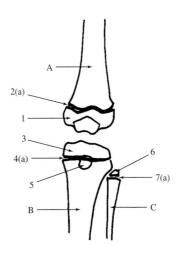

Figure 604   Age 12 weeks male

Figure 604

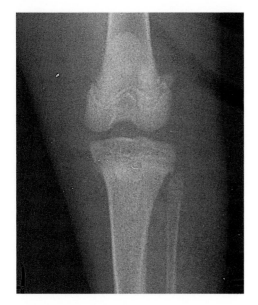

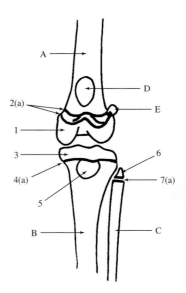

Figure 605   Age 16 weeks male

Figure 605

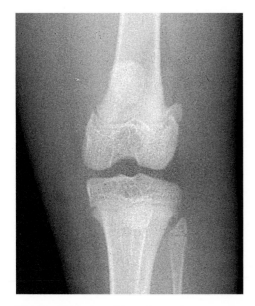

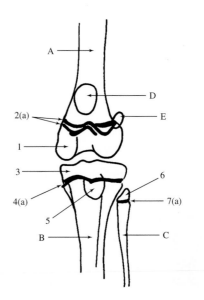

Figure 606   Age 20 weeks male

Figure 606

An Atlas of Interpretative Radiographic Anatomy of the Dog and Cat

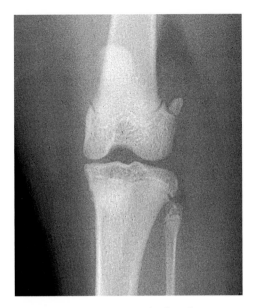

Figure 607   Age 28 weeks female

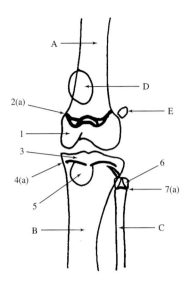

Figure 607

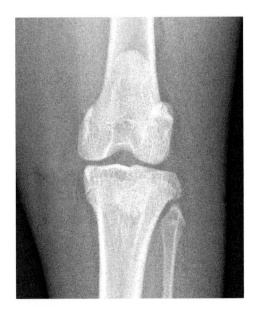

Figure 608   Age 36 weeks female

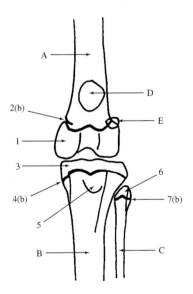

Figure 608

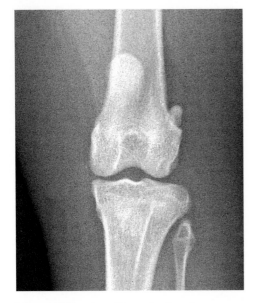

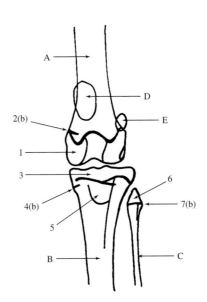

Figure 609   Age 46 weeks female

Figure 609

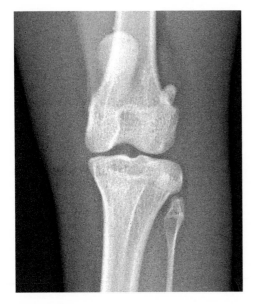

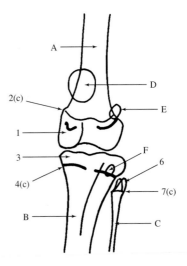

Figure 610   Age 54 weeks female

Figure 610

An Atlas of Interpretative Radiographic Anatomy of the Dog and Cat

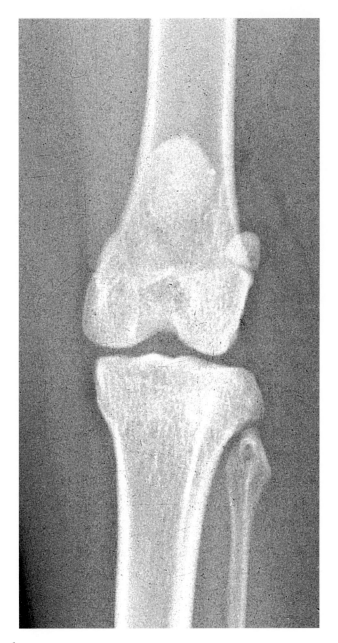

Figure 611   Age 80 weeks female

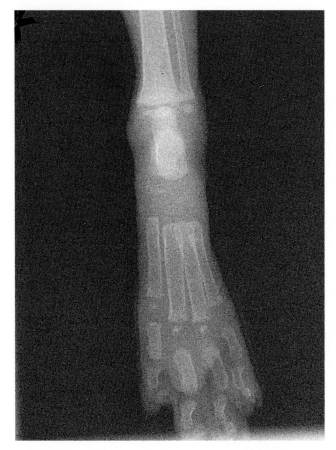

Figure 612

Figure 612   Age 4 weeks male

Figures 612, 613, 614, 615, 616, 617, 618, 619, 620   Dorsoplantar projection of tarsus, metatarsal bones, and phalanges.

British domestic short haired cats at 4 weeks entire male, 8 weeks entire male, 12 weeks entire male, 16 weeks entire female, 20 weeks entire male, 28 weeks entire female, 36 weeks entire female, 40 weeks entire female, and 54 weeks entire female.

Correlating line drawings for all ages except 54 weeks.

A Tibia
  1 Distal epiphysis
  2 Distal growth plate
    2(a) Open
    2(b) Closing

B Fibula
  3 Distal epiphysis
  4 Distal growth plate
    4(a) Open
    4(b) Closing

C Tarsus

D Metatarsal bones 2 and 5 (3 and 4 similar)
  5 Epiphysis.
    Note that there is only a distal epiphysis in these metatarsal bones.
  6 Growth plate
    6(a) Open

    6(b) Closing
    6(c) Remnant
  7 Proximal sesamoid bone

E Proximal phalanx of digits 2 and 5 (3 and 4 similar)
  8 Epiphysis.
    Note that there is only a proximal epiphysis in the proximal phalanx.
  9 Growth plate
    9(a) Open

F Middle phalanx of digits 2 and 5 (3 and 4 similar)

Epiphysis and growth plate similar to proximal phalanx.

G Distal phalanx of digits 2 and 5 (3 and 4 similar)

H Metatarsal bone 1

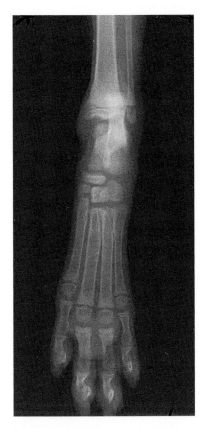

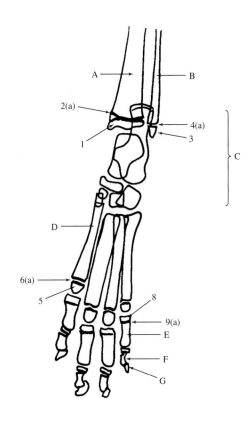

Figure 613   Age 8 weeks male

Figure 613

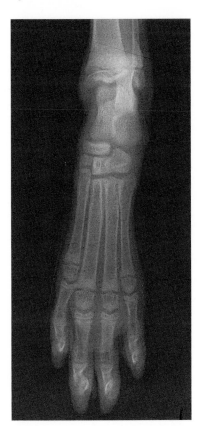

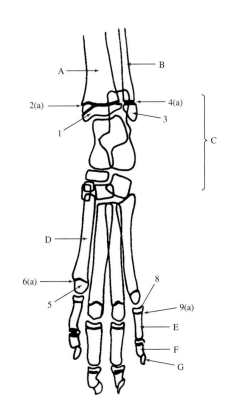

Figure 614   Age 12 weeks male

Figure 614

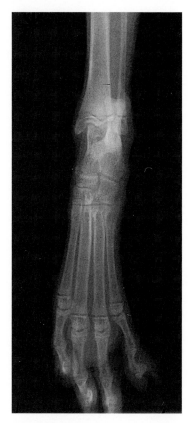

Figure 615   Age 16 weeks female

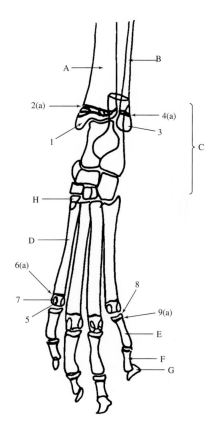

Figure 615

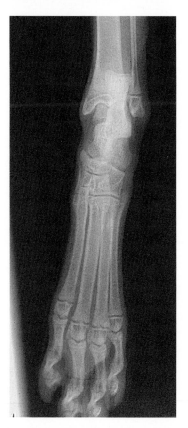

Figure 616   Age 20 weeks male

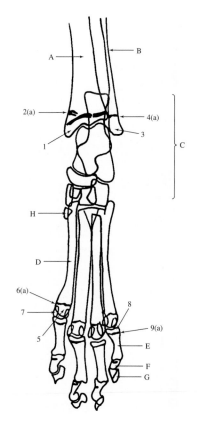

Figure 616

An Atlas of Interpretative Radiographic Anatomy of the Dog and Cat

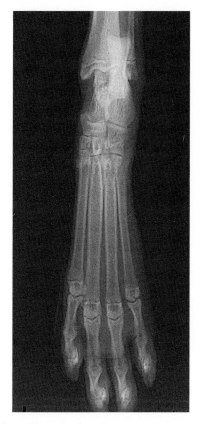

Figure 617   Age 28 weeks female

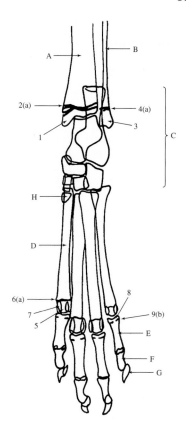

Figure 617

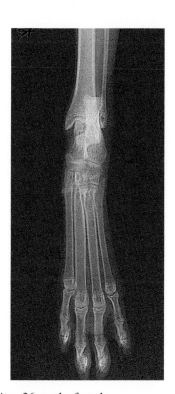

Figure 618   Age 36 weeks female

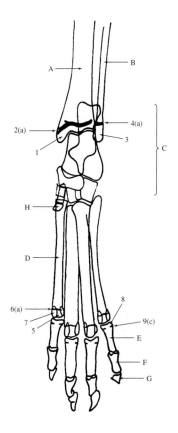

Figure 618

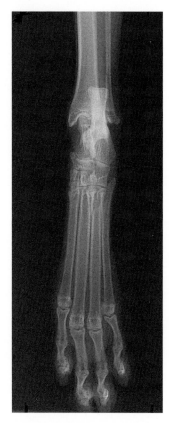

Figure 619   Age 40 weeks female

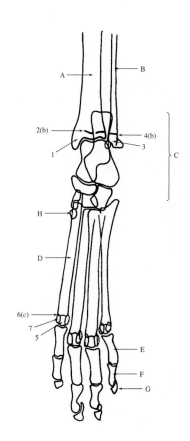

Figure 619

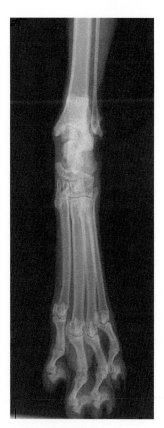

Figure 620   Age 54 weeks female

An Atlas of Interpretative Radiographic Anatomy of the Dog and Cat

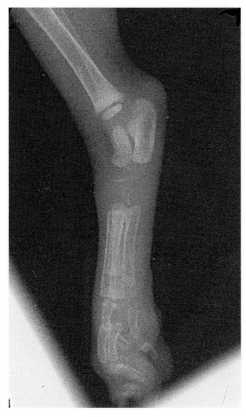

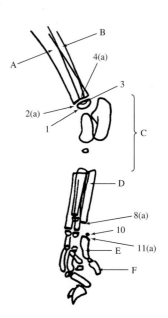

Figure 621   Age 4 weeks male   **Figure 621**

Figures 621, 622, 623, 624, 625, 626, 627, 628, 629   Mediolateral projection of tarsus, metatarsal bones and phalanges. British domestic short haired cats at 4 weeks entire male, 8 weeks entire male, 12 weeks entire male, 16 weeks entire female, 20 weeks entire male, 28 weeks entire female, 36 weeks entire female, 40 weeks entire female, and 54 weeks entire female.

Correlating line drawings for all ages except 54 weeks.

A Tibia
   1 Distal epiphysis
   2 Distal growth plate
      2(a) Open
      2(b) Closing

B Fibula
   3 Distal epiphysis
   4 Distal growth plate
      4(a) Open
      4(b) Closing

C Tarsus
   5 Epiphysis of fibular tarsal bone
   6 Fibular tarsal bone growth plate
      6(a) Open
      6(b) Closing

D Metatarsal bones 2 or 5 (3 and 4 similar)
   7 Epiphysis.
      Note that there is only a distal epiphysis in these metatarsal bones.

8 Growth plate
   8(a) Open
   8(b) Closing
   8(c) Remnant
9 Proximal sesamoid bone

E Proximal phalanx of digit 2 or 5 (3 and 4 similar)
  10 Epiphysis.
  Note that there is only a proximal epiphysis in the proximal phalanx.
  11 Growth plate
     11(a) Open

F Middle phalanx of digit 2 or 5 (3 and 4 similar)

Epiphysis and growth plate similar to proximal phalanx.

G Distal phalanx of digit 2 or 5 (3 and 4 similar)

H Metatarsal bone 1

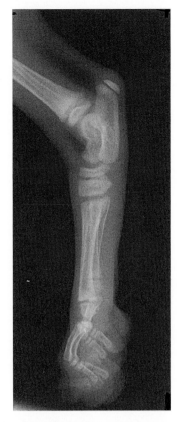

Figure 622   Age 8 weeks male

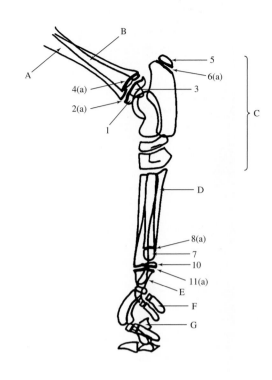

Figure 622

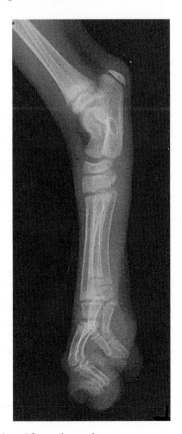

Figure 623   Age 12 weeks male

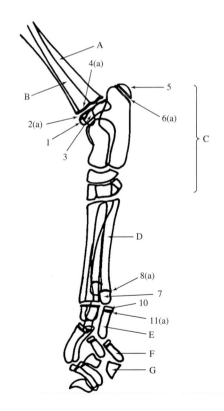

Figure 623

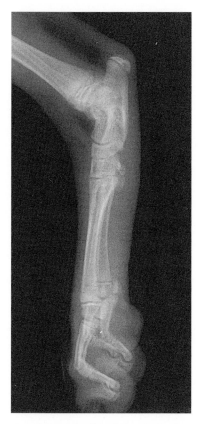

Figure 624 Age 16 weeks female

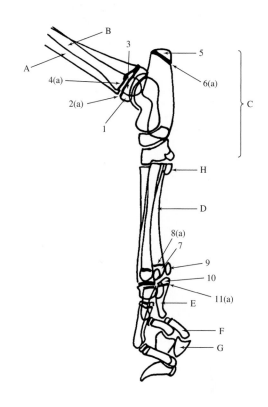

Figure 624

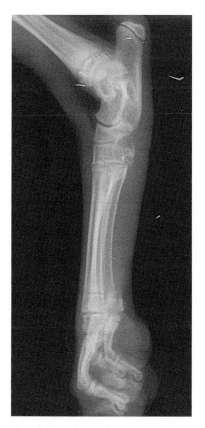

Figure 625 Age 20 weeks male

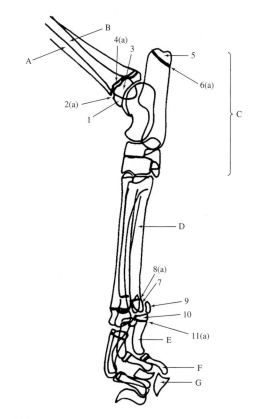

Figure 625

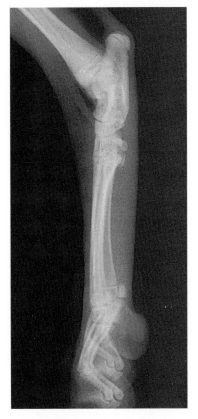

Figure 626   Age 28 weeks female

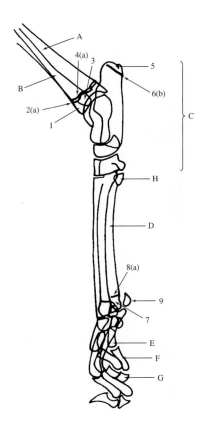

Figure 626

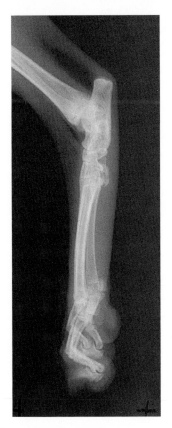

Figure 627   Age 36 weeks female

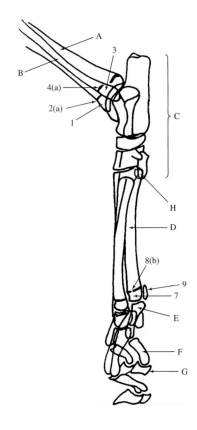

Figure 627

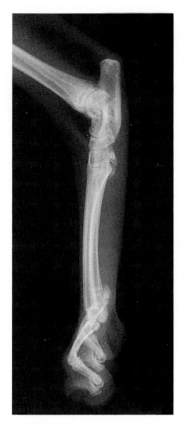

Figure 628   Age 40 weeks female

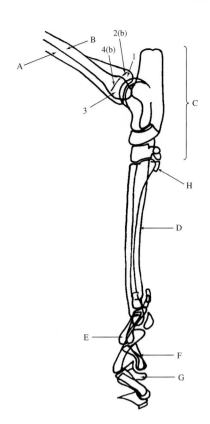

Figure 628

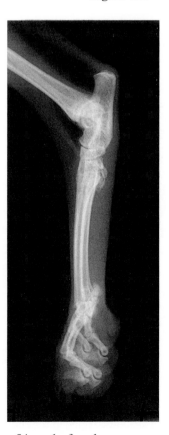

Figure 629   Age 54 weeks female

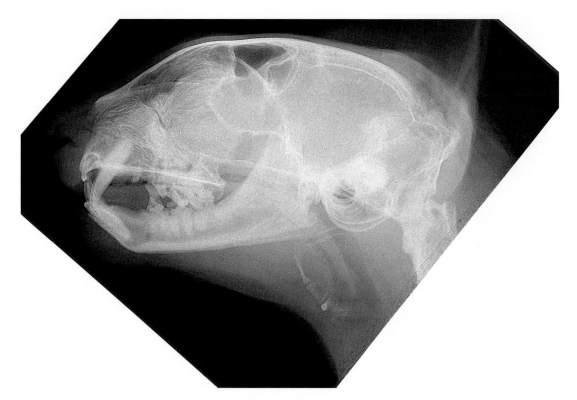

Figure 630   Lateral projection of skull. British domestic short haired cat 4 years old, neutered female.

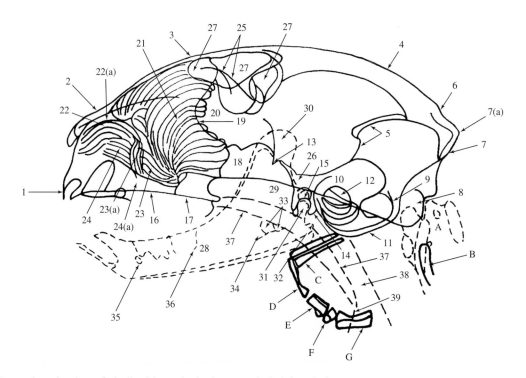

Figure 631   Lateral projection of skull with teeth shadows excluded for clarity.

(631 continued.)

A Atlas

B Axis

C Stylohyoid bone

D Epihyoid bone

E Ceratohyoid bone

F Basihyoid bone

G Thyrohyoid bone
  1 Incisive bone
  2 Nasal bone
  3 Frontal bone
  4 Parietal bone
  5 Osseous tentorium of the cerebellum
  6 Interparietal bone
  7 Occipital bone
    7(a) External occipital protuberance or 'Nuchal crest'
  8 Occipital condyle
  9 Jugular process of occipital bone
  10 Petrous temporal bone or temporal bone;petrosal part
  11 Tympanic bulla of temporal bone or temporal bone; tympanic part
  12 External acoustic meatus of temporal bone
  13 Zygomatic process of temporal bone or temporal bone; squamous part
  14 Retroarticular process of temporal bone
  15 Mandibular fossa of temporal bone
  16 Palatine process of maxilla. The vomer lies dorsally.
  17 Palatine bone. Rostrally the palatine process of maxilla is included.

18 Sphenoid sinus of presphenoid
19 Cribriform plate of ethmoid bone. Rostral limit only is visible.
20 Ethmoidal fossa
21 Ethmoidal conchae
22 Dorsal nasal conchae
    22(a) Dorsal nasal meatus
23 Middle nasal conchae
    23(a) Mass of conchae attached to the ethmoid bone, from the dorsal and middle conchae. Seen as a radiopaque region and must not be mistaken for a foreign body.
24 Ventral nasal conchae
    24(a) Ventral nasal meatus
25 Dorsal orbital margin
26 Basisphenoid bone
27 Frontal sinuses
28 Mandibular body
29 Mandibular ramus
30 Coronoid process of mandible
31 Condyloid or articular process of mandible
32 Angular process of mandible
33 Mandibular foramina
34 Mandibular canal
35 Mental foramen
36 Lamina dura
37 Soft palate
38 Nasopharynx
39 Epiglottis

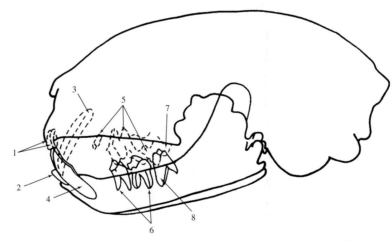

Figure 632 Lateral projection of skull to demonstrate details of teeth excluded in Figure 631.

1 Upper incisors. Total of six.
2 Lower incisors. Total of six.
3 Upper canines. Total of two.
4 Lower canines. Total of two.
5 Upper premolars. Total of six.

6 Lower premolars. Total of four.
7 Upper molars. Total of two.
8 Lower molars. Total of two.

Note that the term upper can be replaced by 'superior' and lower by 'inferior'.

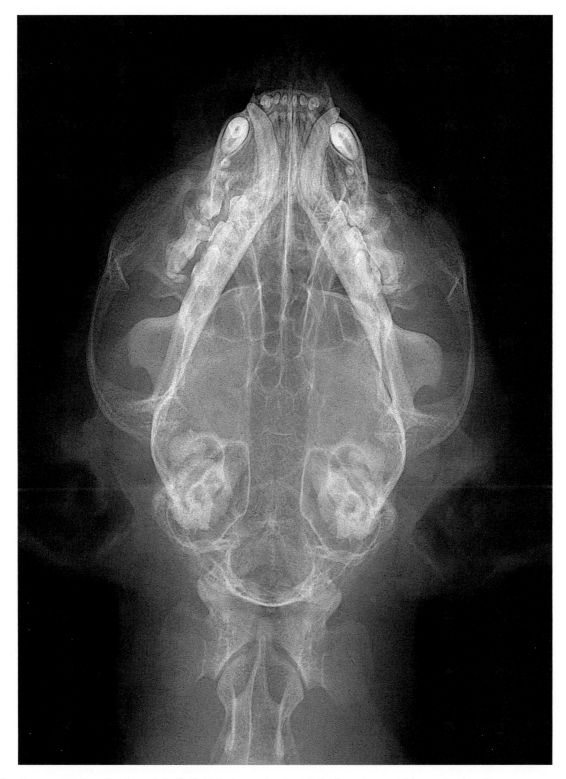

Figure 633   Dorsoventral projection of skull. British domestic short haired cat 1 year old, neutered male.

An Atlas of Interpretative Radiographic Anatomy of the Dog and Cat

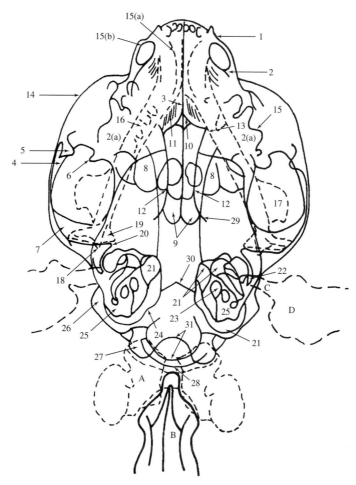

Figure 634 Dorsoventral projection of skull with teeth shadows excluded for clarity.

A Atlas

B Axis

C Cartilaginous ear canal

D Pinna
  1 Incisive bone
  2 Maxilla or maxillary bone
    2(a) Maxillary teeth obscuring bony shadows of maxillary bone (lamina dura seen as radiopaque lines)
  3 Vomer and nasal septum (the osseous part of the nasal septum contributes to the radiopaque line)
  4 Temporal process of zygomatic bone
  5 Frontal process of zygomatic bone
  6 Zygomatic process of frontal bone
  7 Zygomatic process of temporal bone. Forms zygomatic arch with (4).
  8 Frontal sinuses
  9 Sphenoidal sinuses
  10 Cribriform plate of ethmoid enclosing ethmoidal fossa
  11 Ethmoturbinates and dorsal nasal concha (dorsal nasal concha is not seen clearly on this projection)
  12 Border of choanae formed by palatine bone

13 Medial wall of orbit
14 Ventral margin of orbit
15 Lamina dura
  15(a) Mandibular lamina dura
  15(b) Maxillary lamina dura
16 Mandibular body
17 Coronoid process of mandibular ramus
18 Angular process of mandibular ramus
19 Condyloid or articular process of mandibular ramus
20 Retroarticular process of temporal bone
21 Tympanic bulla of temporal bone
22 External acoustic meatus of temporal bone
23 Internal acoustic meatus of temporal bone
24 Jugular foramen
25 Petrous temporal bone
26 Mastoid process of petrous temporal bone
27 Occipital condyle
28 Nuchal crest
29 Hamulus of pterygoid bone
30 Osseous tentorium of cerebellum
31 Foramen magnum

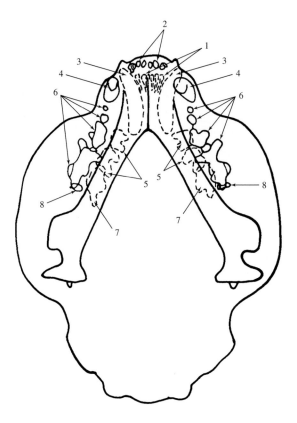

Figure 635   Dorsoventral projection of skull to demonstrate details of teeth shadows excluded in Figure 634.

1 Lower incisors. Total of six.
2 Upper incisors. Total of six.
3 Lower canines. Total of two.
4 Upper canines. Total of two.
5 Lower premolars. Total of four.
6 Upper premolars. (The 1st. premolar in this cat appears to be present, making a total of eight instead of six. (This is unusual.)
7 Lower molars. Total of two.
8 Upper molars. Total of two.

Note that the term lower can be replaced by 'inferior' and upper by 'superior'.

An Atlas of Interpretative Radiographic Anatomy of the Dog and Cat

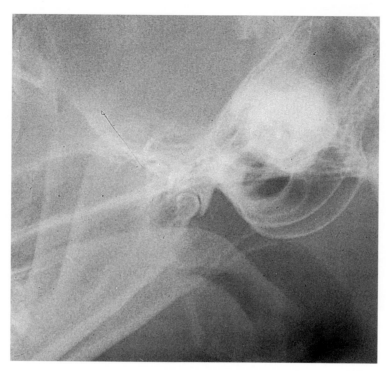

Figure 636   Relaxed lateral skull centred on temporomandibular joint. British domestic short haired cat 2 years old, neutered female.

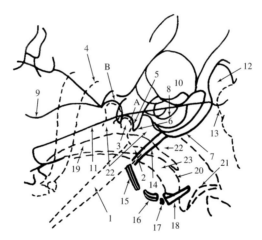

Figure 637   Relaxed lateral skull centred on temporomandibular joint.

A   Temporomandibular joint of recumbent side

B   Temporomandibular joint of non-recumbent side
  1   Body of mandible
  2   Angular process of mandible
  3   Condyloid or articular process of mandible
  4   Coronoid process of mandible
  5   Mandibular fossa of temporal bone
  6   Retroarticular process of temporal bone
  7   Tympanic bulla of temporal bone
  8   External acoustic meatus of temporal bone
  9   Cribriform plate
 10   Petrous temporal bone

11   Cranial base
12   Occipital condyle
13   Atlas
14   Stylohyoid bone
15   Epihyoid bone
16   Ceratohyoid bone
17   Basihyoid bone
18   Thyrohyoid bone
19   Soft palate
20   Epiglottis
21   Rostral limit of arytenoid cartilage
22   Nasopharynx
23   Oropharynx

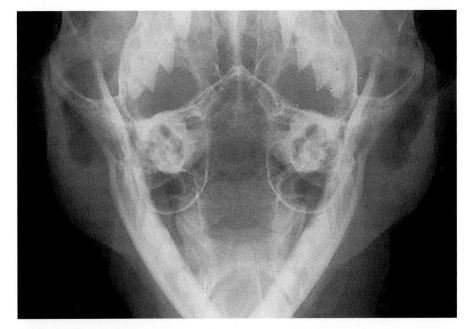

Figure 638   Rostroventral–caudodorsal oblique (open mouth) projection of skull centred on tympanic bullae. British domestic short haired cat 2 years old, neutered female.

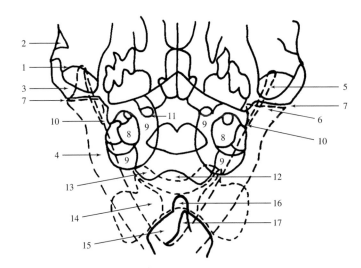

Figure 639   Rostroventral-caudodorsal oblique (open mouth) projection of skull centred on tympanic bullae.

1	Zygomatic bone	10	External acoustic meatus of temporal bone
2	Frontal process of zygomatic bone	11	Canal of auditory tube
3	Zygomatic process of temporal bone	12	Foramen magnum
4	Mandibular body	13	Condyle of occipital bone
5	Coronoid process of mandible	14	Atlas
6	Condyloid or articular process of mandible	15	Axis
7	Temporomandibular articulation	16	Dens of axis
8	Petrous temporal bone	17	Spinous process of axis
9	Tympanic bulla of temporal bone		

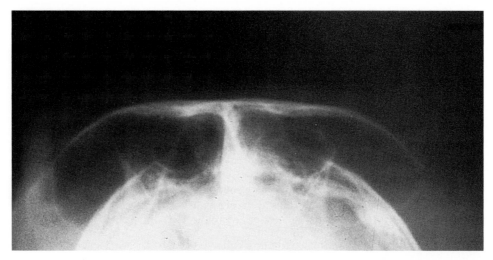

Figure 640 Rostrocaudal projection of skull centred on frontal sinuses. Siamese Cat 15 years old, neutered male.

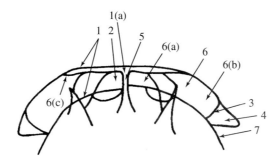

Figure 641 Rostrocaudal projection of skull centred on frontal sinuses.

1 Frontal bone
  1(a) Squamous part of frontal bone
2 Medial surface of frontal bone
3 Lateral surface of frontal bone
4 Zygomatic or supraorbital process of frontal bone. The size of the process varies as the orbital ligament is ossified. It is only 0.3cm long in 'immatures' but 1.3cm long in very old cats when it fuses with the zygomatic arch (Ray Ashdown, unpublished).
5 Septum between right and left frontal sinuses
6 Frontal sinus. The cat has only one sinus on each side.
  6(a) Medial part of frontal sinus containing ethmoidal ectoturbinates 1 and 2
  6(b) Lateral part of frontal sinus extending into the base of the zygomatic or supraorbital process
  6(c) Dorsal part of frontal sinus
The ventral limit of the frontal sinus is in the medial wall of the orbit. It does not reach as far as the sphenoid bone.
7 Parietal bone

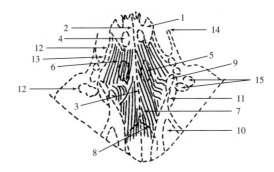

Figure 643 Dorsoventral intraoral projection of nasal chambers with teeth shadows excluded for clarity.

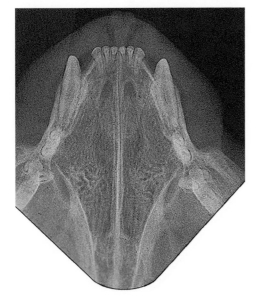

Figure 642 Dorsoventral intraoral projection of nasal chambers. British domestic short haired cat 7 months old, entire female.

1   Incisive bone
2   Incisive bone palatine process
3   Vomer and osseous part of nasal septum. The nasal septum extends rostrally from the ethmoid bone as a perpendicular plate of osseous and cartilaginous tissues.
4   Palatine fissure
5   Dorsal meatus of the nasal cavity
6   Nasal conchae (dorsal, middle and ventral turbinates)
7   Ethmoturbinates and dorsal nasal conchae

8   Cribriform plate of ethmoid enclosing ethmoidal fossa
9   Maxillary recess of maxilla
10 Frontal sinus
11 Medial wall of orbit

Anatomy of alveoli
12 Lamina dura
13 Periodontal membrane. Appears as a radiolucent line between lamina dura and tooth root.
14 Alveolar crest
15 Bony sockets or alveoli of lingual and vestibular roots of premolar 3

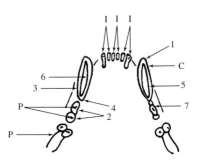

Figure 644 Dorsoventral intraoral projection of nasal chambers to demonstrate details of teeth shadows excluded from Figure 643.

Teeth
I   Upper incisors. Total of six.
C   Upper canine. Total of two.
P   Upper premolar. Total of six.

Upper molars, total of two, are not seen in this radiograph but can be seen in the same projection of a 2.5-year-old cat, Figure 645.

Note that the term upper can be replaced by 'superior'.

Anatomy of teeth
1   Crown
2   Tubercles
3   Root
4   Apex of root (still open at this age)
5   Dentine
6   Pulp cavity (Large in this 7-month-old cat but reduces considerably as cat ages. Compare with the same projection of a 2.5-year-old cat Figure 645.)
7   Enamel

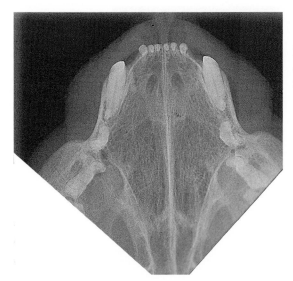

Figure 645 Dorsoventral intraoral projection of nasal chambers. British domestic short haired cat 2.5 years old, neutered female.

This radiograph has been included to illustrate the normal age changes that occur within the nasal chambers and teeth.

The definition of the nasal conchae is reduced as the cat ages but more dramatically teeth pulp cavities become much smaller with advancing years.

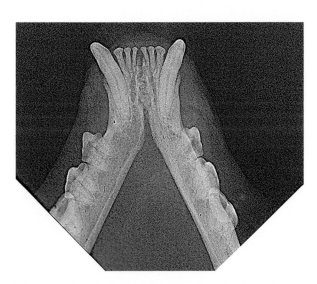

Figure 646 Ventrodorsal intraoral projection of mandibular bodies. British domestic short haired cat 2 years old, neutered female.

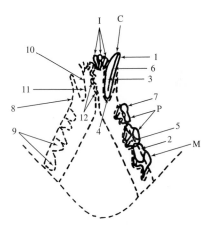

Figure 647 Ventrodorsal intraoral projection of mandibular bodies with teeth shadows excluded from the right mandibular body so that bony features are more easily identified.

Teeth
I   Lower incisors. Total of six.
C   Lower canine. Total of two.
P   Lower premolar. Total of four
M   Lower molar. Total of two.

Note that the term lower can be replaced by 'inferior'.

Anatomy of teeth
1   Crown
2   Tubercle
3   Root
4   Apex of root
5   Dentine

6   Pulp cavity
7   Enamel

Anatomy of alveoli
8   Alveolar crest
9   Bony sockets or alveoli
10 Lamina dura
11 Periodontal membrane. appears as a radiolucent line between lamina dura and tooth root.
12 Mandibular symphysis. Note that this is seen as a radiolucent shadow due to the fibrocartilaginous union present.

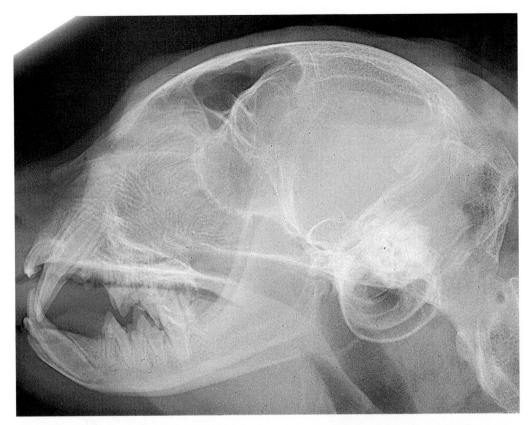

Figure 648   Lateral projection of skull. Persian cat 9 months old, neutered male.

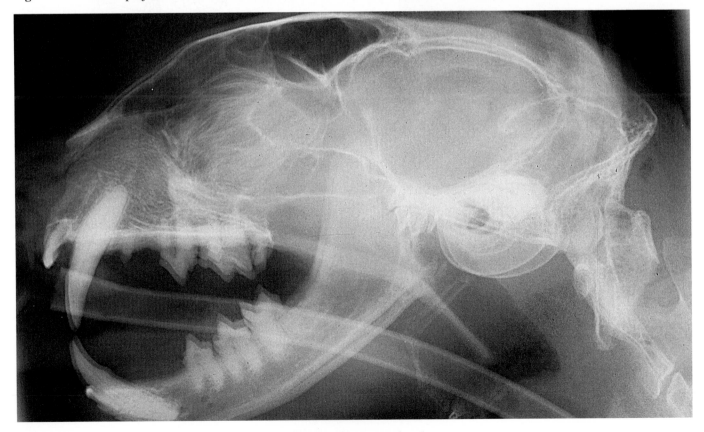

Figure 649   Lateral projection of skull. Siamese cat 9 years old, neutered male.

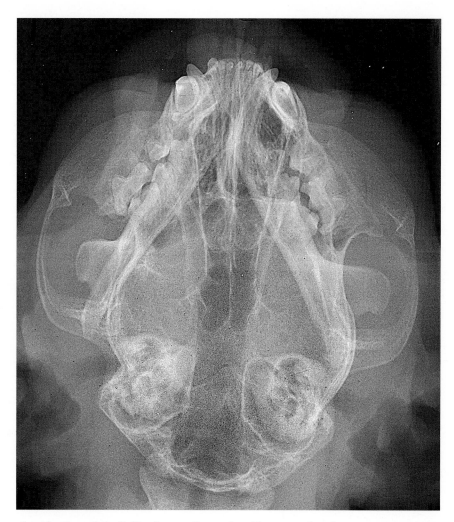

Figure 650 Dorsoventral projection of skull. Persian cat 9 months old, neutered male.

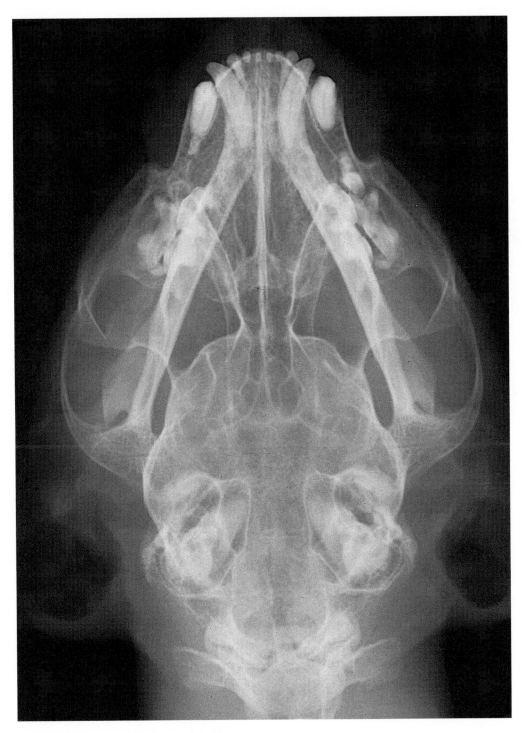

Figure 651   Dorsoventral projection of skull. Russian Blue cat.

An Atlas of Interpretative Radiographic Anatomy of the Dog and Cat

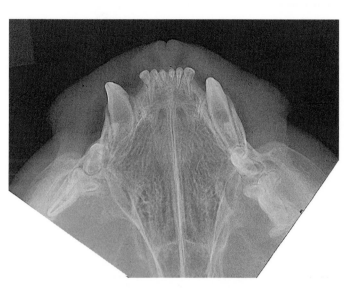

Figure 652 Dorsoventral intraoral projection of nasal chambers. Persian cat 6 months old, neutered male.

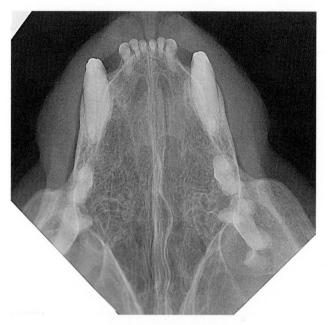

Figure 653 Dorsoventral intraoral projection of nasal chambers. Siamese cat 9 years old, neutered male. The radiograph shows the vomer to have a wavy curvature throughout its entire length. Nasal septum and vomer variations are not uncommon, especially in the cat, but in this case the extent of the curvature is unusual (see also Figure 284, Samoyed dog).

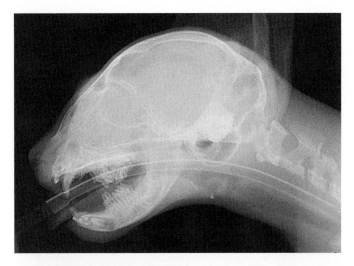

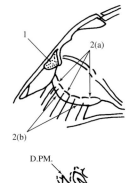

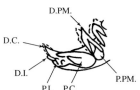

Figure 654   Age 12 weeks male

Figure 654

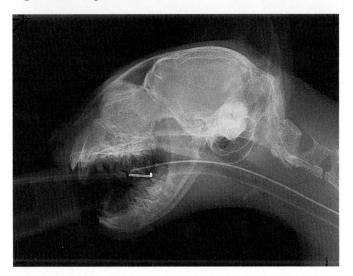

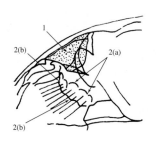

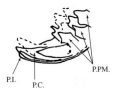

Figure 655   Age 24 weeks male

Figure 655

Figures 654, 655, 656, 657, 658, 659   Lateral projection of skull.
British domestic short haired cats at 12 weeks entire male, 24 weeks entire male, 36 weeks entire female, 46 weeks entire female, 54 weeks entire female, and 68 weeks entire male.

Correlating line drawings for all males at 12, 24 and 68 weeks of age

Drawing to demonstrate frontal sinuses and ethmoidal region

1 Frontal sinuses (Shaded areas)

2 Cribriform plate
   2(a) Caudal limit
   2(b) Rostral limit

Drawing to demonstrate lower or inferior teeth within rostral portion of mandible

D Deciduous teeth
   D.I.   Incisors
   D.C.   Canine
   D.PM. Premolars

P Permanent teeth seen as germs only at 12 weeks of age
   P.I.   Incisors
   P.C   Canine
   P.PM. Premolars
   P.M.   Molar

Dental formulae for the cat

Deciduous teeth	I3	C1	PM3	
	3	1	2	
Permanent teeth	I3	C1	PM3	M1
	3	1	2	1

The premolar teeth in the cat are the equivalent of premolars 2, 3, and 4 in the upper jaw and premolars 3 and 4 in the lower jaw of the dog.

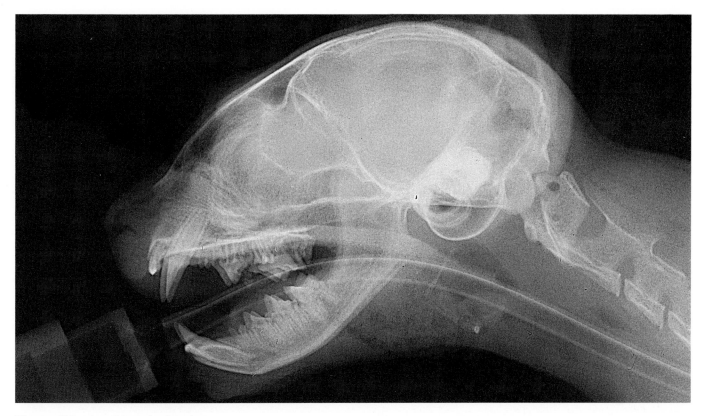

Figure 656   Age 36 weeks female

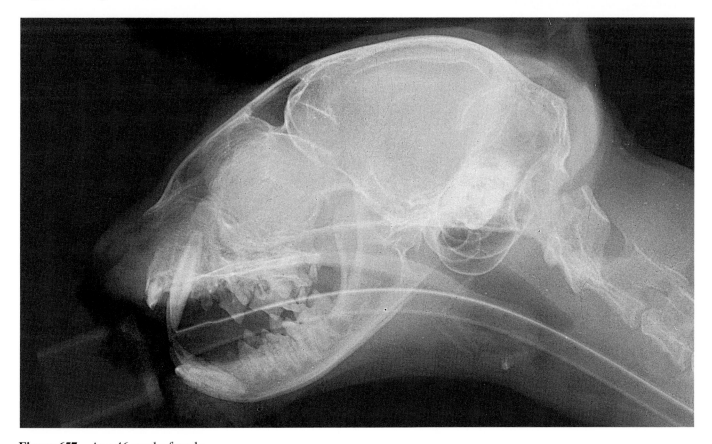

Figure 657   Age 46 weeks female

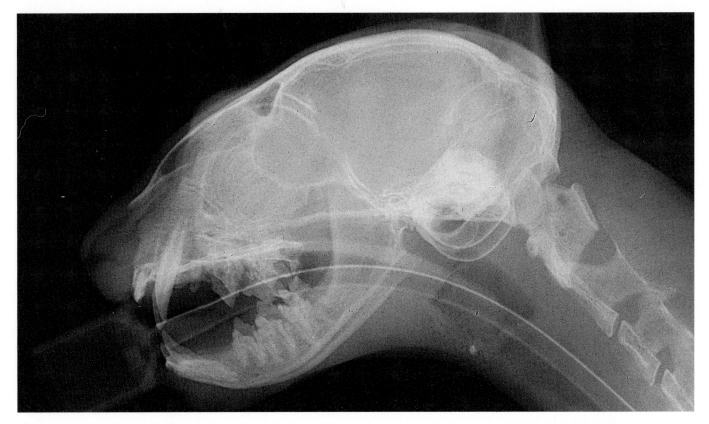

Figure 658   Age 54 weeks female

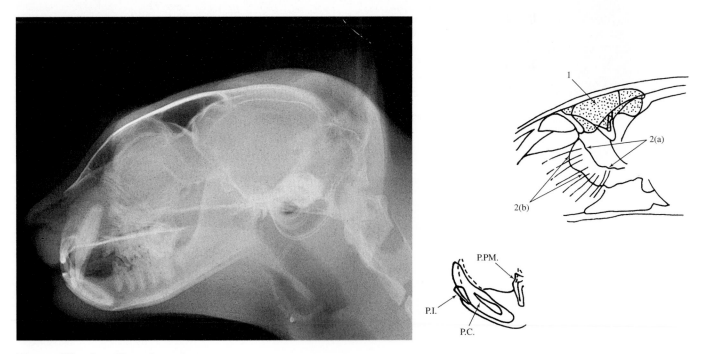

Figure 659   Age 68 weeks male

Figure 659

An Atlas of Interpretative Radiographic Anatomy of the Dog and Cat

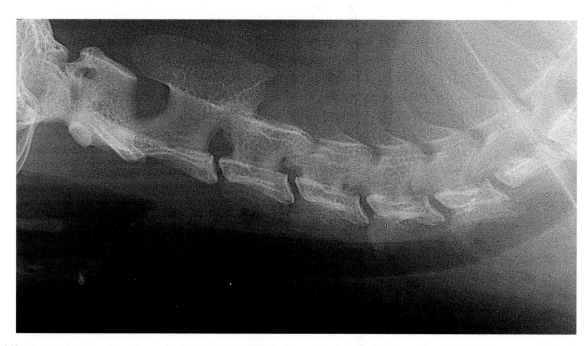

Figure 660   Lateral projection of cervical vertebrae. British domestic short haired cat 18 months old, neutered female.

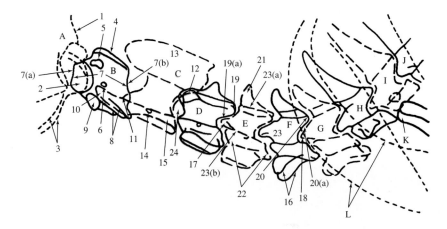

Figure 661   Lateral projection of cervical vertebrae.

A Skull
  1 Occipital bone
  2 Occipital condyle
  3 Tympanic bullae

B Atlas
  4 Dorsal arch
  5 Lateral vertebral foramen
  6 Vascular foramen
  7 Articular foveae
      7(a) Cranial articular fovea rostral edge
      7(b) Caudal articular fovea caudal edge
  8 Wings; transverse processes
  9 Ventral arch; body

C Axis
  10 Dens
  11 Cranial articular surface
  12 Caudal articular surface
  13 Spinous process
  14 Transverse foramen
  15 Transverse process

D 3rd. cervical vertebra

E 4th. cervical vertebra

F 5th. cervical vertebra

G 6th. cervical vertebra

H 7th. cervical vertebra
  16 Transverse processes
  17 Cranial articular surface of 4th. cervical vertebra
  18 Cranial articular surface of 6th. cervical vertebra
  19 Caudal articular surface of 3rd. cervical vertebra
      19(a) Intervertebral synovial joint of 3rd. and 4th. cervical vertebrae
  20 Caudal articular surface of 5th. cervical vertebra
      20(a) Intervertebral synovial joint of 5th. and 6th. cervical vertebrae
  21 Spinous process
  22 Body
  23 Vertebral foramen
      23(a) Dorsal margin
      23(b) Ventral margin
  24 Intervertebral foramen

I 1st. thoracic vertebra

J 2nd. thoracic vertebra

K 1st. rib

L Scapulae

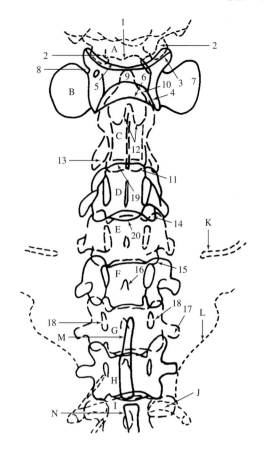

Figure 663   Ventrodorsal projection of cervical vertebrae.

A Skull
   1 Occipital bone
   2 Occipital condyle

B Atlas
   3 Cranial articular fovea
   4 Caudal articular fovea
   5 Ventral arch, body,
     cranial border
   6 Ventral arch, body,
     caudal border
   7 Wing; transverse process
   8 Alar notch

C Axis
   9 Dens
  10 Cranial articular surface
  11 Caudal articular surface
  12 Spinous process
  13 Transverse process

D 3rd. cervical vertebra

E 4th. cervical vertebra

F 5th. cervical vertebra

G 6th. cervical vertebra

H 7th. cervical vertebra
  14 Cranial articular surface
     of 4th. cervical vertebra
  15 Caudal articular surface
     of 4th. cervical vertebra
  16 Spinous process
  17 Transverse process
  18 Lateral margin of
     vertebral foramen
  19 Dorsal cranial margin of
     body of 3rd. cervical
     vertebra
  20 Ventral caudal margin of
     body of 3rd. cervical
     vertebra

I 1st. thoracic vertebra

J 1st. rib

K Clavicle

L Scapula

M Manubrium of sternum

N 2nd. sternebra of sternum

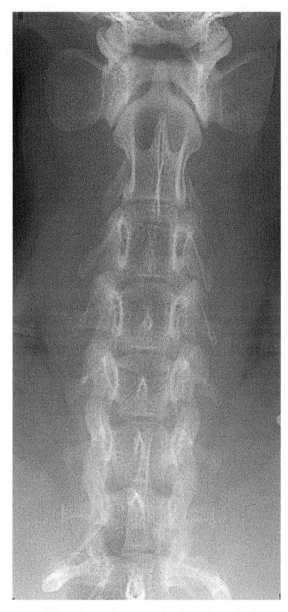

Figure 662   Ventrodorsal projection of cervical vertebrae. British domestic short haired cat 3 years old, neutered female.

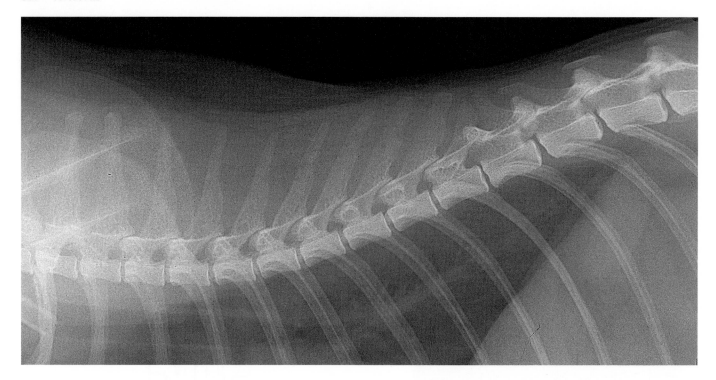

Figure 664   Lateral projection of thoracic vertebrae. British domestic short haired cat 8 years old, neutered female.

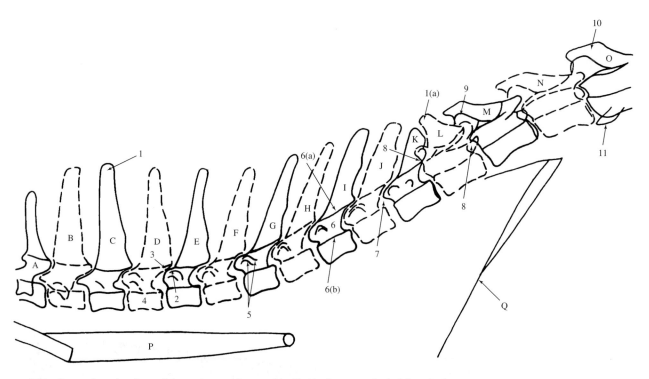

Figure 665   Lateral projection of thoracic vertebrae with rib shadows excluded for clarity.

(665 continued)

A 7th. cervical vertebra

B 1st. thoracic vertebra

C 2nd. thoracic vertebra

D 3rd. thoracic vertebra

E 4th. thoracic vertebra

F 5th. thoracic vertebra

G 6th. thoracic vertebra

H 7th. thoracic vertebra

I 8th. thoracic vertebra

J 9th. thoracic vertebra

K 10th. thoracic vertebra

L 11th. thoracic vertebra. Anticlinal vertebra.

M 12th. thoracic vertebra

N 13th. thoracic vertebra

1 Spinous process
  1(a) Spinous process of anticlinal vertebra; nearly perpendicular to axis
2 Cranial articular process of 4th. thoracic vertebra
3 Caudal articular process of 3rd. thoracic vertebra
4 Body
5 Transverse process
6 Vertebral foramen
  6(a) Dorsal margin
  6(b) Ventral margin
7 Intervertebral foramen
8 Accessory process
9 Mamillary process

O 1st. lumbar vertebra
10 Spinous process
11 Transverse process

P Trachea

Q Diaphragm

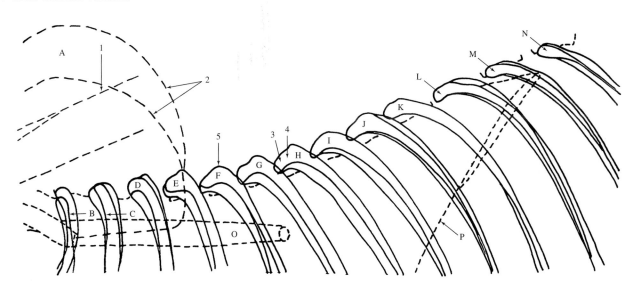

Figure 666 Lateral projection of thoracic vertebrae to demonstrate the rib shadows not seen in Figure 665.

A Scapula
  1 Spine
  2 Dorsal margins

B 1st. rib

C 2nd. rib

D 3rd. rib

E 4th. rib

F 5th. rib

G 6th. rib

H 7th. rib

I 8th. rib

J 9th. rib

K 10th. rib

L 11th. rib

M 12th. rib

N 13th. rib
  3 Head
  4 Neck
  5 Tubercle

O Trachea

P Diaphragm

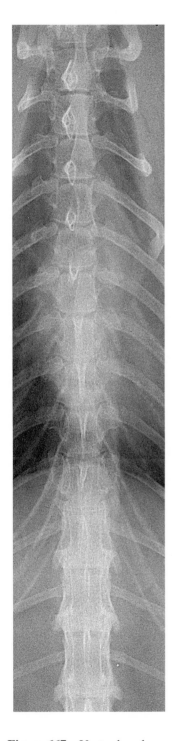

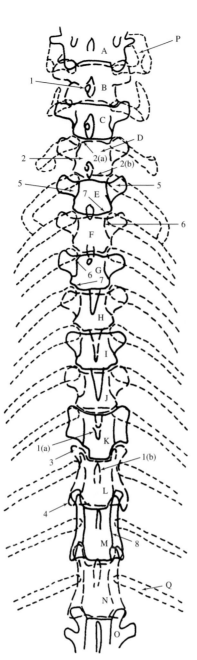

Figure 668 Ventrodorsal projection of thoracic vertebrae with ventral ribs and sternal shadows excluded for clarity.

A 7th. cervical vertebra

B 1st. thoracic vertebra

C 2nd. thoracic vertebra

D 3rd. thoracic vertebra

E 4th. thoracic vertebra

F 5th. thoracic vertebra

G 6th. thoracic vertebra

H 7th. thoracic vertebra

I 8th. thoracic vertebra

J 9th. thoracic vertebra

K 10th. thoracic vertebra

L 11th. thoracic vertebra. Anticlinal vertebra.

M 12th. thoracic vertebra

N 13th. thoracic vertebra
   1 Spinous process of 1st. thoracic vertebra. These processes incline caudally from 1st. to 10th. thoracic vertebrae.
      1(a) Spinous process of 10th. thoracic vertebra
      1(b) Spinous process of 11th. thoracic vertebra
   2 Body
      2(a) Cranial margin
      2(b) Caudal margin
   3 Mamillary process of 11th. thoracic vertebra
   4 Accessory process of thoracic vertebra
   5 Transverse process
   6 Cranial costal fovea of body
   7 Caudal costal fovea of body
   8 Lateral margin of vertebral foramen

O 1st. lumbar vertebra

P 1st. rib

Q 13th. rib

Figure 667 Ventrodorsal projection of thoracic vertebrae. British domestic short haired cat 8 years old, neutered female.

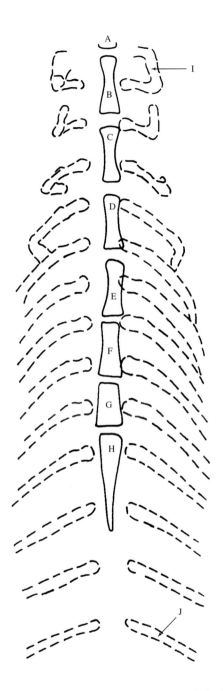

Figure 669   Ventrodorsal projection of thoracic vertebrae to demonstrate sternal shadows not seen in Figure 668.

A Manubrium of sternum

B 2nd. sternebra

C 3rd. sternebra

D 4th. sternebra

E 5th. sternebra

F 6th. sternebra

G 7th. sternebra

H 8th. sternebra

I 1st. rib

J 13th. rib

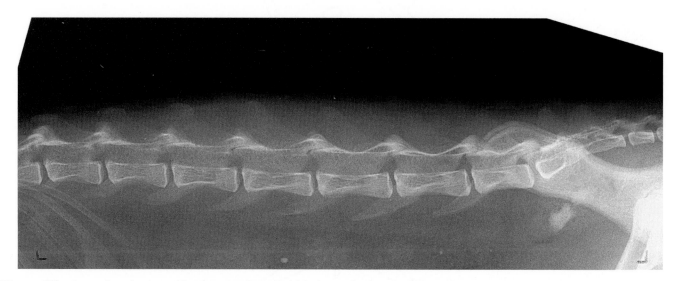

Figure 670 Lateral projection of lumbar vertebrae. British domestic short haired cat 6 years old, neutered male.

An Atlas of Interpretative Radiographic Anatomy of the Dog and Cat

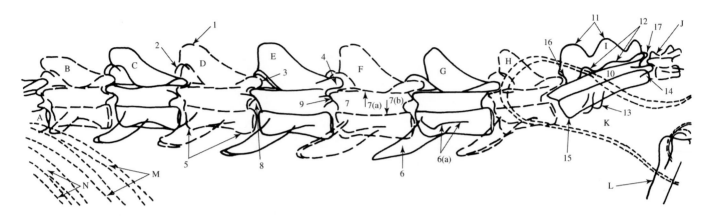

Figure 671   Lateral projection of lumbar vertebrae.

A 13th. thoracic vertebra

B 1st. lumbar vertebra

C 2nd. lumbar vertebra

D 3rd. lumbar vertebra

E 4th. lumbar vertebra

F 5th. lumbar vertebra

G 6th. lumbar vertebra

H 7th. lumbar vertebra
  1 Spinous process
  2 Mamillary process
  3 Cranial articular process of 4th. lumbar vertebra
  4 Caudal articular process of 4th. lumbar vertebra
  5 Body
  6 Transverse process
     6(a) Base of transverse process
  7 Vertebral foramen
     7(a) Dorsal margin
     7(b) Ventral margin
  8 Intervertebral foramen
  9 Accessory process

I Sacrum
  10 Sacral canal
  11 Median sacral crest; spinous processes
  12 Intermediate sacral crest; articular processes
  13 Lateral sacral crest; cranial transverse processes, 1st. and 2nd. sacral segments. Includes the wing which is thought to include two rib elements on each side
  14 Lateral sacral crest; caudal transverse processes, 3rd. sacral segment
  15 Promontory
  16 Cranial articular process of sacrum forming the lumbosacral synovial joint
  17 Caudal articular process of sacrum forming the sacrococcygeal synovial joint

J 1st. coccygeal or caudal vertebra

K Ilium

L Femur

M 13th. ribs

N 12th. ribs

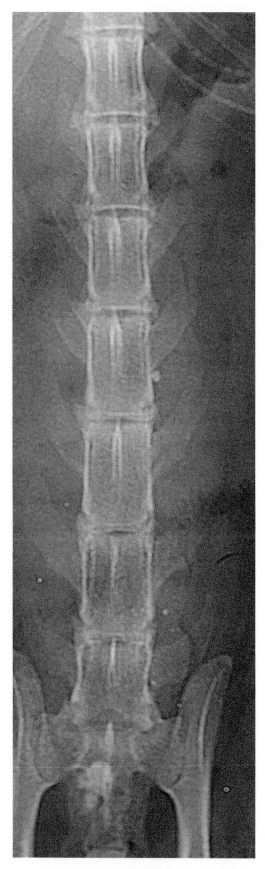

Figure 672 Ventrodorsal projection of lumbar vertebrae. British domestic short haired cat 6 years old, neutered male.

An Atlas of Interpretative Radiographic Anatomy of the Dog and Cat

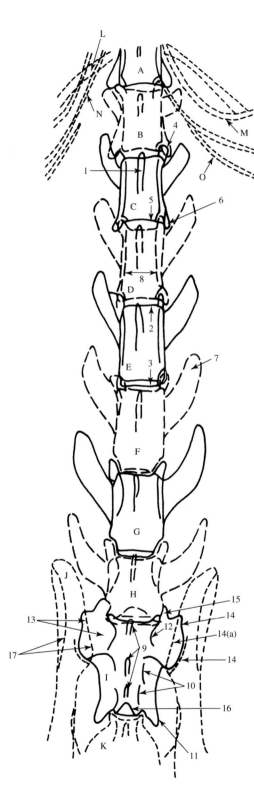

Figure 673 Ventrodorsal projection of lumbar vertebrae.

A 13th. thoracic vertebra

B 1st. lumbar vertebra

C 2nd. lumbar vertebra

D 3rd. lumbar vertebra

E 4th. lumbar vertebra

F 5th. lumbar vertebra

G 6th. lumbar vertebra

H 7th. lumbar vertebra
  1 Spinous process
  2 Cranial margin of body of 4th. lumbar vertebra
  3 Caudal margin of body of 4th. lumbar vertebra
  4 Cranial articular process of 2nd. lumbar vertebra
  5 Caudal articular process of 2nd. lumbar vertebra
  6 Accessory process of 2nd. lumbar vertebra
  7 Transverse process
  8 Lateral margins of vertebral foramen

I Sacrum
  9 Median sacral crest; spinous processes

10 Intermediate sacral crest; articular processes of 1st., 2nd. and 3rd. sacral segments

11 Lateral sacral crest; transverse process of 3rd. sacral segment. Those of 1st. and 2nd. form the sacral wing

12 Lateral margin of sacral canal

13 Wing

14 Sacroiliac joint
  14(a) Ventral limit of sacroiliac joint

15 Cranial articular process

16 Caudal articular process

J Ilium
  17 Tuber sacrale; dorsal iliac spine

K 1st. coccygeal or caudal vertebra

L 13th. rib

M Costal cartilage of 10th. rib (calcified)

N Costal cartilage of 11th. rib (calcified)

O Costal cartilage of 12th. rib (calcified)

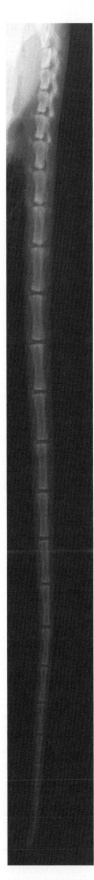

Figure 674 Lateral projection of coccygeal or caudal vertebrae. British domestic short haired cat 6 years old, neutered male.

An Atlas of Interpretative Radiographic Anatomy of the Dog and Cat

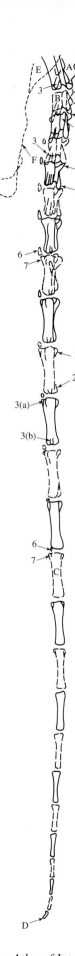

Figure 675 Lateral projection of coccygeal or caudal vertebrae.

A Sacrum

B 1st. coccygeal vertebra

C 13th. coccygeal vertebra

D 24th. coccygeal vertebra
  1 Cranial articular process
  2 Caudal articular process
  3 Transverse process
    3(a) Cranial transverse process
    3(b) Caudal transverse process
  4 Spinous process
  5 Vertebral foramen
  6 Haemal arch
  7 Haemal process

E Ilium

F Ischium

Although this projection would appear simple to achieve note the cranial position of the 1st. coccygeal vertebra. This cranial extent of the 1st. coccygeal vertebra creates an exposure problem when radiography of the whole coccygeal region is required. Often the caudal sacral/proximal coccygeal area is underexposed in order not to overexpose the thinner distal coccygeal vertebrae.

The most common error is to underestimate the cranial position of the 1st. coccygeal vertebra and hence not to include the caudal sacrum/proximal coccygeal area in the primary beam.

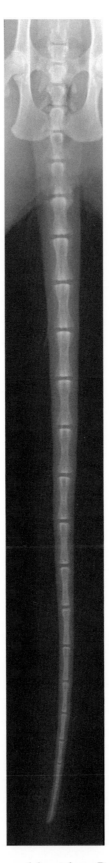

Figure 676   Ventrodorsal projection of coccygeal or caudal vertebrae. British domestic short haired cat 6 years old, neutered male.

An Atlas of Interpretative Radiographic Anatomy of the Dog and Cat

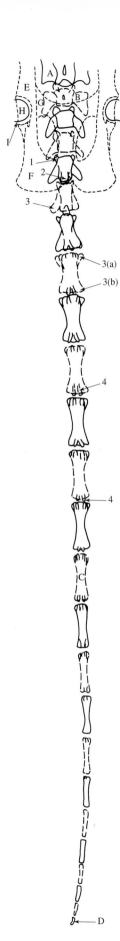

Figure 677   Ventrodorsal projection of coccygeal or caudal vertebrae.

A   Sacrum

B   1st. coccygeal vertebra

C   13th. coccygeal vertebra

D   24th. coccygeal vertebra
   1   Cranial articular process
   2   Caudal articular process
   3   Transverse process
     3(a)   Cranial transverse process
     3(b)   Caudal transverse process
   4   Haemal process

E   Ilium

F   Ischium

G   Pubis

H   Acetabulum

I   Femur

Please see notes about radiography of the lateral projection of coccygeal or caudal vertebrae, Figure 675, as the same applies to this ventrodorsal projection.

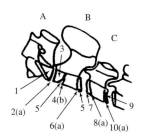

Figure 678

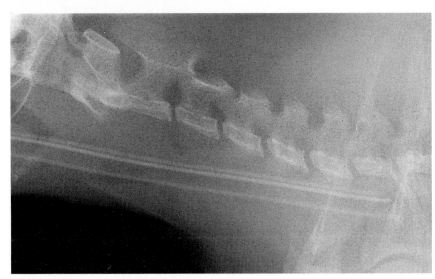

Figure 678   Age 12 weeks male

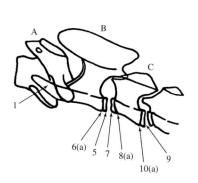

Figure 679

Figure 679   Age 24 weeks male

Figures 678, 679, 680, 681, 682   Lateral projection of cervical vertebrae.
British domestic short haired cats at 12 weeks entire male, 24 weeks entire male, 36 weeks entire female, 46 weeks entire female, and 54 weeks entire female.

Correlating line drawings for all ages except 46 and 54 weeks.

A Atlas. 1st. cervical vertebra.

B Axis. 2nd. cervical vertebra.
  1 Centrum for dens
  2 Growth plate
    2(a) Open
  3 Centrum for cranial epiphysis of body
  4 Cranial growth plate
    4(a) Closing
  5 Caudal epiphysis of body
  6 Caudal growth plate
    6(a) Open
    6(b) Closing

C 3rd. cervical vertebra
  7 Cranial epiphysis
  8 Cranial growth plate
    8(a) Open
    8(b) Closing
  9 Caudal epiphysis
  10 Caudal growth plate
    10(a) Open
    10(b) Closing

  For clarity transverse process shadows have been excluded from all drawings.

An Atlas of Interpretative Radiographic Anatomy of the Dog and Cat

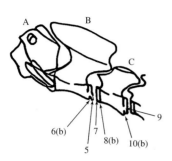

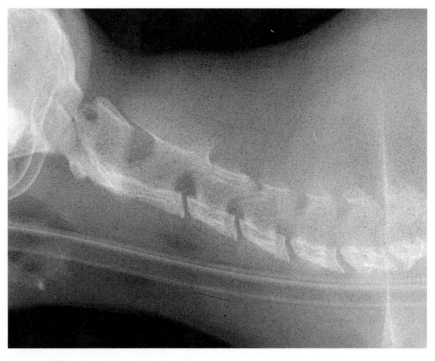

Figure 680

Figure 680   Age 36 weeks female

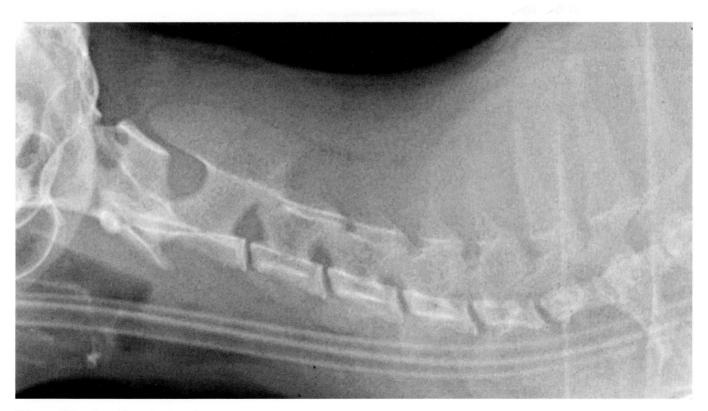

Figure 681   Age 46 weeks female

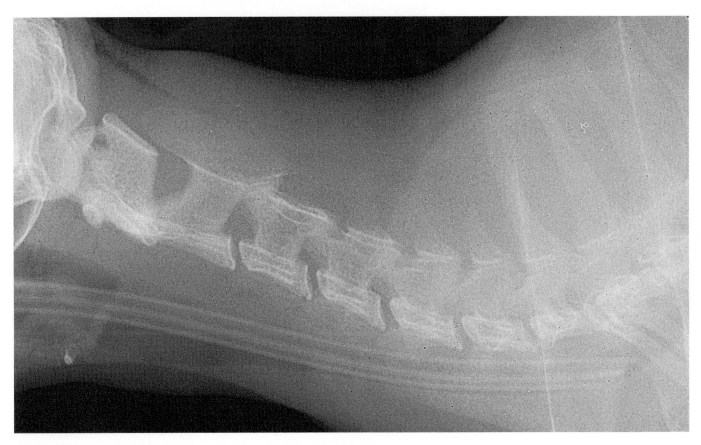

Figure 682   Age 54 weeks female

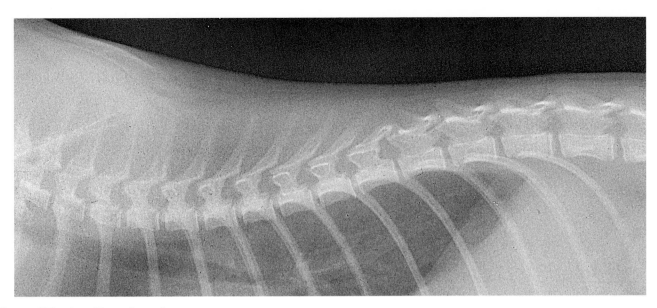

Figure 683   Age 12 weeks male

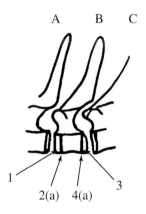

Figure 683

Figures 683, 684, 685, 686, 687   Lateral projection of thoracic vertebrae.
British domestic short haired cats at 12 weeks entire male, 24 weeks entire male, 36 weeks entire female, 46 weeks entire female, and 54 weeks entire female.

Correlating line drawings for all ages except 46 and 54 weeks.

A 3rd. thoracic vertebra

B 4th. thoracic vertebra
   1 Cranial epiphysis of body
   2 Cranial growth plate
      2(a) Open
      2(b) Closing

3 Caudal epiphysis of body
4 Caudal growth plate
   4(a) Open
   4(b) Closing

C 5th. thoracic vertebra

   For clarity the rib shadows have been excluded from all drawings.

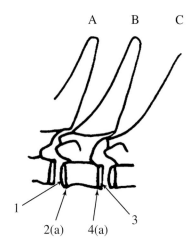

A   B   C

1

2(a)   4(a)

3

Figure 684

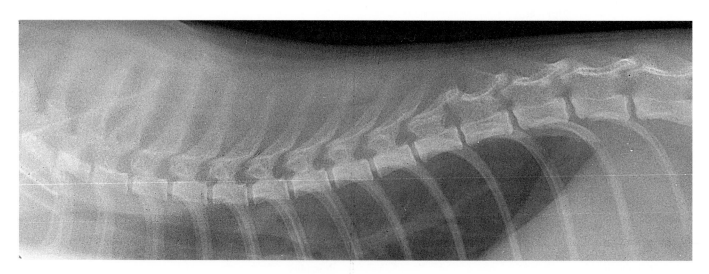

Figure 684   Age 24 weeks male

An Atlas of Interpretative Radiographic Anatomy of the Dog and Cat

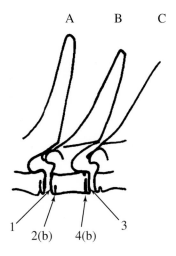

Figure 685

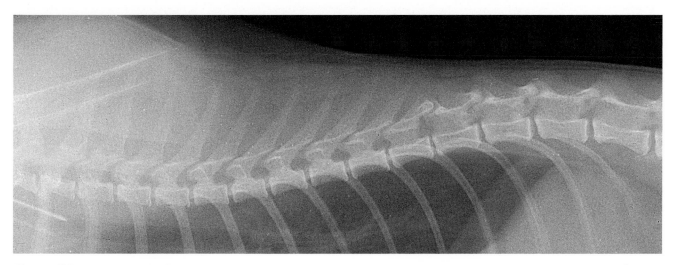

Figure 685   Age 36 weeks female

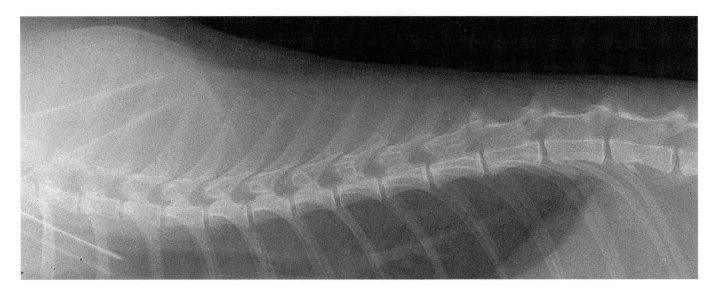

Figure 686   46 weeks female

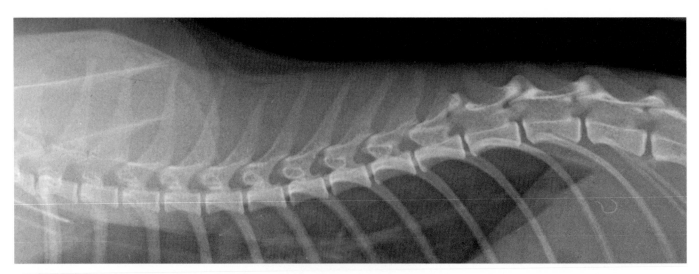

Figure 687   Age 54 weeks female

An Atlas of Interpretative Radiographic Anatomy of the Dog and Cat

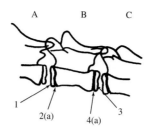

Figure 688

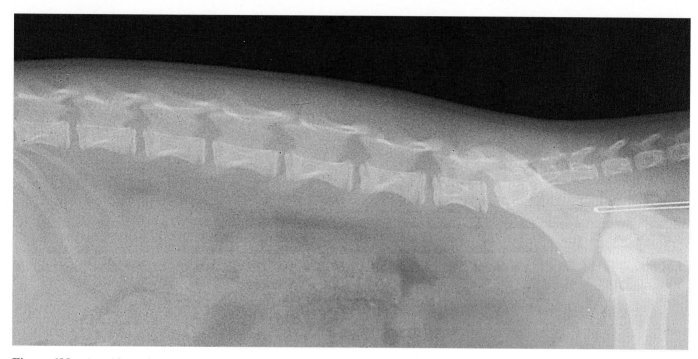

Figure 688   Age 12 weeks male

Figures 688, 689, 690, 691, 692   Lateral projection of lumbar vertebrae. British domestic short haired cats at 12 weeks entire male, 24 weeks entire male, 36 weeks entire female, 46 weeks entire female, 54 weeks entire female.

Correlating line drawings for all ages except 46 and 54 weeks.

A 4th. lumbar vertebra

B 5th. lumbar vertebra
  1 Cranial epiphysis of body
  2 Cranial growth plate
    2(a) Open
    2(b) Closing
  3 Caudal epiphysis of body
  4 Caudal growth plate
    4(a) Open
    4(b) Closing

C 6th. lumbar vertebra

For clarity the transverse process shadows have been excluded from all drawings.

At 24 weeks of age the 3rd. sacral segment, or sacral vertebra, can be seen as a separate segment.

By 36 weeks of age fusion of the 3rd. sacral segment has taken place.

At 36 weeks of age the iliac crest of the pelvis can be seen as a separate ossification centre. This ossification centre was not seen on the ventrodorsal projections of the pelvis.

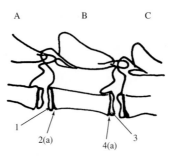

Figure 689

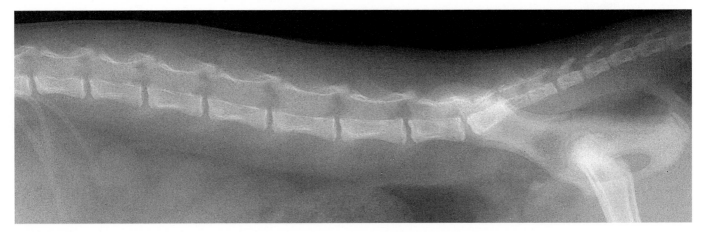

Figure 689   Age 24 weeks male

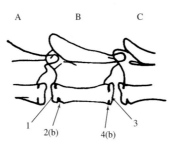

Figure 690

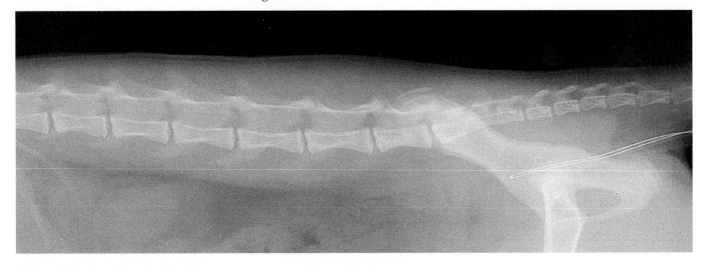

Figure 690   Age 36 weeks female

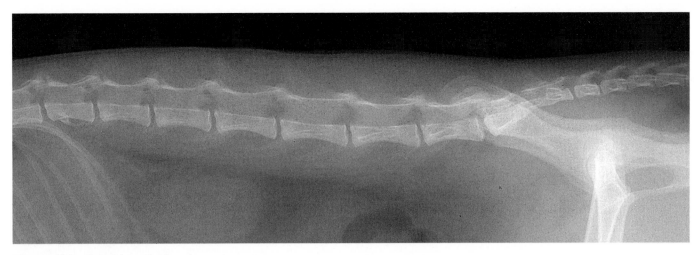

Figure 691   Age 46 weeks female

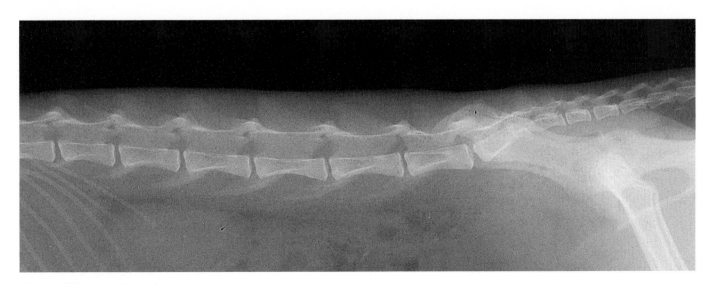

Figure 692   Age 54 weeks female

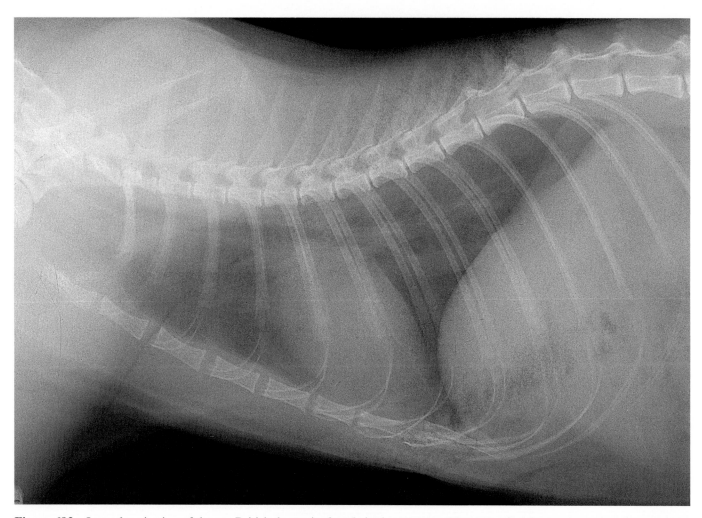

Figure 693   Lateral projection of thorax. British domestic short haired cat 1 year old, neutered male.

An Atlas of Interpretative Radiographic Anatomy of the Dog and Cat

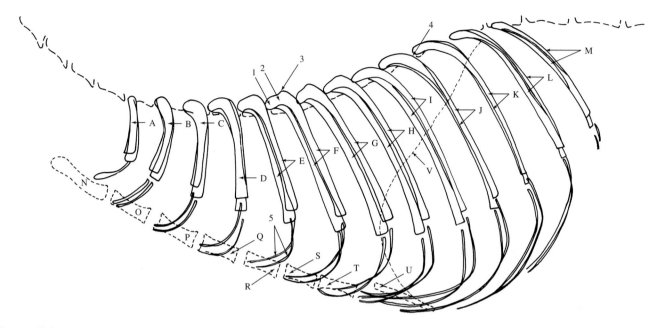

Figure 694 Lateral projection of thorax to demonstrate rib shadows.

A 1st. pair of ribs

B 2nd. pair of ribs

C 3rd. pair of ribs

D 4th. pair of ribs

E 5th. pair of ribs

F 6th. pair of ribs

G 7th. pair of ribs

H 8th. pair of ribs

I 9th. pair of ribs

J 10th. pair of ribs

K 11th. pair of ribs

L 12th. pair of ribs

M 13th. pair of ribs

   1st. to 9th. pairs of ribs are sternal while 10th. to 13th. are asternal. The 13th. pair of ribs is floating.

1 Head of rib
2 Neck of rib
3 Tubercle of rib
4 Angle of rib
5 Costal cartilages. Cartilages of 10, 11 and 12 form the costal arch. The cartilages are calcified except for the most dorsal aspects. 1st. and 13th. rib cartilages are poorly calcified in this cat.

N Manubrium of sternum

O 2nd. sternebra

P 3rd. sternebra

Q 4th. sternebra

R 5th. sternebra

S 6th. sternebra

T 7th. sternebra

U Xiphoid process

V Diaphragm

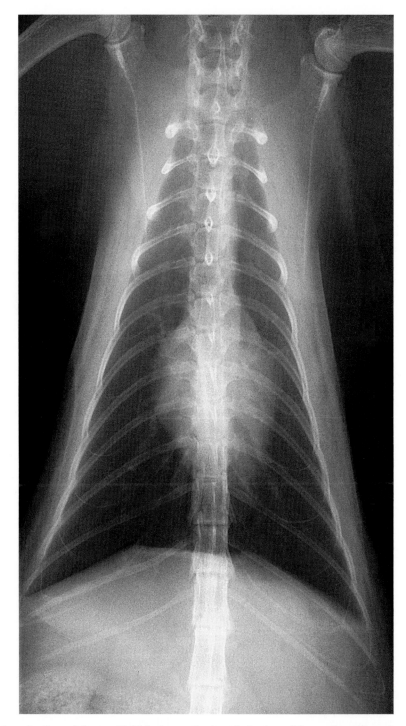

Figure 695   Ventrodorsal projection of thorax. British domestic short haired cat 10 months old, entire female.

An Atlas of Interpretative Radiographic Anatomy of the Dog and Cat

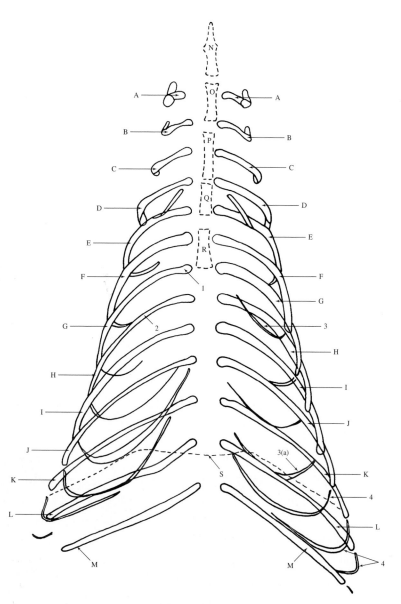

Figure 696   Ventrodorsal projection of thorax to demonstrate rib shadows.

A   1st. pair of ribs

B   2nd. pair of ribs

C   3rd. pair of ribs

D   4th. pair of ribs

E   5th. pair of ribs

F   6th. pair of ribs

G   7th. pair of ribs

H   8th. pair of ribs

I   9th. pair of ribs

J   10th. pair of ribs

K   11th. pair of ribs

L   12th. pair of ribs

M   13th. pair of ribs

1   Head of rib

2   Body of rib

3   Costal cartilage (calcified)

    3(a) Costal cartilage of 9th. rib, last sternal rib

4   Costal cartilages of asternal ribs 10, 11 and 12, which make up the costal arch

N   Manubrium of sternum

O   2nd. sternebra

P   3rd. sternebra

Q   4th. sternebra

R   5th. sternebra

    6th., 7th. and xiphoid process, 8th. sternebra, are not discernible

S   Diaphragm

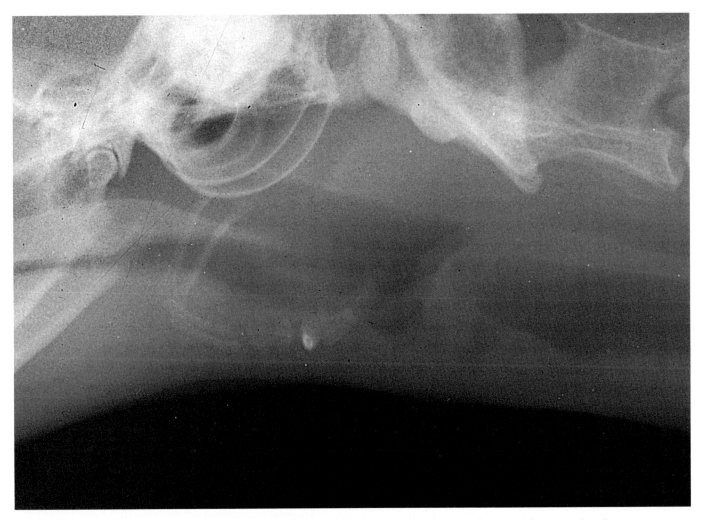

Figure 697 Lateral projection of pharynx and larynx. British domestic short haired cat 6 years old, neutered male.

An Atlas of Interpretative Radiographic Anatomy of the Dog and Cat

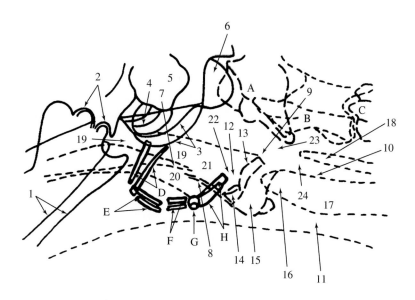

Figure 698   Lateral projection of pharynx and larynx.

1 Mandibular bodies
2 Temporomandibular joints
3 Tympanic bullae of temporal bones
4 External acoustic meatus of temporal bone
5 Petrous temporal bone
6 Occipital condyle

A Atlas

B Axis

C 3rd. cervical vertebra

D Stylohyoid bones

E Epihyoid bones

F Ceratohyoid bones

G Basihyoid bone

H Thyrohyoid bones
   7 Soft palate
   8 Epiglottis

9 Cranial limit of laryngeal part of pharynx
10 Caudal limit of laryngeal part of pharynx. Caudal limit
   is the caudal border of the cricoid cartilage.
11 Caudal limit of larynx
12 Position of the rostral cornu of thyroid cartilage
13 Rostral limit of the arytenoid cartilage. The corniculate
   process of the arytenoid cartilage is missing in
   the cat.
14 Vestibular fold
15 Glottic cleft. The cat lacks lateral ventricles and has
   instead shallow depressions.
16 Infraglottic cavity
17 Trachea
18 Oesophagus
19 Nasopharynx
20 Oropharynx
21 Intrapharyngeal ostium
22 Laryngeal vestibule
23 Thyropharyngeal muscle
24 Cricopharyngeal muscle

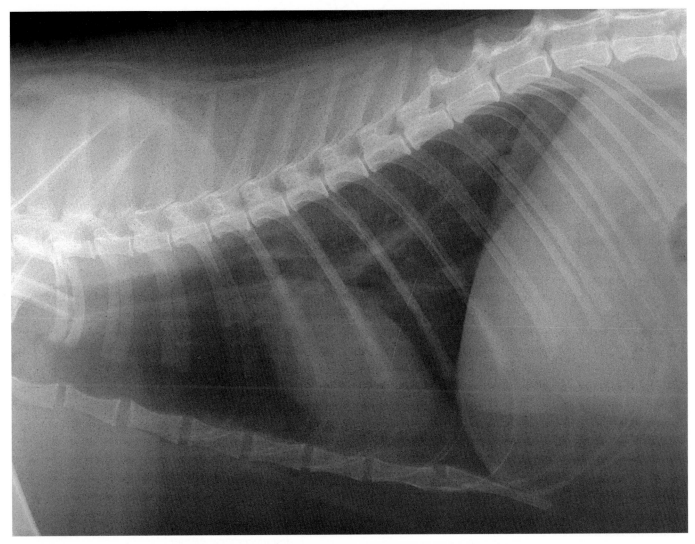

Figure 699   Right lateral recumbent projection of thorax. Radiograph taken during general anaesthesia with inflation of lung lobes. British domestic short haired cat 6 years old, neutered male (same cat as in left lateral recumbent projection of thorax, Figure 713).

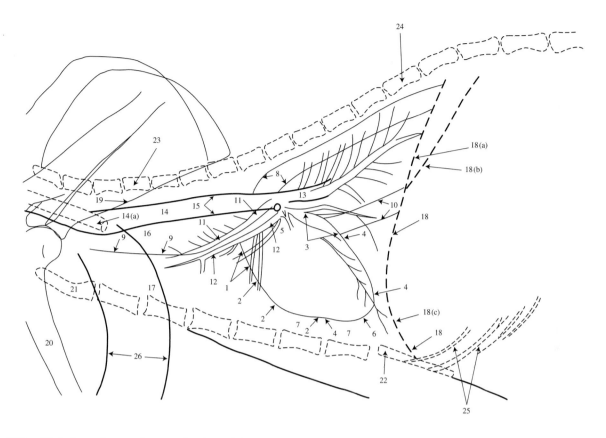

Figure 700   Right lateral recumbent projection of thorax to highlight cardiovascular system.

Pericardium and heart

Cranial border
1   Right auricle
2   Right ventricle

In this projection the aortic arch is not visible but a large aortic arch is more commonly seen in the cat than the dog. It appears as a distinct bulge at the cranial border, at or below the right auricle level, extending into the cranial mediastinum. Where the aortic arch covers the cranial waist the cardiac shadow appears cranially tilted with an increase in sternal contact.

Caudal border
3   Left atrium
4   Left ventricle

Although the cat has a cranial and caudal waistline, as in the dog, using these as a guideline for cardiac enlargement is not as straightforward, particularly for the caudal waistline. Separation of left atrium and left ventricle is more difficult and enlargements often do not affect the waistline.

5   Dorsal base
6   Apex

Fat accumulation within the pericardial sac is only occasionally seen in the cat but care must be taken to differentiate between soft tissue and fat opacities. In this radiograph fat opacity is visible outside the pericardium on the ventral thoracic cavity wall (7).

The right lateral recumbency is preferred for the cardiac shadow, as discussed in the dog section. In addition, the projection should be at full inflation of the lung lobes.

This film is not as fully inflated as the left lateral recumbent projection of thorax of the same cat, Figure 713. As such, the vascular shadows are more prominent and the cardiac shadow is slightly cranially tilted. However, craniocaudal and dorsoventral cardiac measurements for both projections are the same.

Right and left lateral recumbent projections of thoracic cavity in forced inflation, or over-inflation, of lung lobes, Figures 705 and 706, have been included to show the effect of 'loss' of pulmonary radiographic opacity and 'upright' cardiac shadows caused by hyperinflation.

(700 continued.)

Vascular

8 Thoracic aorta.(Aortic arch is not clearly seen as a separate structure in this radiograph.)

9 Ventral limit of cranial vena cava

10 Caudal vena cava

11 Cranial lobe artery

12 Cranial lobe vein

The radiolucent shadow between the paired cranial vessels is the lumen of the cranial lobe bronchus. It should not be mistaken for an air bronchogram. An air bronchogram is a characteristic radiographic feature of an alveolar pattern. The latter occurs in diseases which cause an infiltration into the alveoli. Soft tissue opacity replaces the alveolar air lucency resulting in adjacent air-filled lumens of the bronchi to become visible.

Bronchial walls are not generally visible in the cat unless they are diseased.

13 Pulmonary artery and veins

The arrangement of pulmonary veins is different in the cat as compared to the dog. In the dog the veins are symmetrically arranged as left and right sets of lobar veins.

In the cat there are three groups draining: the two parts of the left cranial lobe; the middle and cranial lobes of the right side; and caudal lobes of the right and left lungs. Each of these groups is of two or three veins and they are not symmetrically arranged. Hence radiographic differentiation of veins in the cat is very difficult.

Non cardiovascular structures

14 Tracheal lumen
    14(a) Endotracheal tube

15 Tracheal walls

16 Cranial mediastinum

17 Ventral mediastinum. (See juvenile section, Figure 721, for appearance in kittens when the thymus occupies the entire cranioventral mediastinum at a level ventral to the cranial vena cava. It also extends 1 to 2 cm cranial to the 1st. ribs into the neck.)

18 Diaphragmatic shadow
    18(a) Right 'crus'
    18(b) Left 'crus'
    18(c) Cupola

In this radiograph the appearance of the right and left 'crura' would suggest left rather than right recumbency. Identification of lateral recumbency is more difficult in the cat than the dog. Often 'crura' are superimposed and, as in this radiograph, are misleading.

Entry of the caudal vena cava is usually unhelpful leaving only the gastric gas, caudal to the left 'crura', as a guide for recumbency analysis. In this radiograph insufficient gas was present to show the presence of the gastric fundus caudal to the left 'crura'.

19 Caudal border of scapula

20 Humerus

21 Manubrium of sternum

22 Xiphoid process

23 1st. thoracic vertebra

24 11th. thoracic vertebra

25 Calcified costal cartilages

26 Skin and muscle masses of forelimbs

'Variations'

It is widely reported that the cat has a fairly standard shape and size for its cardiac shadow, compared to the breed variation seen in dogs.

With this assumption radiographically normal thoracic projections, from clinically normal cats with no evidence of cardiac abnormalities, should have been relatively easy to obtain (see 'normality' in the Introduction). This was not the case as many cats were found to have cardiac 'enlargements' from their radiographic shadows.

A series of radiographs, Figures 709–712, has been included to alert the reader to possible variation in cardiac shadows or, more seriously, latent cardiac disease.

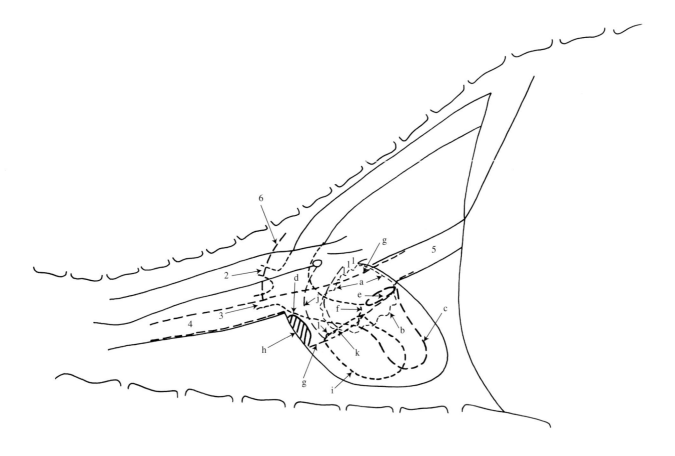

Figure 701 Schematic drawing of right lateral recumbent projection of thorax to illustrate cardiac chambers and major vessels (corresponds to line drawing Figure 700, but with the exclusion of some thoracic cavity details seen in the radiograph).

Left side with associated vessels
a = Left atrium with pulmonary veins (1)
b = Left auricle
c = Left ventricle (drawing does not indicate wall thickness)
d = Aorta with left subclavian artery (2) and brachiocephalic trunk (3). Aortic arch forms the most cranial structure of the 'heart and major vessels'.
e = Left atrioventricular valve; mitral. Length is usually about 25% of the craniocaudal width of the heart.
f = Aortic valve

Right side with associated vessels
g = Right atrium with cranial vena cava (4) and caudal vena cava (5) and azygous vein (6)
h = Right auricle. Right auricle is in contact with aortic arch and almost forms the cranial border of the 'heart' mass at the cardiac base.
i = Right ventricle (drawing does not indicate wall thickness)
j = Pulmonary trunk; main pulmonary artery or pulmonary artery segment
k = Right atrioventricular valve; tricuspid. Length is usually about 50% of the craniocaudal width of the heart. It overlaps both aorta and pulmonary artery.
l = Pulmonary valve

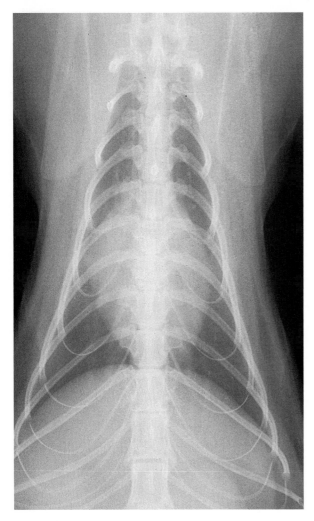

Figure 702 Dorsoventral projection of thorax. Radiograph taken during general anaesthesia with inflation of lung lobes. British domestic short haired cat 10 months old, neutered female (same cat as in ventrodorsal projection of thorax, Figure 716).

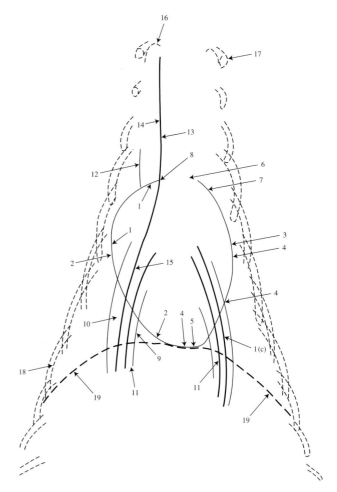

Figure 703 Dorsoventral projection of thorax to highlight cardiovascular system.

Pericardium and heart

Right side
  1 Right atrium
  2 Right ventricle

Left side
  3 Left auricle
  4 Left ventricle
  5 Level of apex; formed by left ventricle. (Unfortunately the apex is not clearly visible in this film due to superimposition of bony shadows of vertebral bodies and ribs.)

Vascular

  6 Level of aortic arch. (The aortic arch and the descending aorta cannot be seen in this film.) In young cats the aortic arch is often obscured by thymic tissue while in aged cats this structure may become enlarged and distorted (see Figure 708).
  7 Pulmonary trunk; main pulmonary artery
  8 Level of cranial vena cava within cranial mediastinum soft tissue opacity. (The soft tissue shadows have been obscured by bony shadows of the thoracic vertebrae, ribs and sternebrae.)

9 Level of caudal vena cava. (The vein is not seen as a separate shadow in this film.) It can be distinguished as a linear soft tissue shadow in the ventrodorsal projection of thorax radiograph, Figure 719.
10 Arteries to caudal lung lobe
11 Veins to caudal lung lobe
12 Right cranial lobe artery. Occasionally the corresponding lobar vein is seen medial to the artery. Between these paired vessels a linear radiolucent shadow is created. As in the lateral recumbent projections the lucent shadow must not be mistaken for an air bronchogram. (Air bronchograms appear in disease as a characteristic radiographic feature of an alveolar pattern. See (12) in right lateral recumbent projection of thorax, Figure 700.)

Non-cardiovascular structures
13 Tracheal lumen
14 Tracheal wall
15 Caudal lobe bronchus
16 Pleural cupola
17 1st. rib
18 8th. rib
19 Diaphragmatic shadow

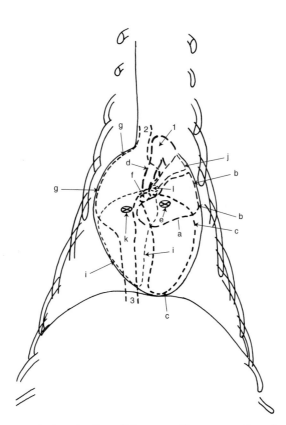

Figure 704 Schematic drawing of dorsoventral projection of thorax to illustrate cardiac chambers and major vessels (corresponds to line drawing Figure 703, but with the exclusion of some thoracic cavity details seen in the radiograph).

Left side with associated vessels
a = Left atrium
b = Left auricle
c = Left ventricle (diagram does not indicate wall thickness)
d = Aorta with aortic arch (1)
e = Left atrioventricular valve; mitral
f = Aortic valve

Right side with associated vessels
g = right atrium with cranial vena cava (2) and caudal vena cava (3)
h = Right auricle
i = Right ventricle (diagram does not indicate wall thickness)
j = Pulmonary trunk; main pulmonary artery
k = Right atrioventricular valve; tricuspid
l = Pulmonary valve

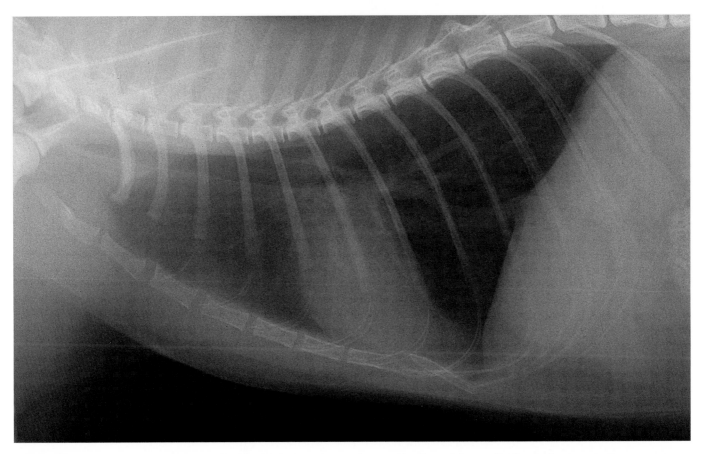

Figure 705   Forced or over-inflation of lungs. Right lateral recumbent projection of thorax. Radiograph taken during general anaesthesia with forced or over-inflation of lung lobes. British domestic short haired cat 10 months old, entire female (same cat as in Figures 706 and 719).

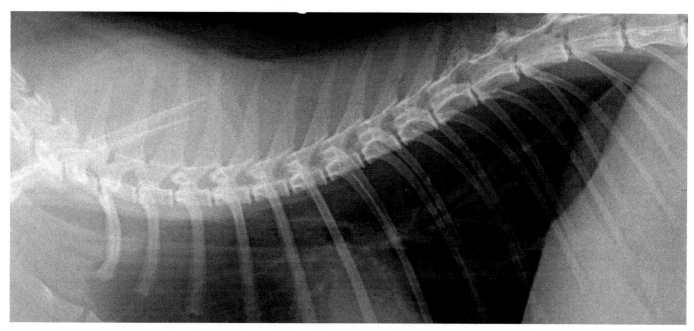

Figure 706 Forced or over-inflation of lungs. Left lateral recumbent projection of thorax. Radiograph taken during general anaesthesia with forced or over inflation of lung lobes. British domestic short haired cat 10 months old, entire female (same cat as in Figures 705 and 719).

These lateral recumbent projections have been included to demonstrate the effect of forced inflation on radiographic opacity and cardiac shadow.

Although when analysing pulmonary features good radiolucency is preferable to poor radiolucency for the lung lobes, the contrast with forced inflation is so high that soft tissue shadows of blood vessels, heart and bronchial walls are less distinct when compared to films in full inflation. The hyperlucency of the lung lobes require bright light illumination for full evaluation of all the lung fields and cardiac outline.

The effect on cardiac shadow is also worthy of note. The cardiac shadow appears overall smaller in area compared to the shadow in full inflation. Also, a caudal rotation occurs changing the cardiac outline to become 'upright' in appearance. This rotation results in an increased dorsoventral measurement, at the maximum cardiac depth, while decreasing the craniocaudal measurement at the maximum cardiac width.

In addition, the diaphragmatic shadow is flattened, especially ventrally, making the cupola indistinguishable as a distinct part of the diaphragmatic shadow.

Radiographic shadows in this cat are normal and the corresponding ventrodorsal projection of thorax can be found in Figure 719.

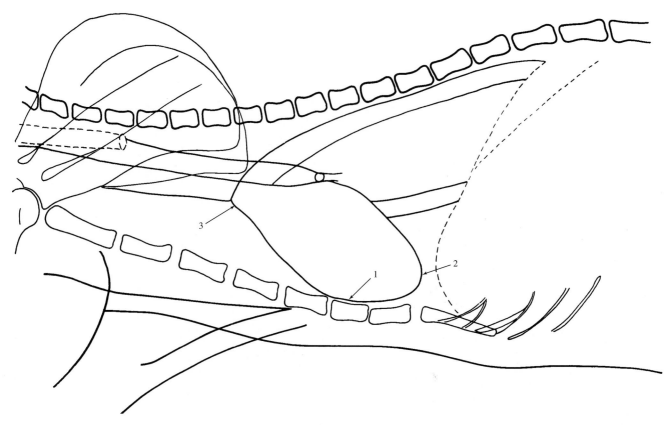

Figure 707 Line drawing to demonstrate cardiovascular changes associated with age in the cat. Left lateral recumbent projection of thorax (Corresponds to original radiograph not included in the book. The radiograph was taken during general anaesthesia and at full inflation of lung lobes.). British domestic short haired cat 14 years old, neutered female. The line drawing corresponds to a radiograph of the 14-year-old cat showing no clinical signs of cardiac disease which was radiographed as a routine in a study of feline rhinitis.

Note the cranial rotation of the cardiac shadow despite full inflation of lung lobes and correct radiographic positioning for the thoracic cavity. The rotation has created an abnormally large craniocaudal measurement for the cardiac shadow, with increase in sternal contact (1).

In addition, the cranial rotation has caused apex (2) to be dorsally elevated. The latter is not a common feature of a diseased heart resulting in left-sided enlargement. Left-sided cardiac enlargement more often shows the apex to be closer to the sternum with an overall increase in cardiac sternal contact. The horizontal position of the cardiac shadow is further exaggerated in this film by the enlarged aortic arch (3).

The cardiac and aortic shadows seen and described in this aged cat are thought to be normal variations in the geriatric cat. However, care must be taken to ensure that cardiac disease is not present. This age group often shows cardiac abnormality, most commonly hypertrophic cardiomyopathy.

The dorsoventral projection of thorax of this cat did not show any evidence of left-sided enlargement. A large, well-defined aortic arch shadow was seen but there was no unusual curvature of the arch or descending aorta.

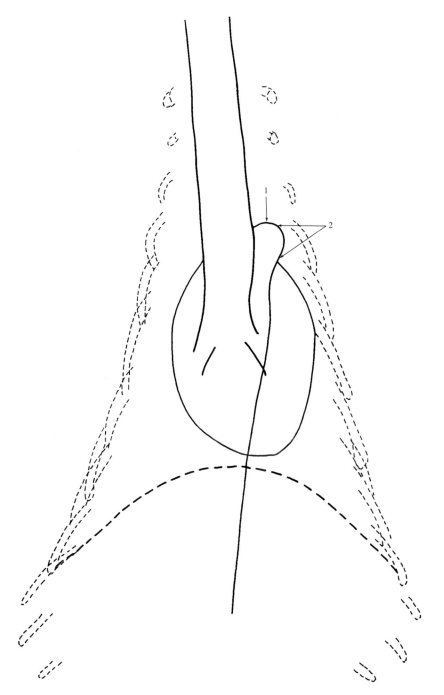

Figure 708   Line drawing to demonstrate cardiovascular changes associated with age in the cat. Dorsoventral projection of thorax (Corresponds to original radiograph not included in the book. The radiograph was taken during general anaesthesia and at full inflation of lung lobes.) British domestic short haired cat 11 years old, neutered male. The line drawing corresponds to a radi-ograph of the 11-year-old cat showing no clinical signs of cardiac disease which was radiographed as a routine in a study of feline rhinitis.

  Note the aortic arch (1) which appears large. A knob or knuckle shape (2) is seen at the junction of the arch and descending aorta; aortic isthmus.

  The appearance of the aorta, as above, is thought to be a normal variation of the aged cat.

  The lateral recumbent projection of thorax of this cat showed similar changes to the 14-year-old cat (Figure 707) with respect to the cardiac and aortic shadows. In addition, a radiopaque appearance of the elongated aortic arch at the level of the aortic isthmus was present.

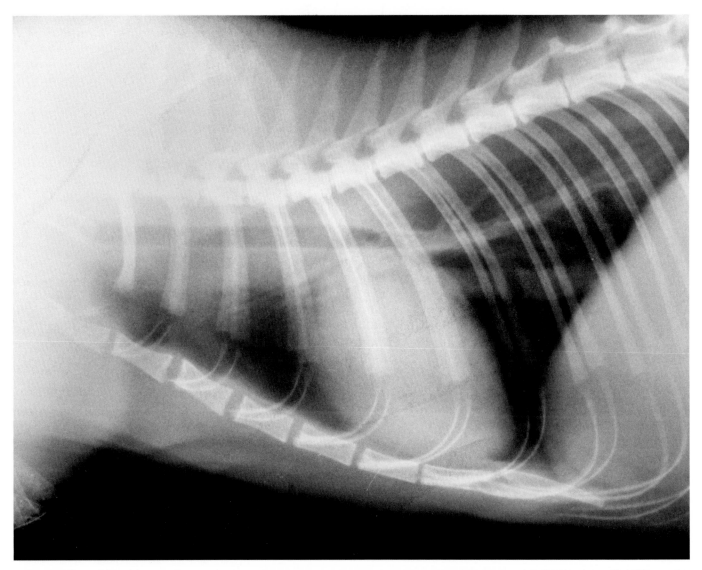

Figure 709 Cardiac 'variations'. Right lateral recumbent projection of thorax. Radiograph taken during general anaesthesia with full inflation of lung lobes. British domestic short haired cat 7 years old, neutered male (same cat as in left lateral recumbent projection of thorax, Figure 710).

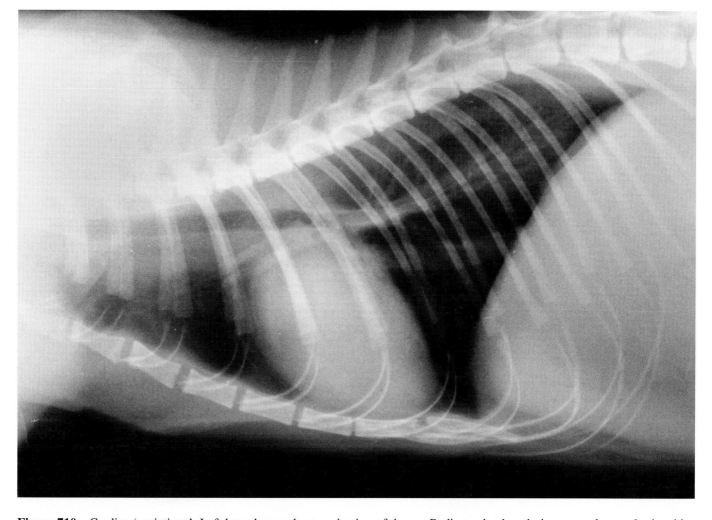

Figure 710 Cardiac 'variations'. Left lateral recumbent projection of thorax. Radiograph taken during general anaesthesia with full inflation of lung lobes. British domestic short haired cat 7 years old, neutered male (same cat as in right lateral recumbent projection of thorax, Figure 709).

These projections have been included to illustrate the comments made about cardiac shadow 'variations' (see text of right lateral recumbent projection of thorax, Figure 700) with reference to latent clinical disease.

They were taken as a screening procedure for possible pulmonary metastasis prior to digital amputation of an osteosarcoma. It was noted that the cardiac shadow appeared larger than expected. No cardiac abnormalities were present from clinical signs and examination. Echocardiography and electrocardiography were not performed at this time.

Following digital amputation the cat made an uneventful recovery but within 18 months was involved in a road traffic accident. The cat was hospitalised after being presented to the emergency duty veterinary surgeon.

Hindlimb bony fractures were an obvious injury but clinical examination of the thorax revealed a systolic cardiac murmur which had not previously been present. The respiration was also abnormal and thoracic radiography revealed pleural effusion. The pleural effusion obscured the cardiac and mediastinal shadows ventrally.

Diaphragmatic shadow appeared intact, although the shadow was lost more ventrally by the pleural effusion. No disturbance of abdominal shadows to suggest a rupture of the diaphragm was present. The rib shadows were intact.

Thoracocentesis showed the effusion to be serous and obstructive in nature. Cardiac failure was suspected as the cause of the effusion but neoplasia was also considered.

Echocardiography using 2D and M mode imaging confirmed that hypertrophic cardiomyopathy was present. No abnormal mediastinal echoes were seen to suggest neoplastic metastasis as the cause of the obstructive effusion. Diaphragmatic line was intact.

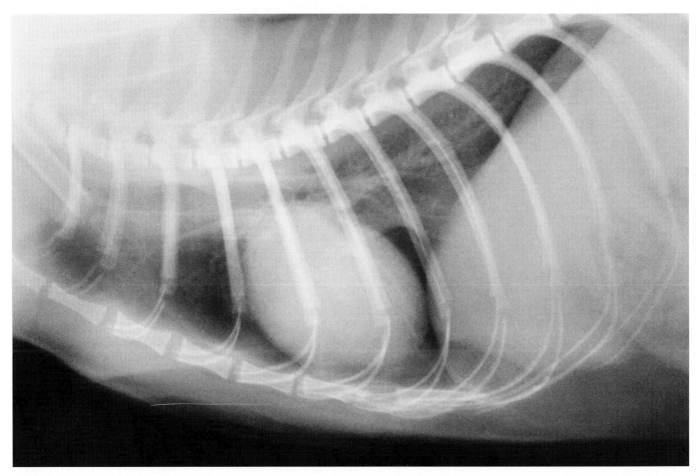

Figure 711   Cardiac 'variations'. Left lateral recumbent projection of thorax. Radiograph taken during general anaesthesia with full inflation of lung lobes. Burmese cat 18 months old, neutered male (same cat as in Figure 712).

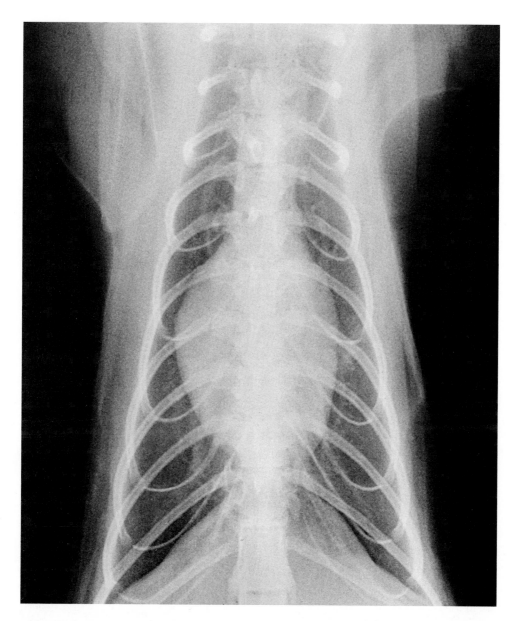

Figure 712 Cardiac 'variations'. Dorsoventral projection of thorax. Radiograph taken during general anaesthesia with full inflation of lung lobes. Burmese cat 18 months old, neutered male (same cat as in Figure 711). Further to the comments made on cardiac shadow 'variation' (see text of right lateral recumbent projection of thorax, Figure 700), the thoracic radiography performed on this young Burmese cat shows that classic normal parameters for cat cardiac shadows do not always apply.

In particular, the lateral projection has a rounded cardiac shadow, as demonstrated by the cranial border and apex. A degree of cardiac enlargement can also be argued although there is a small degree of positional thoracic rotation.

This Burmese cat was showing no clinical signs of cardiac abnormality, radiography being undertaken as part of an investigation into possible pulmonary changes following rhinitis. Unfortunately no further thoracic radiography or clinical history is available for this particular cat and one can only speculate on whether the cardiac shadow was normal or a precursor to overt cardiac disease.

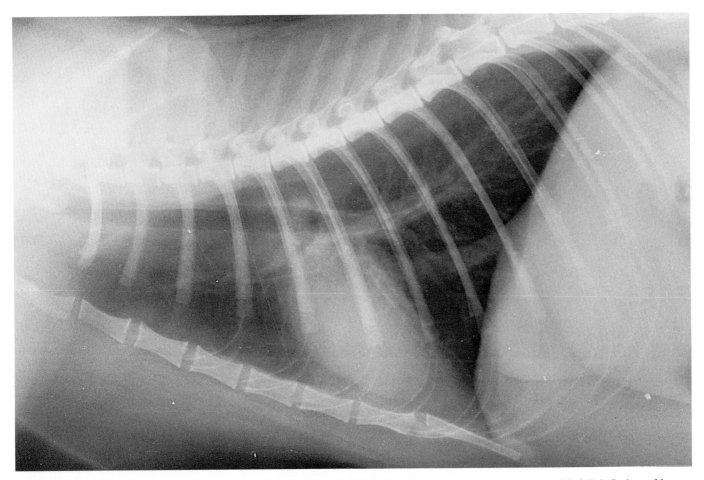

Figure 713   Left lateral recumbent projection of thorax. Radiograph taken during general anaesthesia with full inflation of lung lobes. British domestic short haired cat 6 years old, neutered male (same cat as in right lateral recumbent projection of thorax, Figure 699).

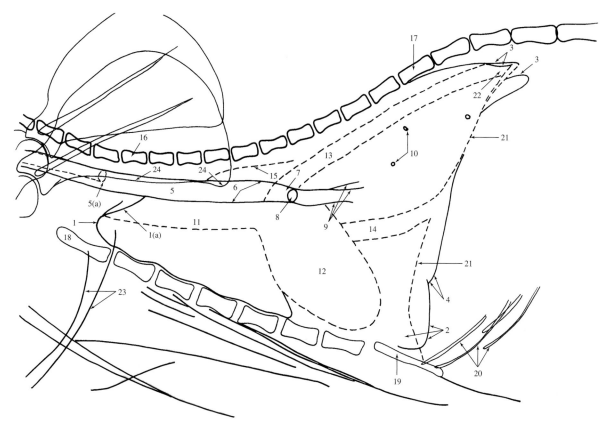

Figure 714 Left lateral recumbent projection of thorax to highlight respiratory system.

1 Cranial limit of the right and left cranial lung lobes. Extension is beyond the 1st. pair of ribs into the pleural cupola in well-inflated lung lobes. Unlike in the dog, the right and left cranial lung lobes in the cat often extend to the same cranioventral level, as in both lateral recumbent projections of this cat, Figures 699 and 713.

   1(a) Craniodorsal limit of right cranial lung lobe

2 Lucent shadow created by middle lobe of right lung. This must not be mistaken for free pleural gas or air. Pulmonary opacities can be seen in the lucent region confirming the identity of lung tissue.

3 Most dorsal parts of caudal lung lobes

4 Ventral limits of caudal lobe, right and left lung. The right caudal lobe extends further ventrally than the left.

5 Tracheal lumen
   5(a) Endotracheal tube

6 Tracheal walls

7 Level of tracheal bifurcation into right and left principal bronchi

8 Radiolucent circular silhouette demonstrating end-on projection of left cranial lung lobe bronchus at bifurcation into bronchus for cranial and caudal parts. The caudal part is often incorrectly termed the middle lobe of the left lung. Only the right lung has a middle lobe.

9 Linear opacities indicating bronchial walls

10 Circular opacities with radiolucent centres indicating bronchial walls; end-on bronchial silhouettes

Although bronchial and interstitial markings are common in dogs from the age of 4 years, and often are dramatic at ages over 10 years, the same does not apply to the cat. A recognisable bronchial and interstitial pattern in the cat indicates present or previous clinical abnormality.

11 Cranial mediastinum
12 Cardiac shadow
13 Aorta
14 Caudal vena cava
15 M.longus colli shadow
16 1st. thoracic vertebra
17 11th. thoracic vertebra
18 Manubrium of sternum
19 Xiphoid process
20 Calcified costal cartilages
21 Diaphragm
22 Lumbodiaphragmatic recess. The position of the recess is very different to the dog and must not be mistaken for abnormality. In this radiograph the dorsal border of the caudal lung lobe is separated from the bony vertebrae by a soft tissue shadow extending from caudal 11th. thoracic vertebra to caudal 13th. thoracic vertebra levels. Such an appearance is normal in the cat and must not be confused with lung retraction due to the presence of pleural effusion.
23 Muscle masses of forelimbs
24 Caudal border of scapula

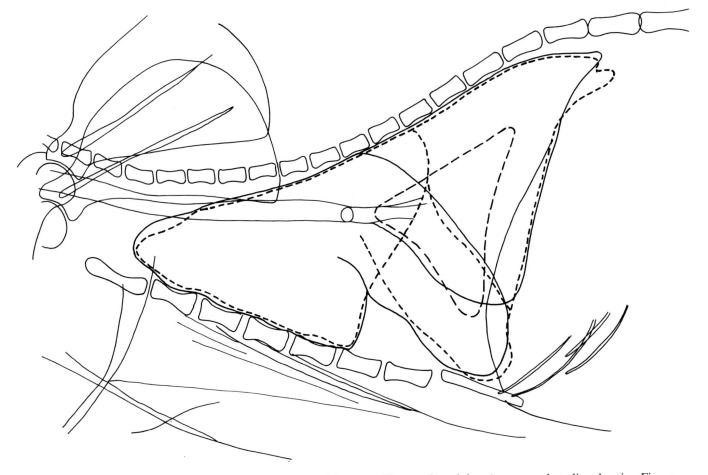

Figure 715 Schematic drawing of left lateral projection of thorax to illustrate lung lobes (corresponds to line drawing Figure 714, but with the exclusion of thoracic cavity details seen in the radiograph).

———— = Left lung. Cranial (cranial and caudal parts) and caudal lobes.

– – – = Right lung. Cranial, middle and caudal lobes.

— — = Accessory lobe

The terms apical, cardiac, diaphragmatic and intermediate lung lobes are no longer in common usage.

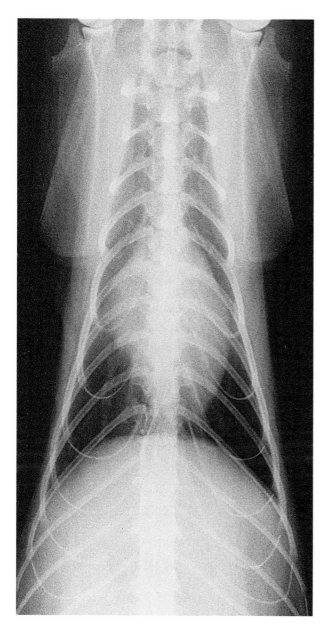

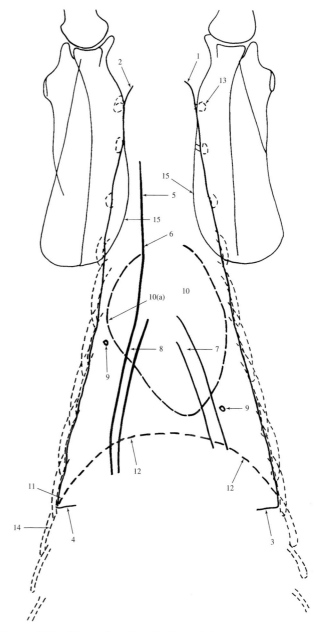

Figure 716 Ventrodorsal projection of thorax. Radiograph taken during general anaesthesia with full inflation of lung lobes. British domestic short haired cat 10 months old, neutered female (same cat as in dorsoventral projection of thorax, Figure 702).

Figure 717 Ventrodorsal projection of thorax to highlight respiratory system.

(717 continued.)

1 Cranial limit of the left cranial lung lobe. Extends beyond the 1st. pair of ribs into pleural cupola in well-inflated lung lobes.
2 Cranial limit of right cranial lung lobe
3 Caudal visible limit of left caudal lung lobe
4 Caudal visible limit of right caudal lung lobe
5 Tracheal wall
6 Tracheal lumen within the cranial mediastinum just right of the midline
7 Left caudal bronchial lumen
8 Right caudal bronchial lumen
9 Circular opacity with radiolucent centre indicating wall with central lumen; end-on bronchial shadow.

The comments on bronchial markings and interstitial opacities made for the left lateral recumbent projection of thorax, Figure 714, also apply to this projection.

Although skin folds do not usually create the same false effect of lung opacity, compared with the dog, it is worth noting that the extreme cranial, and correct, position of the forelimbs in this radiograph has caused superimposition of the bony scapulae over the cranial thoracic cavity. All bony shadows seen in a thoracic cavity radiograph must be traced to their origin to avoid misdiagnosis. The latter is extremely important for rib shadows with their associated calcified costal cartilages.

10 Cardiac shadow. Note the curvature of the right atrium (10a) created by the ventrodorsal positioning.
11 Costodiaphragmatic recess
12 Diaphragmatic shadow
13 1st. rib
14 10th. rib
15 Scapula

The cranial position of the forelimbs makes the thorax appear longer and less triangular than if the legs are positioned to the sides of the thorax.

The ventrodorsal position is the preferred projection for lung shadows but even so dorsoventral projection can show improvement by pulling the forelegs cranially.

A short, triangular thoracic cavity, and hence a reduction of lung shadow, is greatest in the dorsoventral projection with the forelegs at the sides of the thorax.

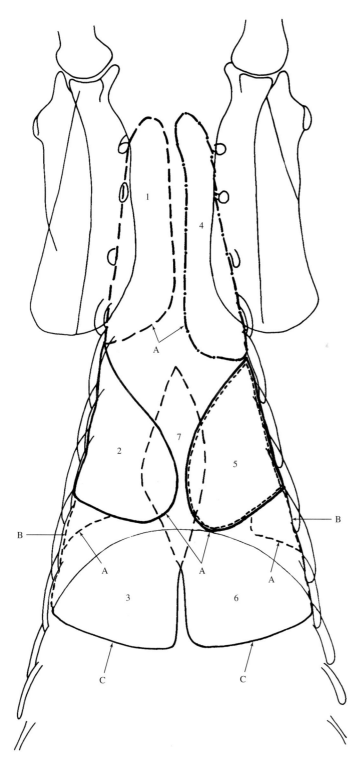

Figure 718 Schematic drawing of ventrodorsal projection of thorax to illustrate lung lobes (corresponds to line drawing Figure 717, but with the exclusion of some thoracic cavity details seen in the radiograph).

1 = Right cranial lung lobe
2 = Right middle lung lobe
3 = Right caudal lung lobe
4 = Left cranial lung lobe, cranial part
5 = Left cranial lung lobe, caudal part
6 = Left caudal lung lobe
   A = Most ventral parts of right and left lung lobes

B = Most lateral parts of right and left caudal lung lobes
C = Most dorsal parts of right and left caudal lung lobes
7 = Accessory lung lobe
The terms apical, cardiac, diaphragmatic and intermediate lung lobes are no longer in common usage.

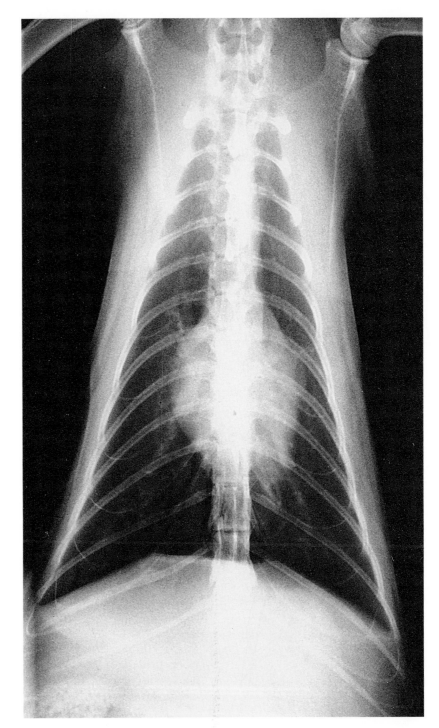

Figure 719 Ventrodorsal projection of thorax. Radiograph taken during general anaesthesia with forced or over-inflation of lung lobes. British domestic short haired cat 10 months old, entire female (same cat as in right and left lateral recumbent projections of thorax, Figures 705 and 706).

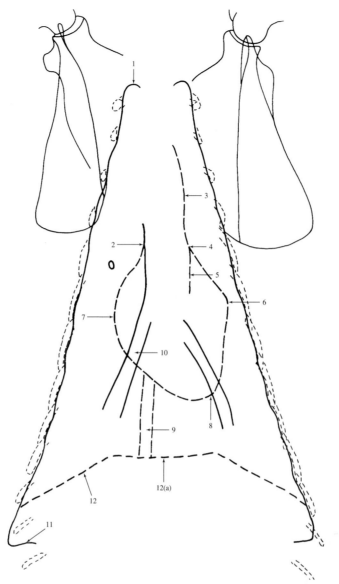

Figure 720   Ventrodorsal projection of thorax to highlight the effects of forced or over-inflation on cardiac and diaphragmatic shadows.

The effect of forced or over inflation compared to full inflation was discussed in the right and left lateral recumbent projection of thorax, Figures 705 and 706. Considering the ventrodorsal projection note the increased radiolucency of the lung lobes and flattening of the central and peripheral parts of the diaphragmatic shadow.

   Although the cardiac shadow is reduced in area with forced inflation, evaluation of this shadow cannot be accurately made on any ventrodorsal projection. This is because the heart rotates craniodorsally creating a space between the cardiac and diaphragmatic shadows. The rotation often distorts the position of the cardiac shadow within the thorax. Also, the curved cranial cardiac borders may become more prominent. Compare with Figures 702 and 716 of the same cat in dorsoventral and ventrodorsal projections.

  1 Pleural cupola
  2 Tracheal wall
  3 Cranial mediastinal shadow
  4 Aortic arch
  5 Aorta
  6 Left auricle
  7 Right atrium

Numbers 6 and 7 appear 'enlarged' due to positional effect

  8 Cardiac apex; left ventricle wall
  9 Caudal vena cava
 10 Caudal bronchial lumen
 11 Caudal limit of lung lobe
 12 Diaphragmatic shadow. The central part of the diaphragm (12(a)) is markedly flattened due to forced or over-inflation of the lung lobes.

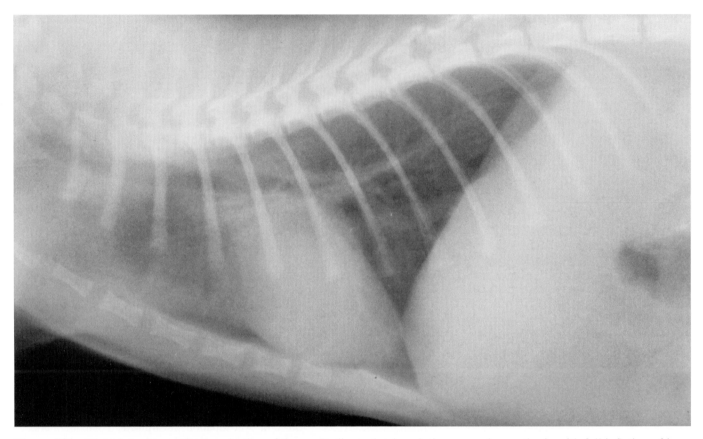

Figure 721 Right lateral recumbent projection of thorax. Radiograph taken during general anaesthesia with full inflation of lung lobes. British domestic short haired cat 12 weeks old, entire male.

The radiograph shows the opaque linear pattern seen in the young animal thought to be due to interstitial fluid not present in adults. The opacity in this cat has considerably reduced the clarity of the vascular pattern with the aorta being barely visible.

The cardiac shadow is typically large and rounding of the borders, especially the cranial, with increase in sternal contact is evident.

A diffuse soft tissue shadow with a well-defined ventral margin is seen in the cranial thorax, its caudal border merging with the cranial cardiac border. This opacity is the thymus within the ventral mediastinum. Radiographically the thymic presence is clearly defined in the lateral projection of the thoracic cavity of very young cats.

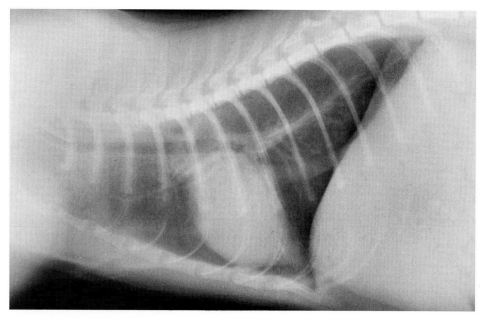

Figure 722   Right lateral recumbent projection of thorax. Radiograph taken during general anaesthesia with full inflation of lung lobes. British domestic short haired cat 24 weeks old, entire male.

The radiograph shows a reduction in lung opacity compared to 12 weeks of age (see Figure 721) but still a very fine linear interstitial pattern is present.

The cardiac shadow has changed little in appearance, with the rounded border still being visible.

The cranial thymic opacity seen at 12 weeks of age has almost disappeared. Only an indistinct soft tissue shadow is evident at the 1st. and 2nd. rib levels.

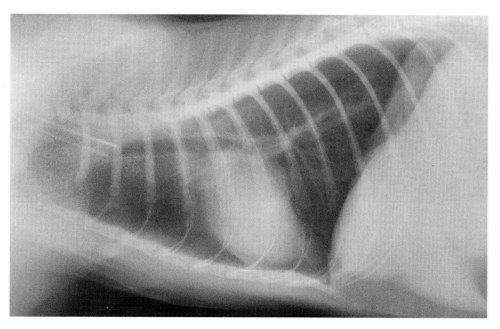

Figure 723   Right lateral recumbent projection of thorax. Radiograph taken during general anaesthesia with full inflation of lung lobes. British domestic short haired cat 36 weeks old, entire female.

The radiograph, compared to 24 weeks of age, Figure 722, now shows pulmonary, ventral mediastinal and cardiac shadows similar to those of an adult cat.

The lung opacity seen previously at the younger ages has been lost and lucent shadows of lung tissue replace the thymic soft tissue opacity at the 1st. and 2nd. rib levels. Reduction in the rounding of the cardiac shadow has given the cranial border a normal contour.

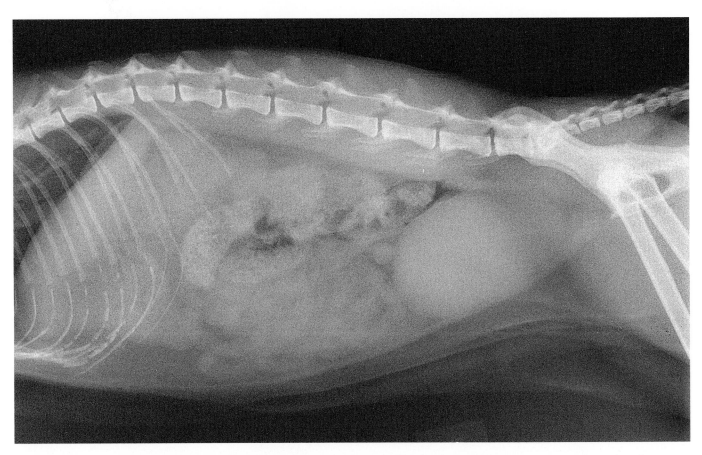

Figure 724   Left lateral recumbent projection of abdomen. British domestic short haired cat 8 years old, neutered female (same cat as in right lateral recumbent projection of abdomen, Figure 726).

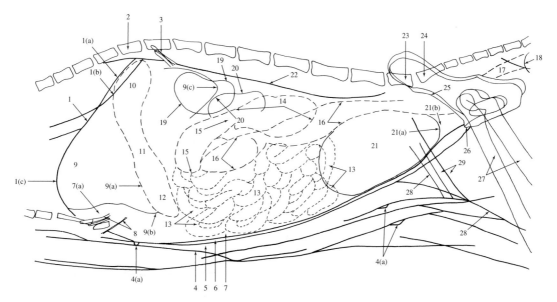

Figure 725 Left lateral recumbent projection of abdomen.

1 Diaphragmatic shadow
 1(a) Left 'crus'
 1(b) Right 'crus'
 1(c) Cupola
2 12th. thoracic vertebra
3 13th. rib
4 Skin margin
 4(a) Soft tissue shadows of nipples (only just visible)
5 Subcutaneous fat
6 M.rectus abdominis
7 Intraperitoneal fat
 7(a) Falciform ligament of liver, mainly fat
8 Calcified costal cartilages
9 Soft tissue shadow of liver. Caudally this shadow creates a positive silhouette sign with the soft tissue shadow of the pyloric part of the gastric shadow 9(a).
 9(b) Caudoventral margin of liver; left lateral lobe
 9(c) Caudodorsal margin of liver; caudate process of caudal lobe
10 Gastric fundus
11 Gastric body
12 Pyloric part of gastric shadow

The lack of gastric gas is causing poor definition of the gastric shadow parts numbers 10 to 12. Shadows of cardia and pylorus are not seen.

13 Jejunum and ileum (seen as tubular soft tissue shadows)

Jejunum and ileum cannot be differentiated on non-contrast films, or even clearly on contrast studies. Generally the diameter of all small intestinal bowel is equal; 'rule of thumb' maximum diameter is normally equal to height of lumbar vertebral body.

14 Ascending colon (caecum cannot be seen as a separate structure on this film)
15 Transverse colon. In the cat it is a very small portion of bowel and is only rarely seen in abdominal projections.

16 Descending colon
17 Rectum
18 Anus
19 Right kidney
20 Left kidney

Cats' kidneys are more variable in their location than dogs' kidneys. They tend to be more caudoventral and overlap on the lateral projections. In addition, the most caudally located kidney is not always right, hence requiring a ventrodorsal or dorsoventral projection for an accurate kidney analysis. Kidney shape is similar to the dog but they are smaller in size, being twice the length of the 2nd. lumbar vertebral body. Kidneys and ureters, not visible on plain radiographs, are retroperitoneal.

21 Urinary bladder.
 21(a) Bladder neck. The cat bladder has a long narrow neck so that the bladder's radiographic position is 2 to 3 cm cranial to the pubis. This is in contrast to the dog where the position is immediately cranial to the pubis in the female and cranial to the prostate in the male.
 21(b) Urethra located in the fat caudal to the bladder neck. The urethra in the cat is very narrow and usually requires contrast material to demonstrate its position.
22 Sublumbar muscles. Although the muscles in the cat are similar to those in the dog their volume is greater, so creating a very distinct soft tissue shadow. In non-domestic predatory cats the muscle mass is very large at the 4th. lumbar vertebral level.
23 7th. lumbar vertebra
24 Sacrum. Only two sacral segments are present in this cat.
25 Body of ilium
26 Pubic tubercle
27 Femoral bodies
28 Skin margin of hind leg
29 Muscles of hind leg

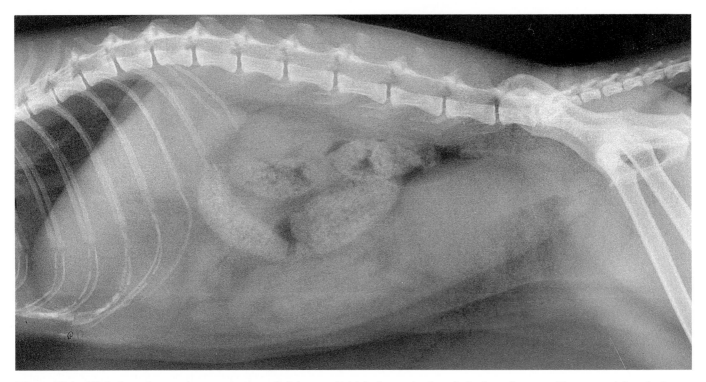

Figure 726 Right lateral recumbent projection of abdomen. British domestic short haired cat 8 years old, neutered female (same cat as in left lateral recumbent projection of abdomen, Figure 724).

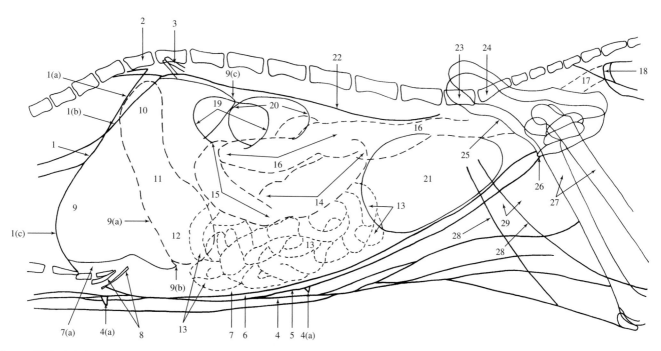

Figure 727 Right lateral recumbent projection of abdomen.

For a routine survey radiograph of the abdomen, a right lateral recumbency is often preferred by many radiographers and radiologists. The most important factor is being consistent with one's radiographic approach and hence radiographic appraisal and interpretation.

1 Diaphragmatic shadow
  1(a) Left 'crus'
  1(b) Right 'crus'
  1(c) Cupola
2 12th. thoracic vertebra
3 13th. rib
4 Skin margin
  4(a) Soft tissue shadows of nipples (just visible)
5 Subcutaneous fat
6 M.rectus abdominis
7 Intraperitoneal fat
  7(a) Falciform ligament of the liver, mainly fat
8 Calcified costal cartilages
9 Soft tissue shadow of liver. Caudally creating a positive silhouette sign with the soft tissue shadow of the pyloric part of gastric shadow 9(a).
  9(b) Caudoventral margin of liver; left lateral lobe
  9(c) Caudodorsal margin of liver; caudate process of caudal lobe
10 Gastric fundus
11 Gastric body
12 Pyloric part of gastric shadow

Right lateral recumbency has caused gravitational filling of these ventrally positioned gastric areas (numbers 11 and 12).

Notice the large shadow compared to the left lateral recumbent projection line drawing, Figure 725.

13 Jejunum and ileum (Seen as tubular soft tissue shadows. See text in left lateral recumbent projection, Figure 725.)
14 Ascending colon. (Note the more 'normal' ventral position compared to left lateral recumbent projection line drawing, Figure 725.)
15 Transverse colon
16 Descending colon
17 Rectum
18 Anus
19 Right kidney. In the right lateral recumbency the right kidney is more caudally positioned than in the left lateral recumbency.
20 Left kidney
21 Urinary bladder
22 Sublumbar muscles

For numbers 19 to 22 see corresponding numbers in the left lateral recumbent projection of abdomen, Figure 725.

23 7th. lumbar vertebra
24 Sacrum. Only two sacral segments are present in this cat.
25 Body of ilium
26 Pubic tubercle
27 Femoral bodies
28 Skin margin of hind leg
29 Muscles of hind legs

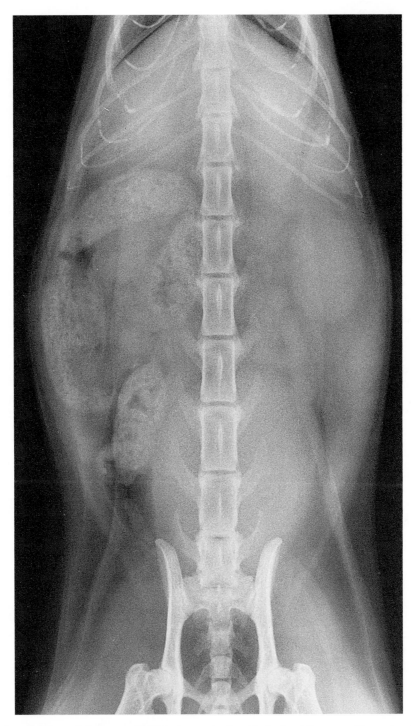

Figure 728 Ventrodorsal projection of abdomen. British domestic short haired cat 8 years old, neutered female (same cat as in left and right lateral recumbent projections of abdomen, Figures 724 and 726).

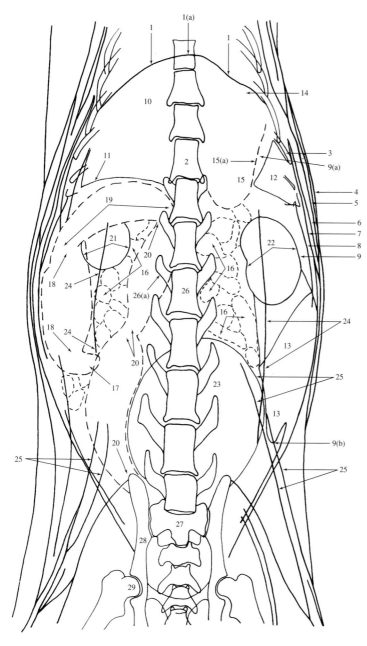

Figure 729 Ventrodorsal projection of abdomen.

1 Diaphragmatic shadow
 1(a) Cupola
2 13th. thoracic vertebra
3 11th. rib
4 Skin margin
5 Subcutaneous fat
6 M.obliquus externus abdominis
7 Fat layer overlying the superficial surface of the caudal ribs. This layer usually serves to separate the m.obliquus externus abdominis from the m.obliquus internus abdominis and m.transversus abdominis.
8 M.obliquus internus abdominis and m.transversus abdominis. Seen as a single soft tissue line from the caudal margin of the rib cage.
9 Retroperitoneal fat surrounding kidney shadow
 9(a) Fat in gastrosplenic part of greater omentum attaching greater curvature to spleen
 9(b) Peritoneal cavity fat
10 Soft tissue shadow of liver
11 Right lateral lobe of liver
12 Dorsal extremity of spleen
13 Ventral extremity of spleen
14 Gastric fundus
15 Gastric body
 15(a) Greater curvature

The lack of gastric gas is causing poor definition of the gastric shadow parts

numbers 10 to 12. Gastric fundus is poorly defined and positions of cardia and pyloric parts are not seen.

16 Jejunum and ileum (seen as tubular soft tissue shadows)
17 Caecum. In the cat this structure is rarely seen without the aid of contrast media but in this cat a distinct caecal shadow is present. Unlike the dog the cat has no separate caecocolic junction or compartments.
18 Ascending colon
19 Transverse colon
20 Descending colon. Usually found on the left side not midline. In this cat it is on the right side of the abdomen. The distal third of the descending colon varies considerably in position.
21 Right kidney
22 Left kidney
23 Urinary bladder
24 Sublumbar muscles. The sublumbar muscle mass extends laterally to a greater degree than in the dog.
25 Skin folds
26 3rd. lumbar vertebra
 26(a) Transverse process
27 Sacrum. Only two sacral segments are present in this cat.
28 Body of ilium
29 Femoral head

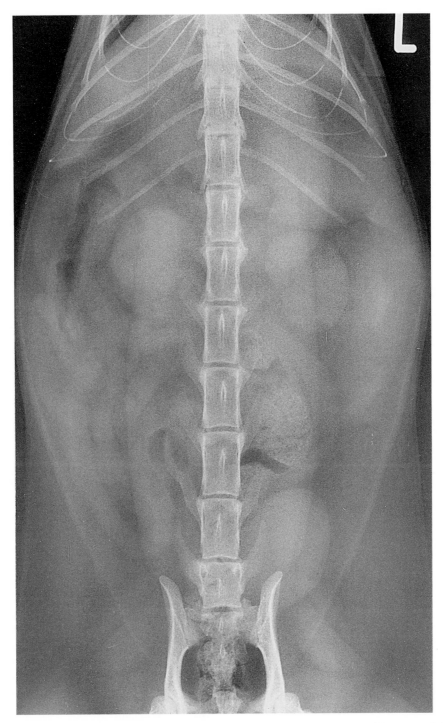

Figure 730 Dorsoventral projection of abdomen. British domestic short haired cat 4 years old, neutered female (same cat as in ventrodorsal projection of abdomen, Figure 732).

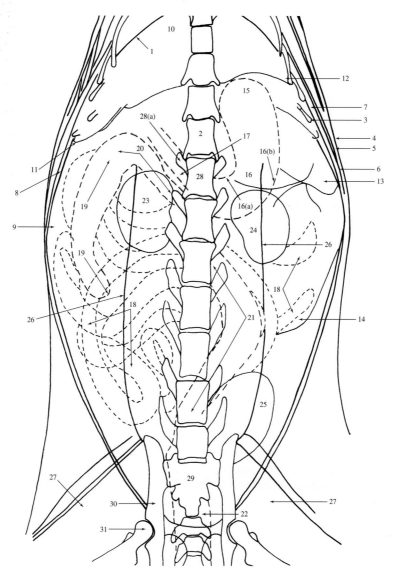

Figure 731   Dorsoventral projection of abdomen.

1 Diaphragmatic shadow
2 13th. thoracic vertebra
3 11th. rib
4 Skin margin
5 Subcutaneous fat
6 M.obliquus externus abdominis
7 Fat layer overlying the superficial surface of the caudal ribs
8 M.obliquus internus abdominis and m.transversus abdominis
9 Intraperitoneal fat
10 Soft tissue shadow of liver
11 Right lateral lobe of liver
12 Left lateral lobe of liver
13 Dorsal extremity of spleen
14 Ventral extremity of spleen
15 Gastric fundus
16 Gastric body
    16(a) Lesser curvature
    16(b) Greater curvature

17 Pyloric part
18 Jejunum and ileum (mainly seen as soft tissue shadows but a few gas-filled loops are present caudally)
19 Ascending colon
20 Transverse colon
21 Descending colon
22 Rectum
23 Right kidney
24 Left kidney
25 Urinary bladder
26 Sublumbar muscles
27 Hind limb muscles
28 1st. lumbar vertebra
    28(a) Transverse process
29 Sacrum
30 Body of ilium
31 Femoral head

An Atlas of Interpretative Radiographic Anatomy of the Dog and Cat

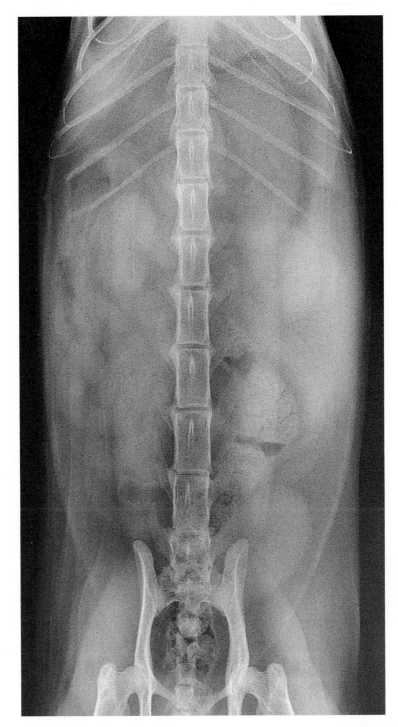

Figure 732 Ventrodorsal projection of abdomen. British domestic short haired cat 4 years old, neutered female (same cat as in dorsoventral projection of abdomen, Figure 730).

The radiographic shadows are very similar to the corresponding dorsoventral projection of abdomen in this cat. Kidney shadows are usually more well defined in the ventrodorsal projection while the dorsal extremity of the spleen is less clear.

Gastric and intestinal shadows are virtually unchanged in these ventrodorsal and dorsoventral projections of the abdomen. This is due to the absence of recognisable lumenal gas shifting with alterations of abdominal positioning.

Please see the differences in the dog ventrodorsal and dorsoventral projections of abdomen, Figures 464–469 and 471–475.

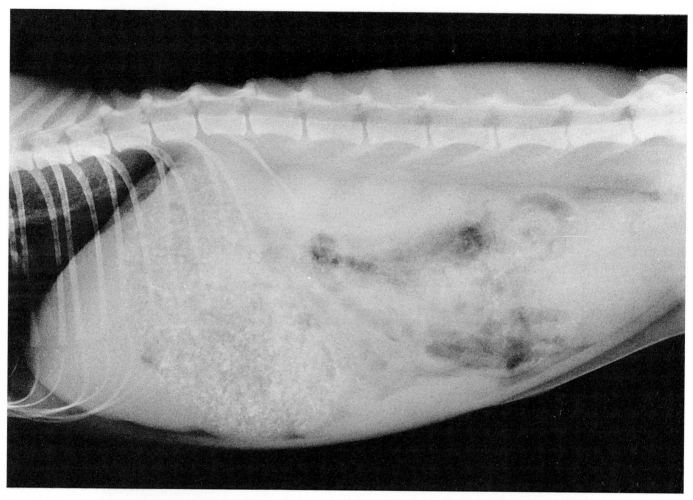

Figure 733 Right lateral recumbent projection of abdomen. British domestic short haired cat 6 years old, entire male (same cat as in dorsoventral projection of abdomen, Figure 734).

The gastric shadow shows gross distension of the gastric lumen with recent ingesta. Notice how large the cat's stomach can stretch without clinical signs of dilation. The degree of distension has caused displacement of the ventral extremity of the spleen, making it appear more elongated and readily visible.

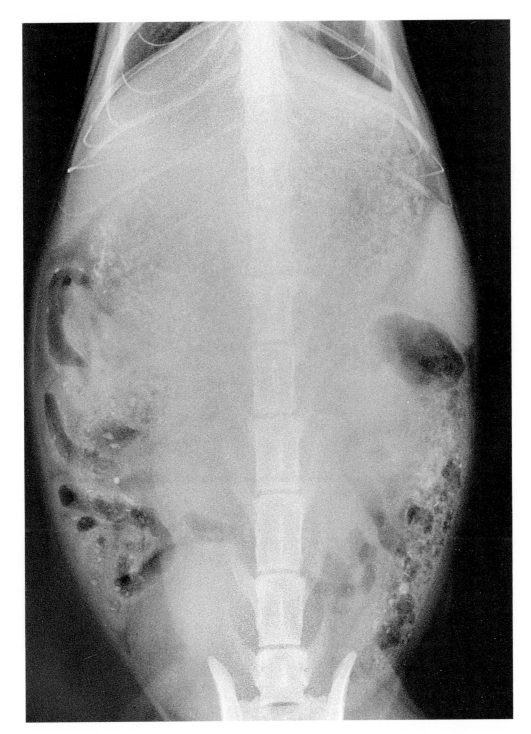

Figure 734 Dorsoventral projection of abdomen. British domestic short haired cat 6 years old, entire male (same cat as in right lateral recumbent projection of abdomen, Figure 733).

The gastric shadow is grossly distended with recent ingesta. The degree of lumenal distension has displaced the caudal body and pyloric parts of the stomach to the right side of the abdomen.

When the stomach is empty or moderately filled the body usually lies to the left and the pyloric parts lie in the midline of the abdomen. This radiograph demonstrates the changes brought about by normal gastric distension in the cat. Gastric enlargement has resulted in the splenic shadow being obscured at the ventral extremity but the dorsal extremity is highlighted.

The descending colon can be seen on the left side of the abdomen, which is the more frequent anatomical position in both the dog and cat.

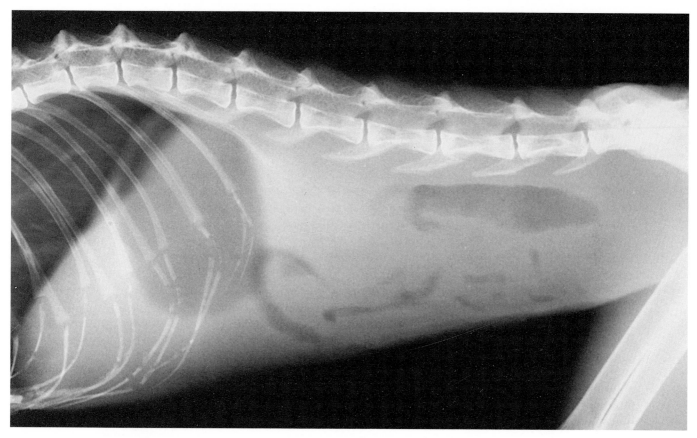

Figure 735 Left lateral recumbent projection of abdomen. Extreme loss of abdominal fat contrast. British domestic short haired cat 13 years old, neutered female.

The radiograph shows gross loss of a well-defined inner surface of abdominal wall, serosal surface of bowel and organ soft tissue shadows such as liver, kidneys and bladder. Abdominal shadows are limited to gas-filled structures surrounded by a homogeneous soft tissue opacity. The appearance is due to excessive loss of the grey opacity fat tissue, in this case secondary to hyperthyroidism. Identification of different soft tissue shadows within the abdomen is only possible in the presence of fat tissue and hence fat is vital for abdominal contrast.

The reduction in abdominal contrast seen in this radiograph must not be mistaken for free abdominal fluid. The latter also causes a loss of contrast as the fluid has the same radiographic opacity as soft tissue. Differentiation from free abdominal fluid or ascites is aided by the long, shallow appearance of the abdomen, together with the absence of subcutaneous fat.

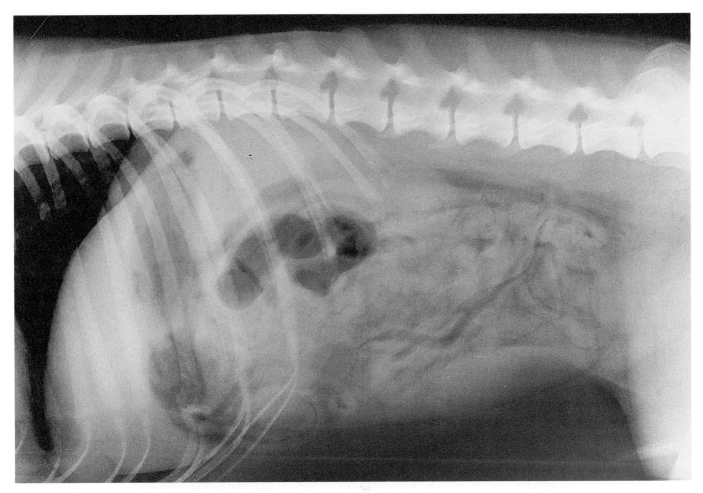

Figure 736   Right lateral recumbent projection of abdomen. Plain survey film.

Figures 736–751   Barium meal; barium in the gastrointestinal tract. Comprises, routinely, serial lateral recumbent and ventrodorsal radiographs of the abdomen and shows the appearance of liquid barium sulphate passing through the gastrointestinal tract over a period of up to 24 hours.

Restraint is by positioning aids, e.g. sandbags, and tranquillisation where necessary.

Note that the appearance of the stomach can vary with species and dog breed conformation, the degree of distension and the ratio of fluid to gas. The distribution of fluid and gas depends on the radiographic projection being used.

Also, the gastric emptying and general transit times through the bowel can vary considerably according to the temperament of the animal, the type of any chemical restraint used and whether there is residual ingesta in the tract.

Right lateral recumbent and ventrodorsal projections of abdomen. Barium meal in the dog. Radiographs taken during restraint with sandbags before and following oral administration of liquid barium sulphate. Beagle dog adult, entire male (same dog in all figures for barium meal).

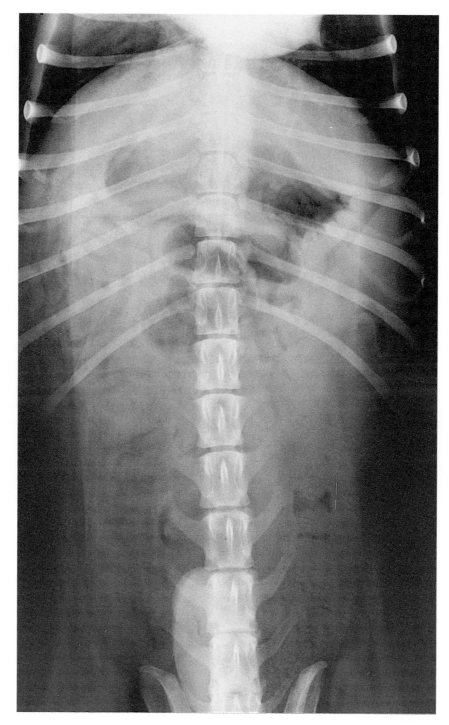

Figure 737   Ventrodorsal projection of abdomen. Plain survey film.

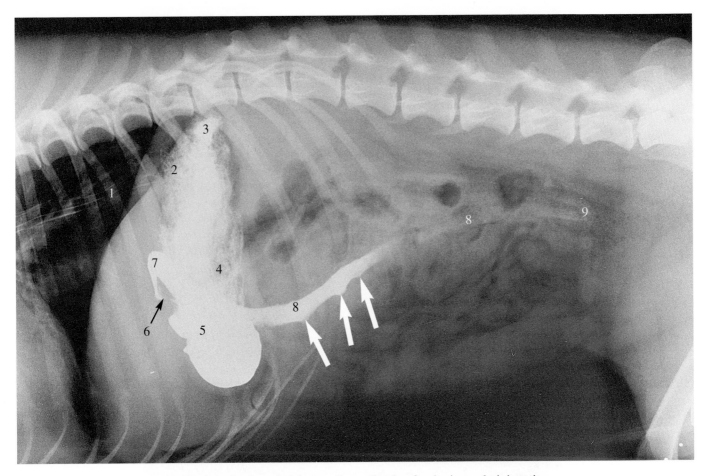

Figure 738   Right lateral recumbent projection of abdomen. Immediately after barium administration.

Streaks of barium show within the mucosal folds of the oesophagus whilst barium is already passing along the descending portion of the duodenum.

Open arrows indicate 'pseudoulcers' in the duodenum (see also Figure 739).

1 Oesophagus
2 Cardia of the stomach
3 Fundus of the stomach
4 Body of the stomach
5 Pyloric antrum
6 Pyloric canal
7 Cranial flexure of the duodenum
8 Descending portion of the duodenum
9 Caudal flexure of the duodenum

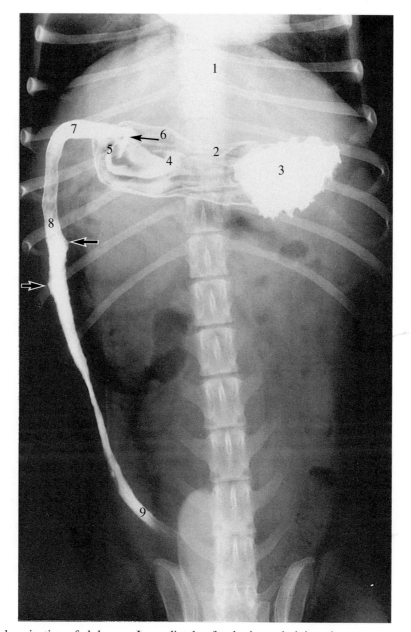

Figure 739 Ventrodorsal projection of abdomen. Immediately after barium administration.

Streaks of barium within the oesophagus are more difficult to see in this projection because of the superimposition of the spine.
   Barium is pooled in the fundus of the stomach (compared with a dorsoventral projection see Figure 754).
   Open arrows indicate 'pseudoulcers' in the duodenum (see also Figure 738).

1 Oesophagus
2 Cardia of the stomach
3 Fundus of the stomach
4 Body of the stomach
5 Pyloric antrum
6 Pyloric canal
7 Cranial flexure of the duodenum
8 Descending portion of the duodenum
9 Caudal flexure of the duodenum

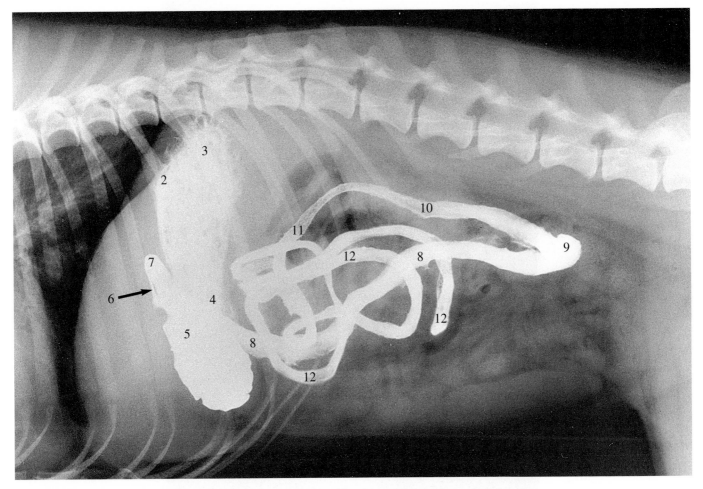

Figure 740 Right lateral recumbent projection of abdomen. 30 minutes after barium administration.

2 Cardia of the stomach
3 Fundus of the stomach
4 Body of the stomach
5 Pyloric antrum
6 Pyloric canal
7 Cranial flexure of the duodenum
8 Descending portion of the duodenum
9 Caudal flexure of the duodenum
10 Ascending portion of the duodenum
11 Duodenojejunal flexure
12 Loops of jejunum and ileum

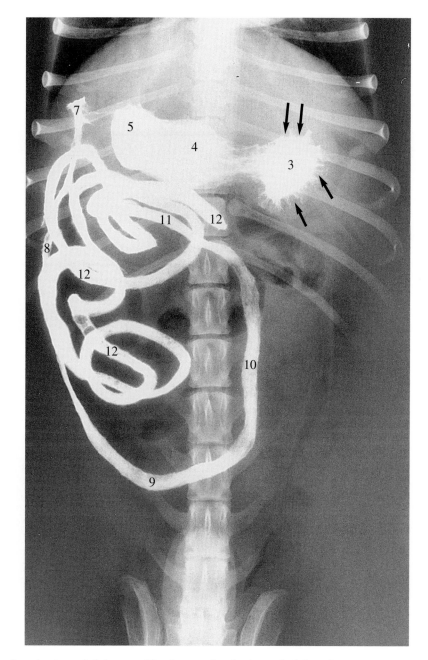

Figure 741   Ventrodorsal projection of abdomen. 30 minutes after barium administration.

Rugal folds of the stomach wall are well seen here, in cross-section (arrows).
   Bubbles of gas are highlighted by the barium within jejunal loops.

   3 Fundus of the stomach
   4 Body of the stomach
   5 Pyloric antrum
   7 Cranial flexure of the duodenum
   8 Descending portion of the duodenum
   9 Caudal flexure of the duodenum
  10 Ascending portion of the duodenum
  11 Duodenojejunal flexure
  12 Loops of jejunum and ileum

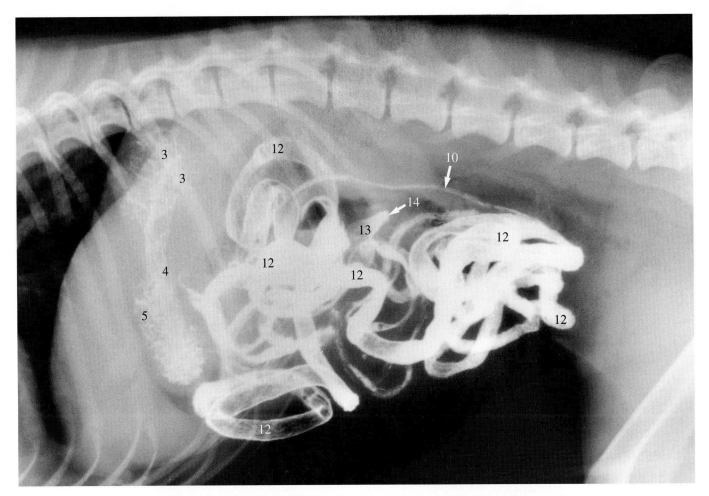

Figure 742   Right lateral recumbent projection of abdomen. 1 hour after barium administration.

The column of barium has reached the ileocolic junction.

 3 Fundus of the stomach
 4 Body of the stomach
 5 Pyloric antrum
10 Ascending portion of the duodenum
12 Loops of jejunum and ileum
13 Terminal portion of the ileum
14 Ileocolic junction

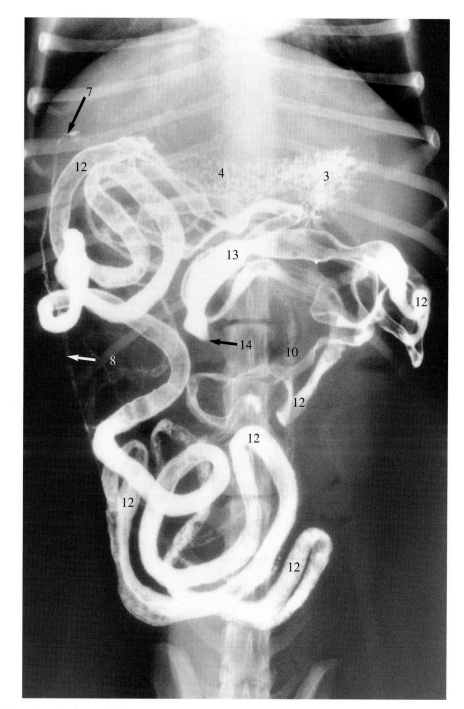

Figure 743 Ventrodorsal projection of abdomen. 1 hour after barium administration.

The column of barium has reached the ileocolic junction.

  3 Fundus of the stomach
  4 Body of the stomach
  7 Cranial flexure of the duodenum
  8 Descending portion of the duodenum
10 Ascending portion of the duodenum
12 Loops of jejunum and ileum
13 Terminal portion of the ileum
14 Ileocolic junction

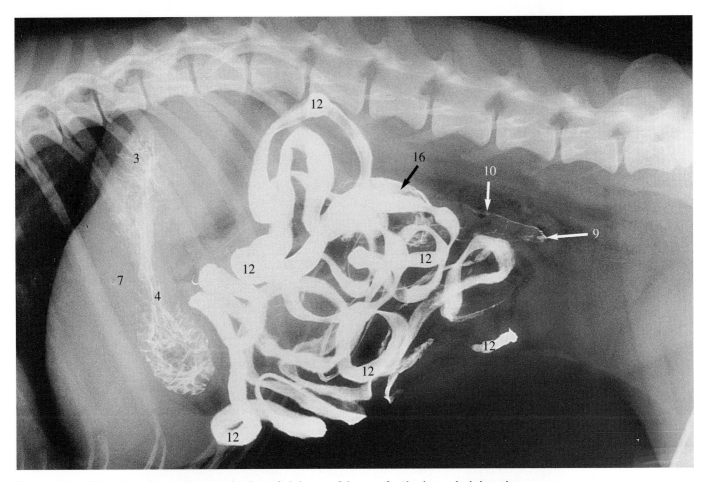

Figure 744   Right lateral recumbent projection of abdomen. 2 hours after barium administration.

Barium is starting to pass through the ileocolic sphincter.

 3 Fundus of the stomach
 4 Body of the stomach
 7 Cranial flexure of the duodenum
 9 Caudal flexure of the duodenum
10 Ascending portion of the duodenum
12 Loops of jejunum and ileum
16 Ascending portion of the colon

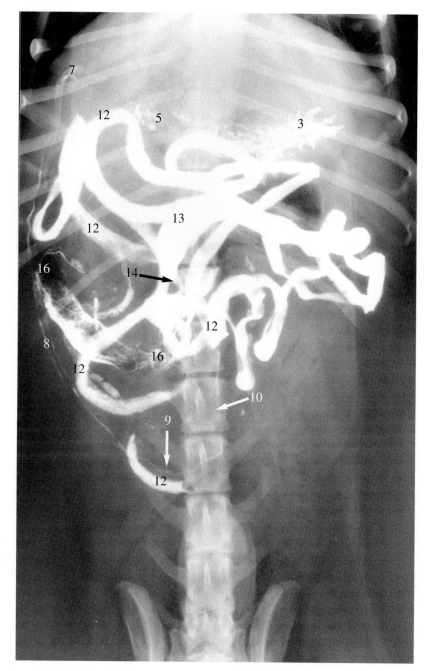

Figure 745   Ventrodorsal projection of abdomen. 2 hours after barium administration.

Barium is starting to pass into the ascending portion of the colon.

   3 Fundus of the stomach
   5 Pyloric antrum
   7 Cranial flexure of the duodenum
   8 Descending portion of the duodenum
   9 Caudal flexure of the duodenum
  10 Ascending portion of the duodenum
  12 Loops of jejunum and ileum
  13 Terminal portion of the ileum
  14 Ileocolic junction
  16 Ascending portion of the colon

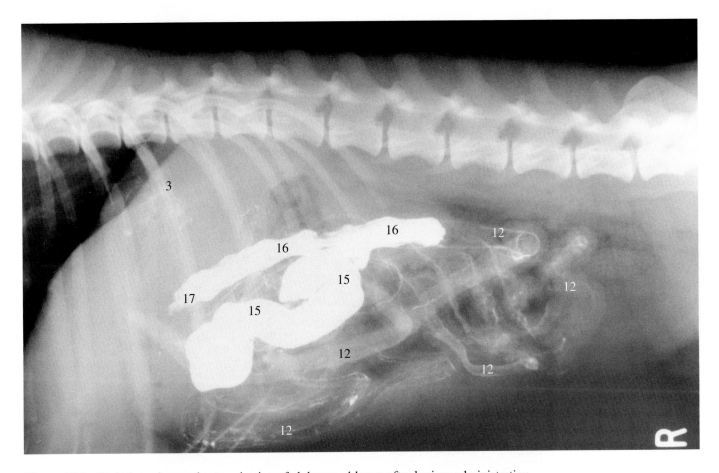

Figure 746 Right lateral recumbent projection of abdomen. 4 hours after barium administration.

The caecum has filled as well as the ascending portion of the colon.

 3 Fundus of the stomach
12 Loops of jejunum and ileum
15 Caecum
16 Ascending portion of the colon
17 Right colic flexure or hepatic flexure of the colon

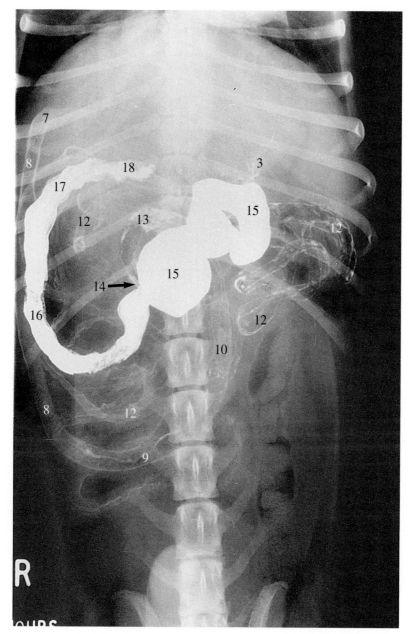

Figure 747   Ventrodorsal projection of abdomen. 4 hours after barium administration.

Much of the barium has collected in the caecum, well demonstrated in this projection.

3 Fundus of the stomach
7 Cranial flexure of the duodenum
8 Descending portion of the duodenum
9 Caudal flexure of the duodenum
10 Ascending portion of the duodenum
12 Loops of jejunum and ileum
13 Terminal portion of the ileum
14 Ileocolic junction
15 Caecum
16 Ascending portion of the colon
17 Right colic flexure or hepatic flexure of the colon
18 Transverse portion of the colon

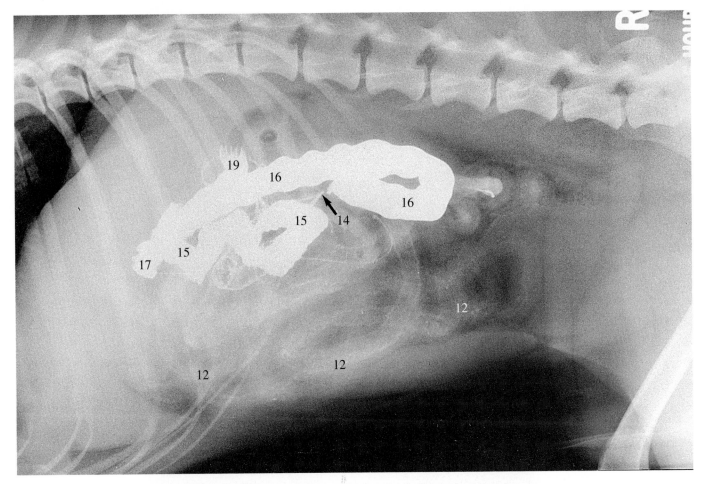

Figure 748 Right lateral recumbent projection of abdomen. 6 hours after barium administration.

Most of the barium is now within the colon.

12 Loops of jejunum and ileum
14 Ileocolic junction
15 Caecum
16 Ascending portion of the colon
17 Right colic flexure or hepatic flexure of the colon
19 Left colic flexure or splenic flexure of the colon

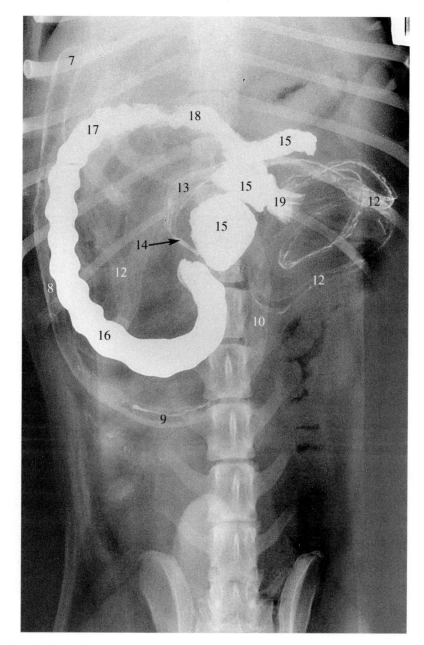

Figure 749 Ventrodorsal projection of abdomen. 6 hours after barium administration.

The caecum is emptying and barium has just reached the left colic flexure.

 7 Cranial flexure of the duodenum
 8 Descending portion of the duodenum
 9 Caudal flexure of the duodenum
10 Ascending portion of the duodenum
12 Loops of jejunum and ileum
13 Terminal portion of the ileum
14 Ileocolic junction
15 Caecum
16 Ascending portion of the colon
17 Right colic flexure or hepatic flexure of the colon
18 Transverse portion of the colon
19 Left colic flexure or splenic flexure of the colon

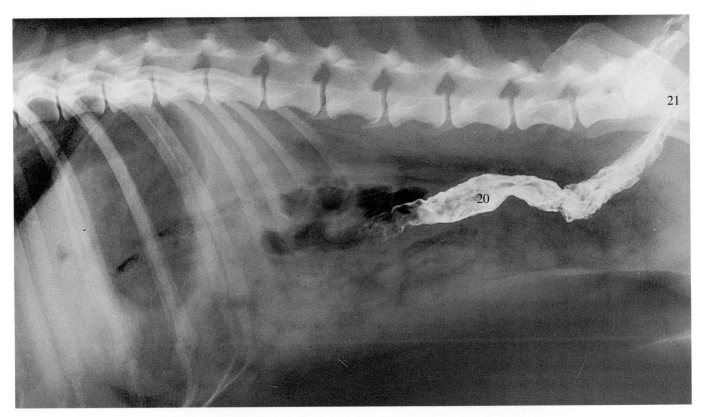

Figure 750   Right lateral recumbent projection of abdomen. 24 hours after barium administration.

Some barium still remains in the descending portion of the colon and the rectum.

20 Descending portion of the colon
21 Rectum

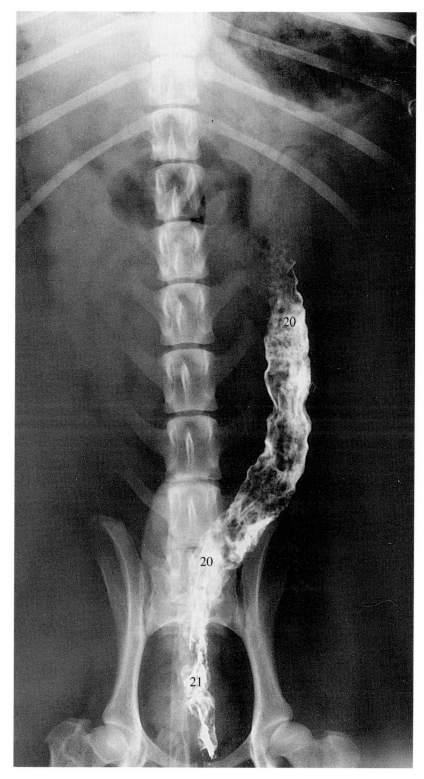

Figure 751 Ventrodorsal projection of abdomen. 24 hours after barium administration.

Some barium still remains in the descending portion of the colon and the rectum.

20 Descending portion of the colon
21 Rectum

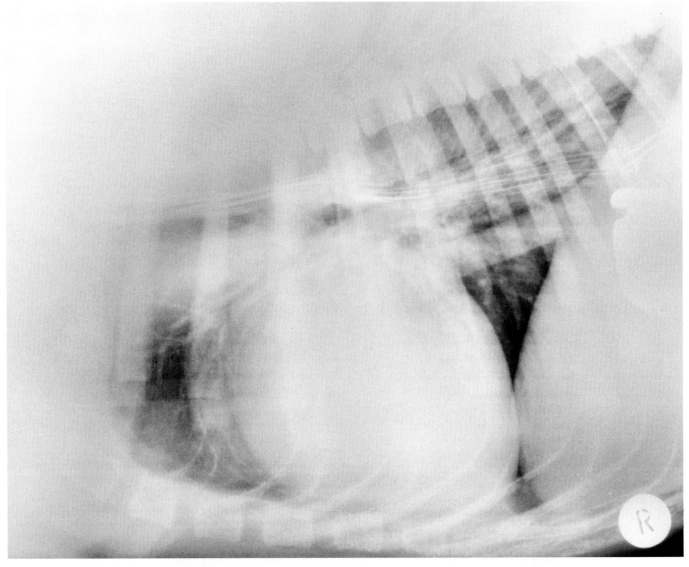

Figure 752 Right lateral recumbent projection of thorax. Normal appearance of liquid barium sulphate within the thoracic oesophagus of the dog.

Radiograph taken during restraint with sandbags immediately following oral administration of liquid barium sulphate as part of a barium meal investigation.

German Shepherd dog 9 years old, entire male.

The normal striped appearance of barium in the longitudinal mucosal folds of the oesophageal wall is seen, together with the dorsal elevation of the oesophageal shadow at the 4th. intercostal space level over the base of the heart (dorsal to the circular radiolucent shadow of the left cranial lobe, caudal part, bronchus).

A repeat radiograph, approximately 10 minutes post-administration of the liquid barium, should reveal no traces of barium in the normal oesophagus.

The cardiac shadow appears an abnormal size and shape.

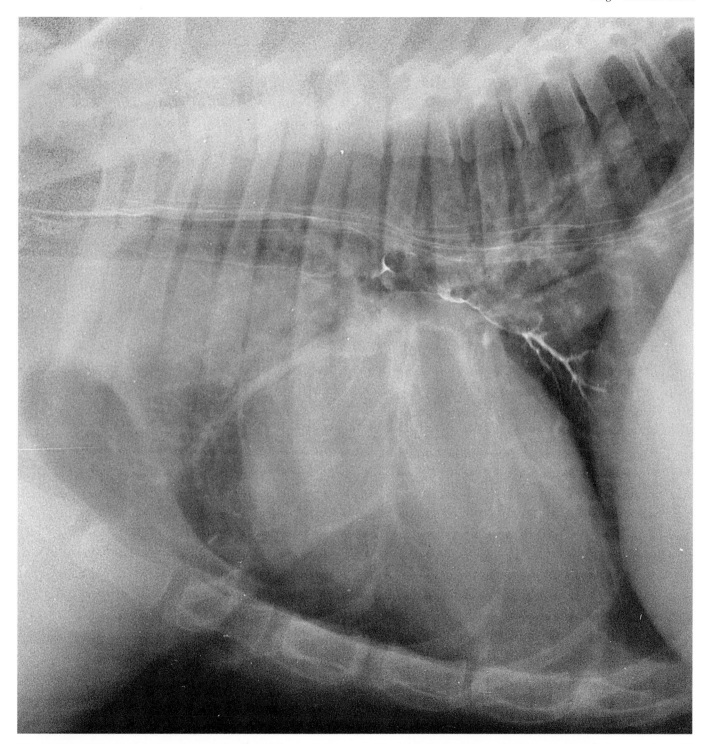

Figure 753 Right lateral recumbent projection of thorax. Inhalation of liquid barium sulphate. Radiograph taken during restraint with sandbags immediately following oral administration of liquid barium sulphate. German Pointer dog 7 years old, entire male.

Accidental inhalation of the contrast material is shown.

Cranially the tracheal lumen is outlined, and more caudally the contrast has entered the right caudal lobe bronchus. The contrast has gravitated into the smaller bronchioles and traces of this will remain within the lung tissue for many years.

It is worth noting that compared with Figure 752, which shows contrast in the normal oesophagus, the deviation at the 4th. intercostal space level is a ventral dipping rather than a dorsal elevation. This anomaly has been caused by positional rotation of the thorax resulting in a 'loss' of the normal dorsal elevation of the oesophagus at the left cranial lung lobe, caudal part, bronchus.

Incidental findings are the shot gun pellets and their transit track fragments.

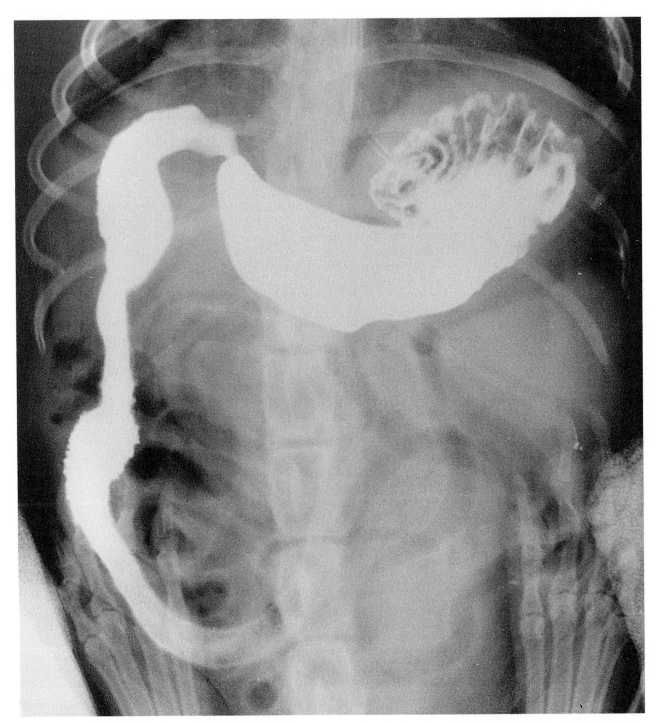

Figure 754   Dorsoventral projection of abdomen. Normal appearance of liquid barium sulphate within the stomach in the dorsoventral projection. Radiograph taken during restraint with sandbags immediately following oral administration of liquid barium sulphate as part of a barium meal investigation of the stomach. Miniature Poodle dog 7 years old, entire female.

   Note the positional gravitation of the contrast medium into the body of the stomach and the pyloric antrum compared with the ventrodorsal projection, Figure 739, where it is in the fundus. The shape is more of a shallow 'U' with the pylorus more medial.

   For a routine barium meal evaluation of the stomach, both right and left lateral recumbencies, ventrodorsal and dorsoventral projections of the abdomen are required.

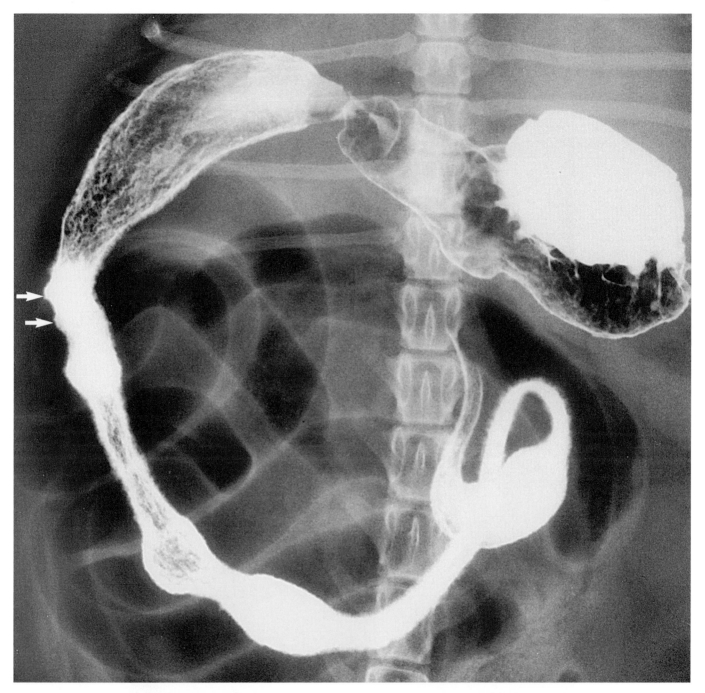

Figure 755 Ventrodorsal projection of abdomen. Duodenal pseudoulcers and small intestinal fimbriation in the dog. Radiograph taken during restraint with sandbags 5 minutes after oral administration of liquid barium sulphate as part of a barium meal investigation. Crossbred dog adult, entire female.

Small out-pouchings (arrows) of the barium column in the descending duodenum may sometimes be seen. They are termed pseudoulcers and occur where the mucosa thins out over submucosal lymph follicles. They should not be confused with pathological ulcers.

A finely villous appearance of the mucosal surface, varying in extent along the small intestine, may also be evident. This is called fimbriation and is generally considered to be due to barium separating individual mucosal villi. Other factors are also involved. Fimbriation is reduced with increased bowel distension but mucus, clumping of villi and regional differences in mucosal movement all play a part.

Differentiation of normal fimbriation from diseased mucosa must be made by studying other radiographic signs and clinical history. Here the whole of the duodenal mucosal surface is involved.

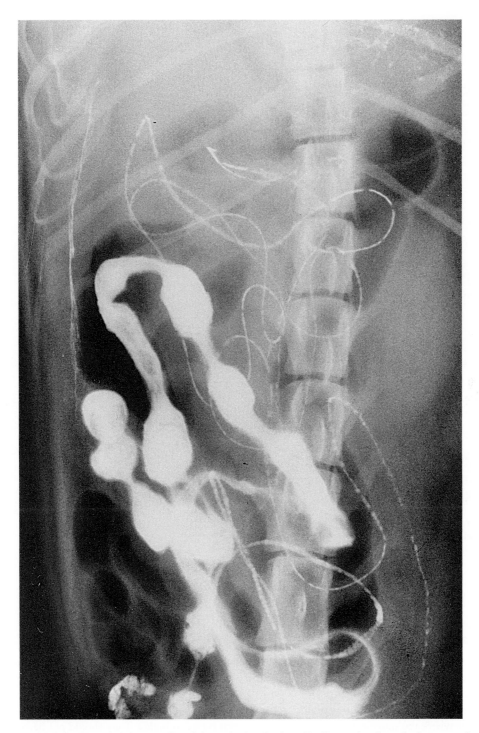

Figure 756   Ventrodorsal projection of abdomen. Small intestinal stringing. Radiograph taken during restraint with sandbags 1 hour after oral administration of liquid barium sulphate as part of a barium meal investigation. Crossbred dog adult, entire female.

 Finely narrowed columns of contrast may be seen, caused by lengthy, segmental contractions of the small intestine. Serial radiographs will confirm their transient nature.

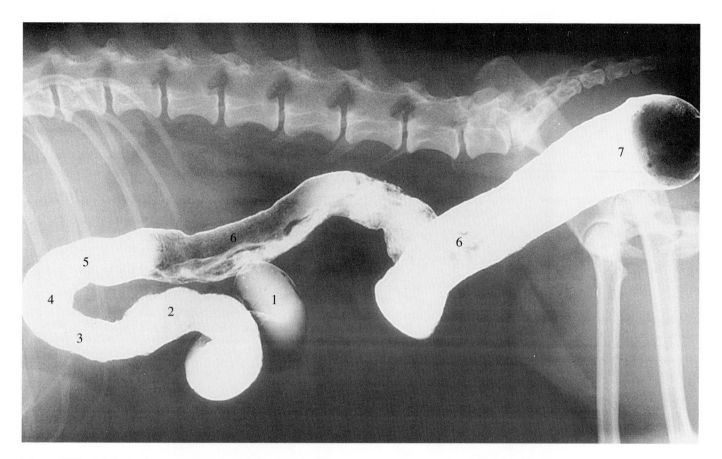

Figure 757 Right lateral recumbent projection of abdomen. Barium enema. Radiograph taken during general anaesthesia following rectal administration of liquid barium sulphate. Jack Russell Terrier dog 2 years old, entire female (same dog as in Figure 758).

1 Caecum
2 Ascending portion of the colon
3 Right colic flexure, or hepatic flexure of the colon
4 Transverse portion of the colon
5 Left colic flexure, or splenic flexure of the colon
6 Descending portion of the colon
7 Rectum

Note that repeat radiographs would demonstrate the temporary, peristaltic nature of the flexure apparently present here in the distal third of the descending portion of the colon.

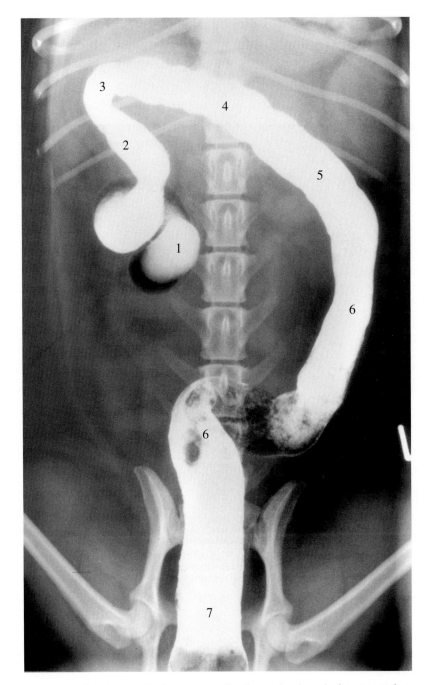

Figure 758 Ventrodorsal projection of abdomen. Barium enema. Radiograph taken during general anaesthesia following rectal administration of liquid barium sulphate. Jack Russell Terrier dog 2 years old, entire female (same dog as in Figure 757).

1 Caecum
2 Ascending portion of the colon
3 Right colic flexure, or hepatic flexure of the colon
4 Transverse portion of the colon
5 Left colic flexure, or splenic flexure of the colon
6 Descending portion of the colon
7 Rectum

Note that repeat radiographs would demonstrate the temporary, peristaltic nature of the flexure apparently present here in the distal third of the descending portion of the colon.

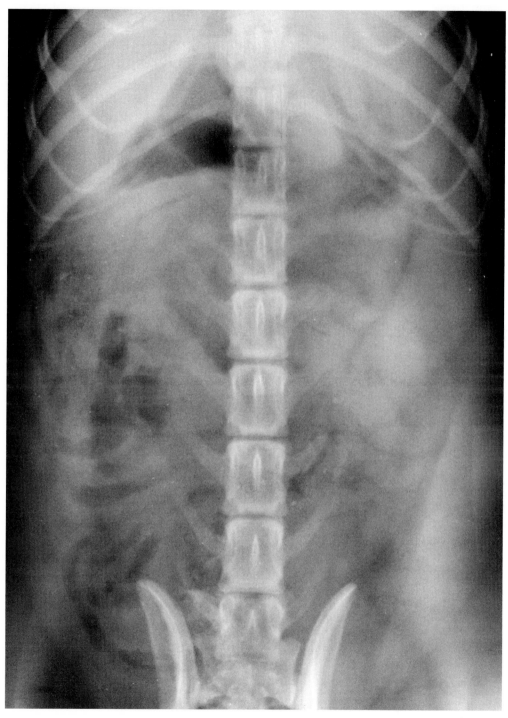

Figure 759 Ventrodorsal projection of abdomen. Intravenous urography (I.V.U.). Radiograph taken during general anaesthesia. Plain survey film. Beagle dog adult, entire female (same dog as in Figures 760, 761 and 762). Right kidney not apparent, left kidney only partly discernible.

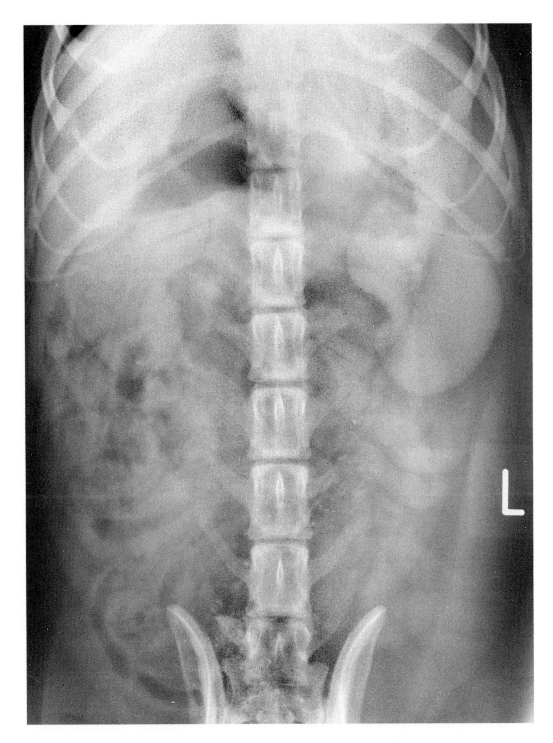

Figure 760 Ventrodorsal projection of abdomen. Intravenous urography (I.V.U.). Radiograph taken during general anaesthesia 1 minute after injection of an iodine-based, water-soluble contrast medium. Beagle dog adult, entire female (same dog as in Figures 759, 761 and 762).

Nephrogram phase of I.V.U.
Sufficient contrast has reached the kidneys to show their size, shape and position.

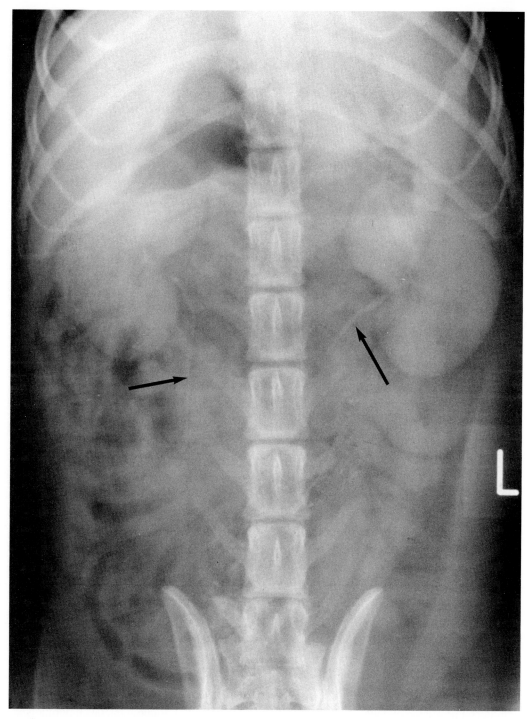

Figure 761 Ventrodorsal projection of abdomen. Intravenous urography (I.V.U.). Radiograph taken during general anaesthesia 3 minutes after injection of an iodine-based, water-soluble contrast medium. Beagle dog adult, entire female (same dog as in Figures 759, 760 and 762).

Pyelogram phase of I.V.U.
The renal pelves, though in this case not the pelvic recesses (see Figure 763), and the cranial ureters are visible (arrows).

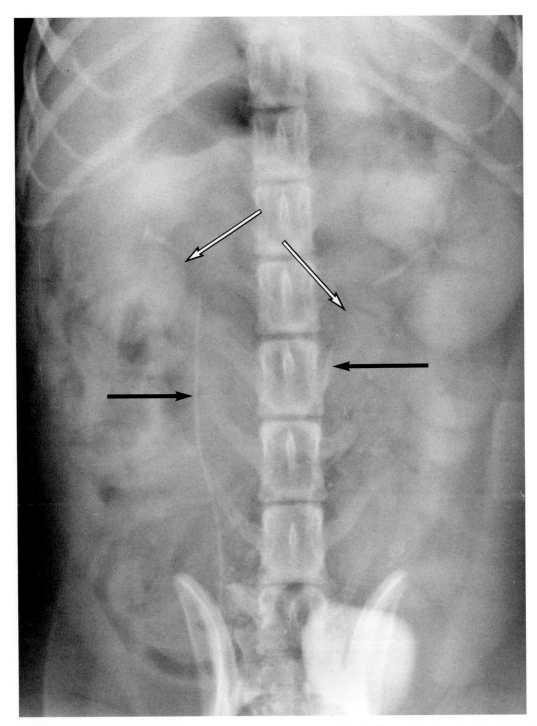

Figure 762   Ventrodorsal projection of abdomen. Intravenous urography (I.V.U.). Radiograph taken during general anaesthesia 8 minutes after injection of an iodine-based, water-soluble contrast medium. Beagle dog adult, entire female (same dog as in Figures 759, 760 and 761).

   Pyelogram phase of I.V.U.
   Normal peristaltic contractions cause segmental gaps (open arrows) in the contrast columns (closed arrows) of the ureters. Contrast is already appearing in the urinary bladder.

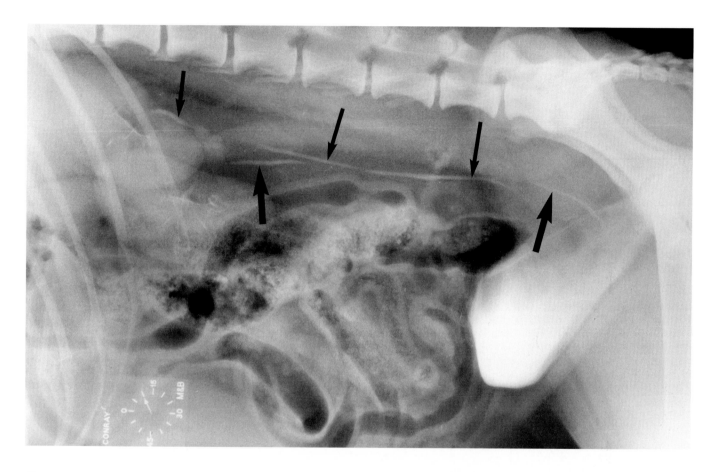

Figure 763 Lateral recumbent projection of abdomen. Intravenous urography (I.V.U.) with pneumocystography. Radiograph taken during general anaesthesia 10 minutes after injection of an iodine-based, water-soluble contrast medium with prior insertion of air into urinary bladder. Irish Setter adult, entire female.

Pyelogram phase of I.V.U.

The renal pelves and the pelvic recesses are outlined. Tracing, and identifying separately, the individual ureters along their length can be particularly difficult in the lateral projection because of the effects of peristalsis and superimposition. The right ureter is marked with thin arrows while the left ureter is labelled with thick arrows.

The ureterovesical junctions are more likely to be clearly seen than in the ventrodorsal projection where the pelvis overlies. Clarity may be enhanced by the use of pneumocystography.

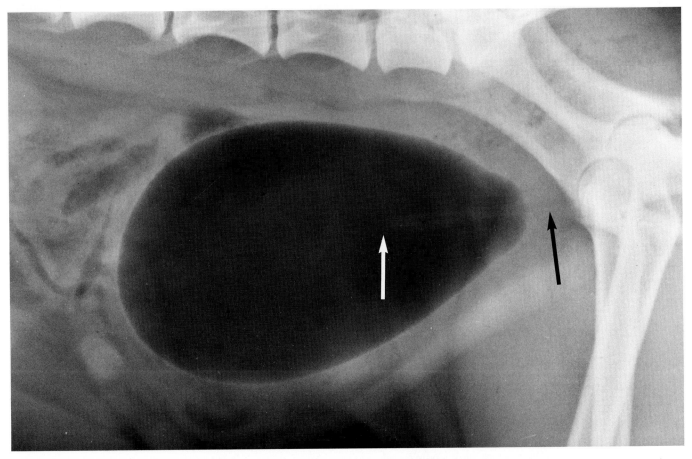

Figure 764 Lateral recumbent projection of caudal abdomen. Pneumocystography. Radiograph taken during general anaesthesia after insertion of air into urinary bladder until full distension was reached. Crossbred dog adult, entire female.

The urinary bladder is distended with air; the urinary catheter is still in place and projecting from the urethra an acceptable distance into the bladder lumen. The catheter shaft is labelled with a black arrow while the catheter tip has a white arrow.

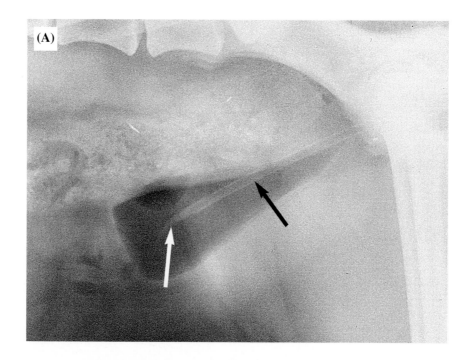

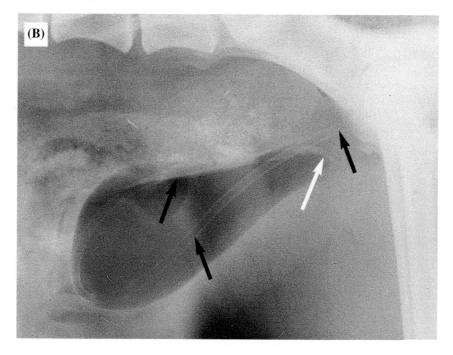

Figures 765A and 765B   Lateral recumbent projections of caudal abdomen. Pneumocystography. Different volumes of air in the same urinary bladder. Labrador dog adult, entire female.

(A) Radiograph taken during general anaesthesia after insertion of 100 ml of air into the urinary bladder.
The inadequate distension of the bladder results in a questionable shape cranially.

(B) Radiograph taken during general anaesthesia after insertion of 200 ml of air into the urinary bladder
The urinary bladder is more adequately distended, demonstrating a more normal shape than in radiograph 765A. However, the urinary catheter has now been inserted far too cranially so that it curves back on itself within the bladder lumen. Also, its tip is distorting the shape of the bladder neck ventrally. Ease of extraction could be a problem.

The catheter shaft is labelled with arrows. The catheter tip is marked with an open/white arrow.

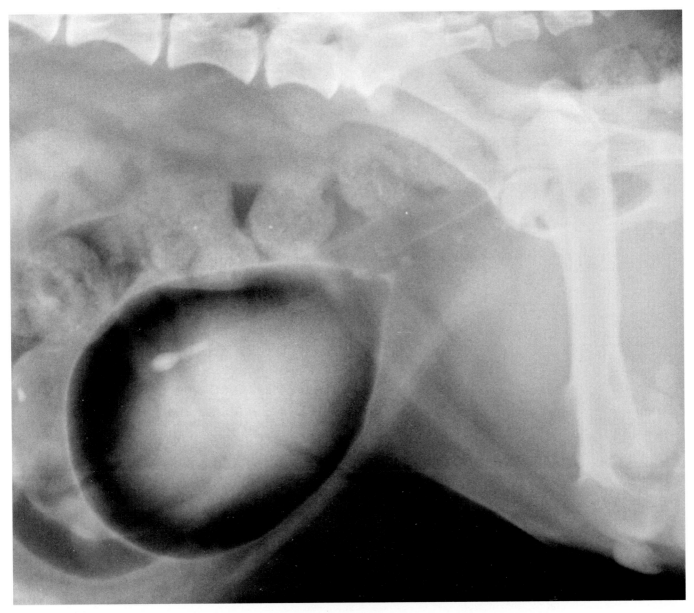

Figure 766 Lateral recumbent projection of caudal abdomen. Double contrast cystography. Radiograph taken during general anaesthesia after insertion of an iodine-based, water-soluble contrast medium followed by air into the urinary bladder until full distension was reached. Miniature Dachshund adult, entire female.

This bladder lies more cranially than in the previous cases illustrated. Note the faecal boluses present in the descending colon and the rectum.

The linear opacity just visible parallel and dorsal to the urethra in the caudal abdomen is the cranial vagina containing a small amount of the positive contrast medium.

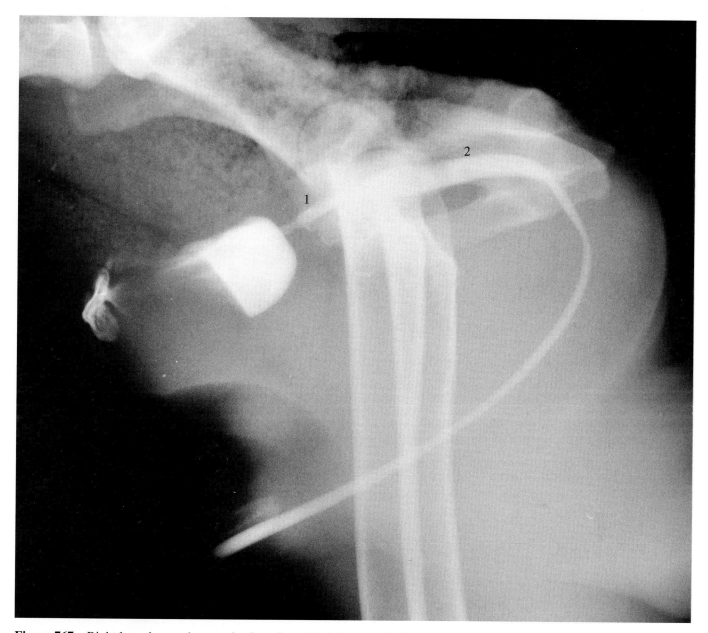

Figure 767 Right lateral recumbent projection of caudal abdomen with hind legs cranially extended. Retrograde urethrography in the male dog. Radiograph taken during general anaesthesia after insertion of an iodine-based, water-soluble contrast medium into the urethra. German Shepherd dog 1.5 years old, entire male.

Radiography is performed immediately after filling the urethra with the contrast media via a catheter whose tip is lodged in the distal urethral lumen. Distension of the lumen, particularly that of the prostatic portion of the urethra, is aided by a full bladder. An apparently narrow prostatic portion is not necessarily abnormal and contrast may show as longitudinal streaks within the folds of the lining mucous membrane.

In this radiograph some of the contrast medium has passed into the bladder. The prostatic portion (1) of the pelvic urethra is not as distended as the caudal portion (2). Globular lucencies within the latter are air bubbles.

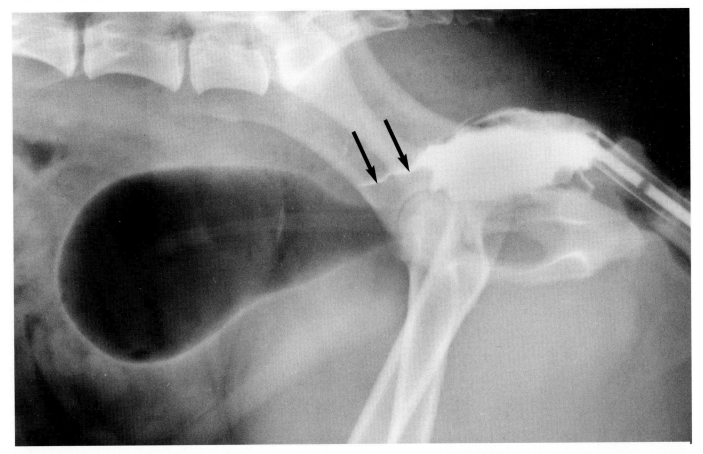

Figure 768   (Please see text referring to Figures 768 and 769.) Right lateral recumbent projection of caudal abdomen. Retrograde vaginography with pneumocystography. Springer Spaniel crossbred dog 2 years old, entire female.

The caudal vagina is only moderately distended so that some of the longitudinal folds appear, dorsally, as filling defects. Further distension with contrast would eliminate them.

The cranial vagina is just apparent, with a suggestion of the shapes of the dorsomedian fold and the vaginal cervix (arrows).

Figures 768 and 769   Right lateral recumbent projections of caudal abdomen. Retrograde vaginography and vaginourethrography in the female dog.

Radiographs are taken after filling the vagina, or vestibule, vagina and urethra, with water-soluble contrast medium via a catheter whose tip is lodged at the vaginovestibular junction, or just within the vestibule. The length and the diameter of the vagina vary with the body size and breed of the subject as well as the hormonal status.

The caudal, or plicate, intrapelvic section has longitudinal folds and is easily distended, the folds smoothing out.

The cranial, or paracervical, intra-abdominal section is much more restricted with a 'U'-shaped lumen and one fold always present, the dorsomedian fold, lying caudal to the vaginal cervix.

With only a small amount of contrast the cranial vagina may show simply as a fine horizontal line, whereas more complete filling will define, caudally, the crescent-shaped lower border of the dorsomedian fold and, cranially, the protrusion of the cervix into the vagina.

Radiography is performed during general anaesthesia.

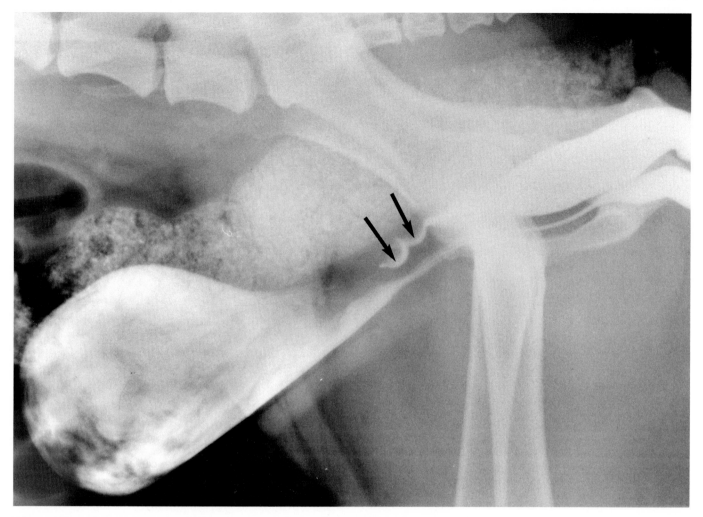

Figure 769 (Please see text referring to Figures 768 and 769.) Right lateral recumbent projection of caudal abdomen. Retrograde vaginourethrography (urine left in bladder). Golden Labrador Retriever dog 4 years old, entire female.

The dorsomedian fold and the vaginal cervix are outlined in the cranial vagina (arrows).
Note that the diameter of the urethra widens considerably towards the external orifice.
Some contrast has passed into the bladder to mix with the urine.

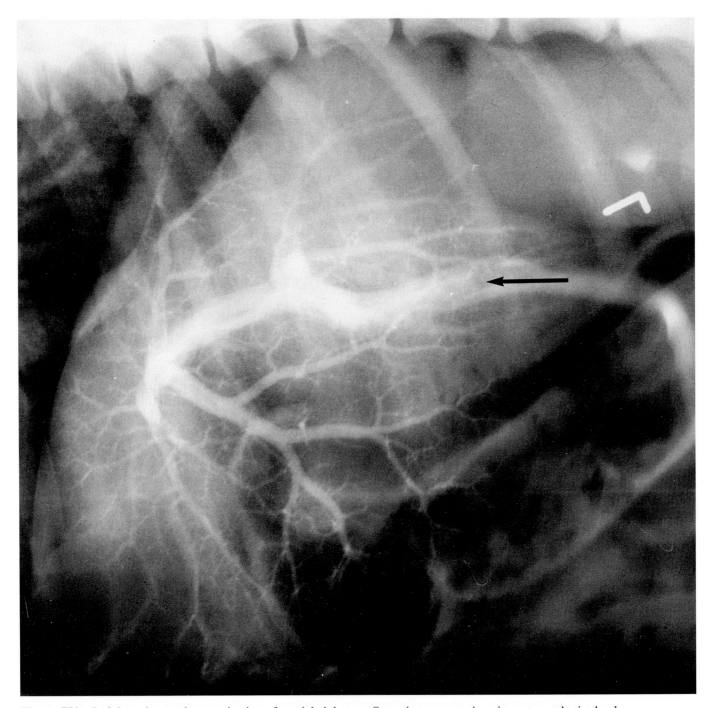

Figure 770 Left lateral recumbent projection of cranial abdomen. Operative mesenteric vein portography in the dog. Radiograph taken during ventral midline laparotomy as the final millilitre of water-soluble contrast medium is injected into the portal vein via a catheter inserted into a contributory jejunal vein. Munsterlander dog 6 months old, entire male (same dog as in Figure 771).

Direction of flow of contrast in the portal vein is indicated by the arrow.

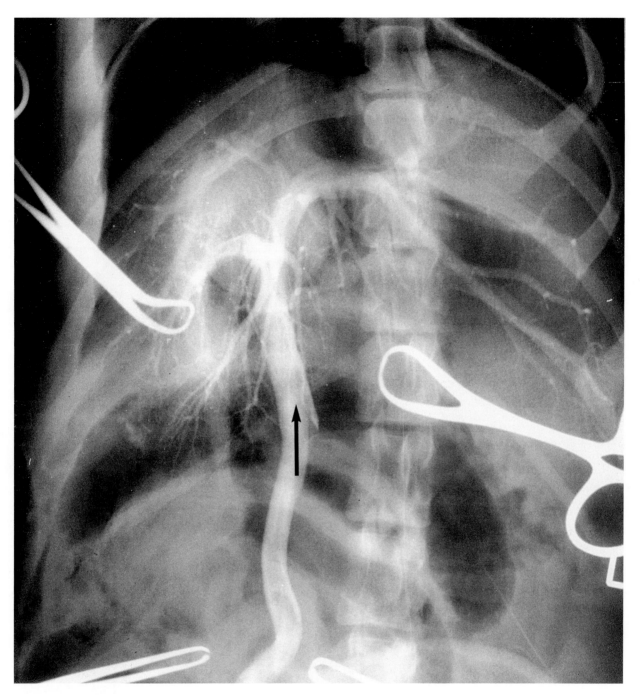

Figure 771 Ventrodorsal oblique projection of cranial abdomen. Operative mesenteric vein portography in the dog. Radiograph taken during ventral midline laparotomy as the final millilitre of water-soluble contrast medium is injected into the portal vein via a catheter inserted into a contributory jejunal vein. Munsterlander dog 6 months old, entire male (same dog as in Figure 770).

The direction of flow of the contrast in the portal vein is indicated by the arrow.
The rotation of the abdomen enhances the picture by avoiding superimposition of the spine.

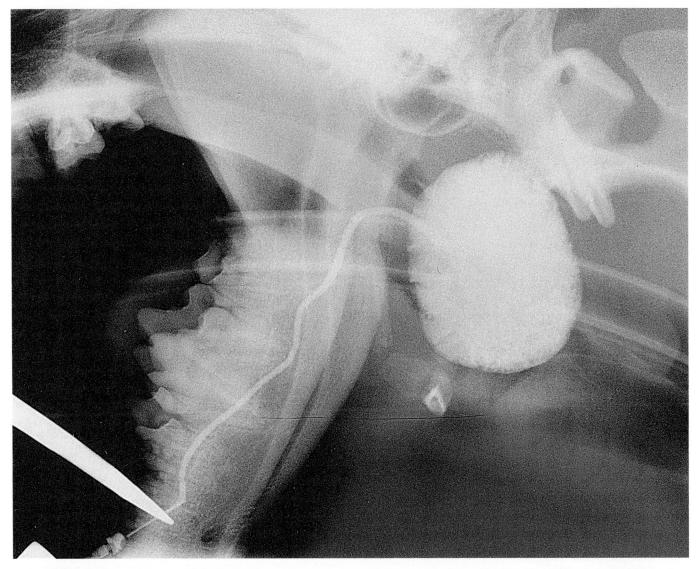

Figure 772   Lateral projection (open mouth) of pharynx and larynx. Sialography of mandibular salivary gland. Radiograph taken during general anaesthesia after catheterisation of the mandibular salivary gland duct and injection of a water-soluble contrast medium into the gland. Bull Terrier dog 1.5 years old, entire male.

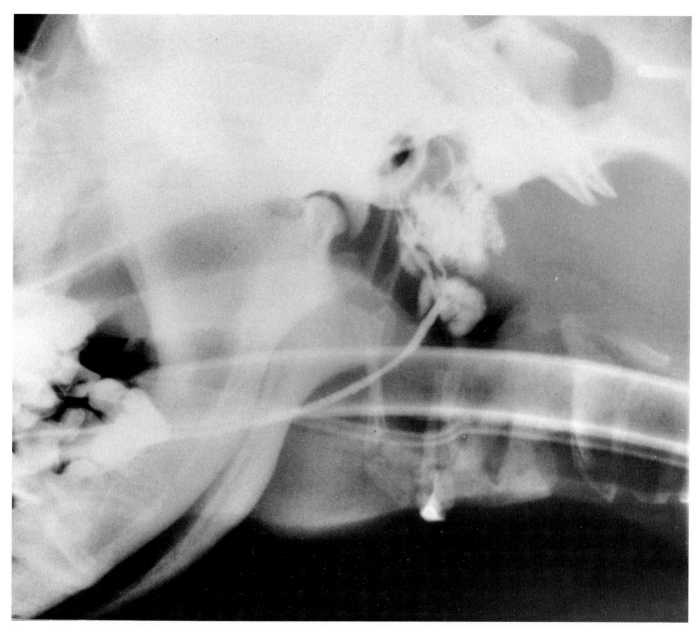

Figure 773 Lateral projection of pharynx and larynx. Sialography of parotid salivary gland. Radiograph taken during general anaesthesia after catheterisation of the parotid salivary gland duct and injection of a water-soluble contrast medium into the gland. Labrador dog 1 year old, entire male.

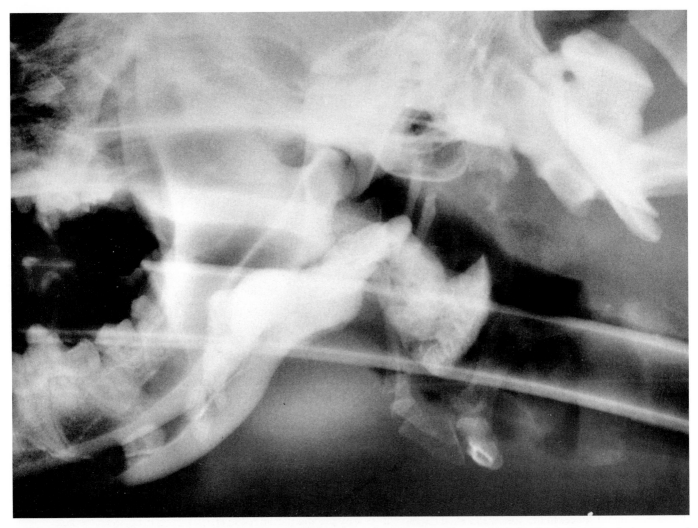

Figure 774 Lateral projection of pharynx and larynx. Sialography of sublingual salivary gland. Radiograph taken during general anaesthesia after catheterisation of the sublingual salivary gland duct and injection of a water-soluble contrast medium into the gland. Weimaraner dog 4 years old, entire male.

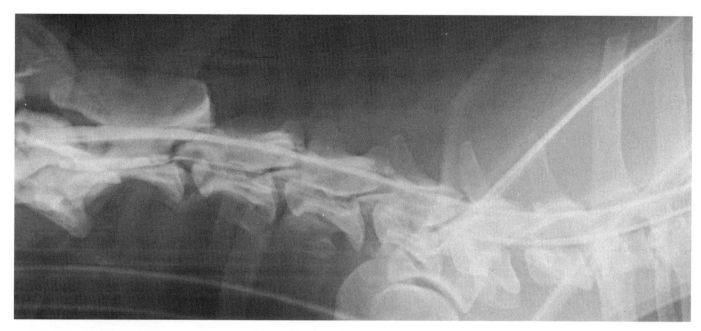

Figure 775 Right lateral recumbent projection of cervical and upper thoracic vertebrae (1st. cervical vertebra to 3rd. thoracic vertebra). Myelography in the dog. Radiograph taken during general anaesthesia immediately following the injection of water-soluble contrast medium into the cisterna magna. Labrador dog adult (same dog as in Figure 777).

The subarachnoid space is at its widest through the 1st. and 2nd. cervical vertebrae. The ventral column of contrast not infrequently bends slightly dorsally, as well as narrowing, at the 2nd. to 3rd. cervical intervertebral disc space. Slight narrowing of the ventral column with minor indentations may also occur over each of the subsequent intervertebral disc spaces.

The spinal cord is at its widest in the lower cervical region where it gives rise to the nerves of the brachial plexus. Through the 5th. and 6th. cervical vertebrae the ventral column often appears raised from the floor of the canal.

The use of a tilting table for this contrast technique enables positioning of the head and neck at an angle of 5 to 10 degrees from the horizontal in a dorsocranial–ventrocaudal direction, which encourages the caudal flow of the contrast medium along the subarachnoid space. In the absence of such a table temporarily placing the animal in sternal recumbency with the head moderately elevated has a similar effect.

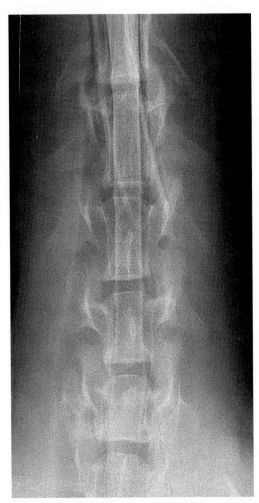

Figure 776 Ventrodorsal projection of cervical vertebrae (2nd. to 7th. cervical vertebrae).
Myelography in the dog. Radiograph taken during general anaesthesia following the injection of water-soluble contrast medium into the cisterna magna. Doberman dog. Linear opacities representing the walls of the endotracheal tube can be seen superimposed on the 2nd. and 3rd. cervical vertebrae and on the cranial part of the 4th. In some cases such shadows create confusion in the interpretation of the myelogram.

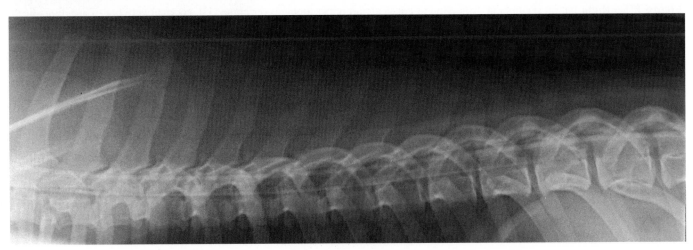

Figure 777 Right lateral recumbent projection of thoracic vertebrae (1st. to 13th. thoracic vertebrae). Myelography in the dog. Radiograph taken during general anaesthesia 3 minutes after injection of water-soluble contrast medium into the cisterna magna. Labrador dog adult (same dog as in Figure 775).

There is a gradual re-distribution of the contrast in the caudal thoracic subarachnoid space, resulting in a well-filled dorsal column and a thinner ventral column.

Considerable tilting of the long axis of the spine in a dorsocranial–ventrocaudal direction was necessary in this case to further the flow of contrast medium beyond the caudal cervical region.

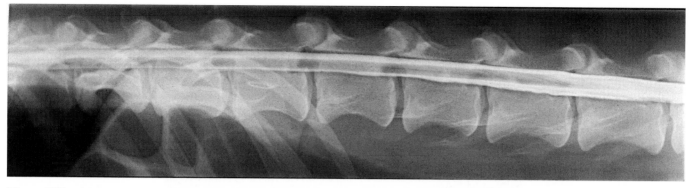

Figure 778   Right lateral recumbent projection of thoracolumbar vertebrae (11th. thoracic vertebra to 5th. lumbar vertebra). Myelography in the dog. Radiograph taken during general anaesthesia 10 minutes after injection of a water-soluble contrast medium into the cisterna magna. Great Dane dog 2.5 years old, entire male (same dog as in Figures 779 and 780).

In the caudal thoracic region the dorsal column of contrast is much wider than the ventral. Through the cranial lumbar vertebrae the ventral column increases again in width. From the 4th. lumbar vertebra the columns begin to converge as the spinal cord tapers into the cauda equina. Radiolucent linear filling defects obliquely crossing the cord at the 4th. lumbar vertebra are caused by the emerging spinal nerve roots and confirm the subarachnoid distribution of the contrast medium (as opposed to epidural deposition; see lumbar puncture myelogram, Figure 781).

Shallow undulations of the ventral column, lifting over the intervertebral spaces, are frequently seen in the lumbar region, occasionally with a slight break in the contrast.

Some widening of the cord at the 4th. and 5th. lumbar vertebrae, the origin of the nerves of the sacral plexus, may be apparent.

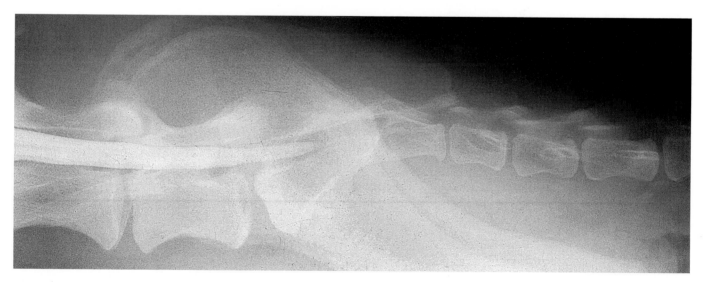

Figure 779   Right lateral recumbent projection of lumbosacral and upper coccygeal vertebrae (6th. lumbar vertebra to 3rd. coccygeal vertebra). Myelography in the dog. Radiograph taken during general anaesthesia 15 minutes after the injection of water-soluble contrast medium into the cisterna magna. Great Dane dog 2.5 years old, entire male (same dog as in Figures 778 and 780).

The contrast tapers caudally through the 6th. and 7th. lumbar vertebrae around the cauda equina, to terminate within the spinal canal of the 1st. sacral segment.

The shape, length and position of the contrast image at the lumbosacral junction should not alter with either flexion or extension of the vertebrae.

An Atlas of Interpretative Radiographic Anatomy of the Dog and Cat

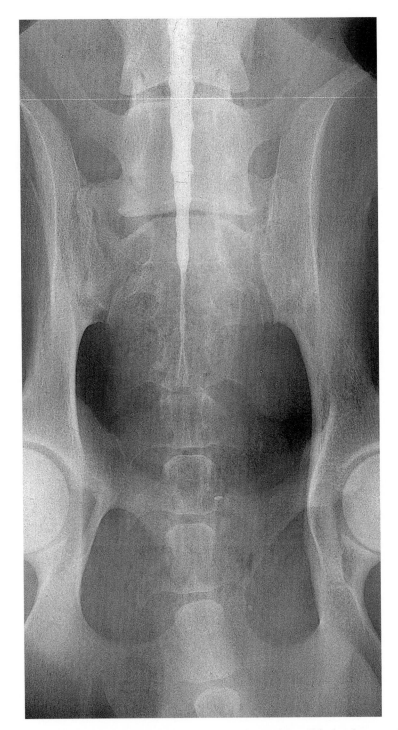

Figure 780 Ventrodorsal projection of lumbosacral and upper coccygeal vertebrae (6th. lumbar vertebra to 5th. coccygeal vertebra). Myelography in the dog. Radiograph taken during general anaesthesia 20 minutes after the injection of water-soluble contrast medium into the cisterna magna (corresponding projection to right lateral recumbent projection of lumbosacral and upper coccygeal vertebrae, Figure 779).

Great Dane dog 2.5 years old, entire male (same dog as in Figures 778 and 779).
The subarachnoid contrast column tapers around the cauda equina to terminate within the sacrum.

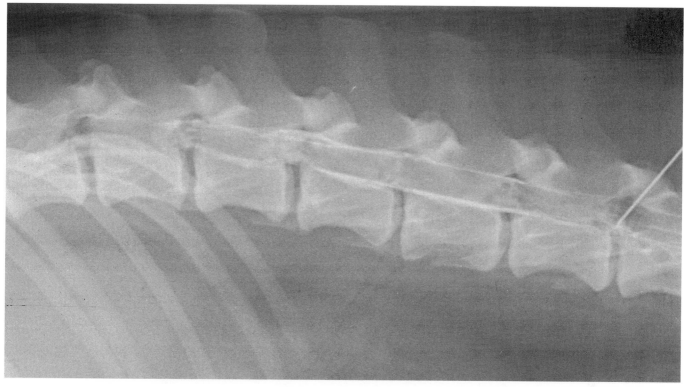

Figure 781 Right lateral recumbent projection of lumbar vertebrae (13th. thoracic vertebra to 6th. lumbar vertebra). Myelography in the dog. Radiograph taken during general anaesthesia following lumbar puncture between the 5th. and 6th. lumbar vertebrae with the injection of water-soluble contrast medium. Labrador dog 8.5 years old, entire male.

Some contrast has entered the subarachnoid space to be seen as thin straight linear opacities along the spinal canal while the rest has been deposited epidurally, resulting in secondary, undulating and thicker linear opacities following the upper and lower bony limits of the spinal canal and lifting, ventrally, over the emerging spinal nerves at the intervertebral foramina. The resulting pattern is best seen on this film at the 3rd and 4th. lumbar vertebrae.

Such an epidural pattern, not uncommon with lumbar myelography, should not be mistaken for abnormality.

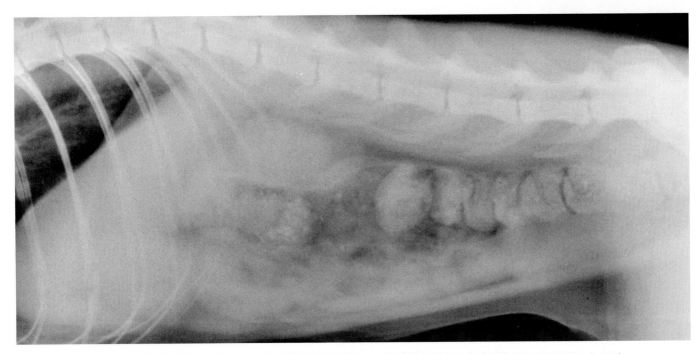

Figure 782   Right lateral recumbent projection of abdomen. Plain survey film. Faecal boluses are present in the colon.

Figures 782–787   Right lateral recumbent and ventrodorsal projections of abdomen. Barium meal in the cat. Radiographs taken during restraint with sandbags before and following oral administration of liquid barium sulphate. British domestic short haired cat adult (same cat in all figures for barium meal).

This barium meal series was not followed beyond the transverse colon. Note that the caecum is not identifiable in any of the films; in the cat it is a very small, simple sac compared with that of the dog.

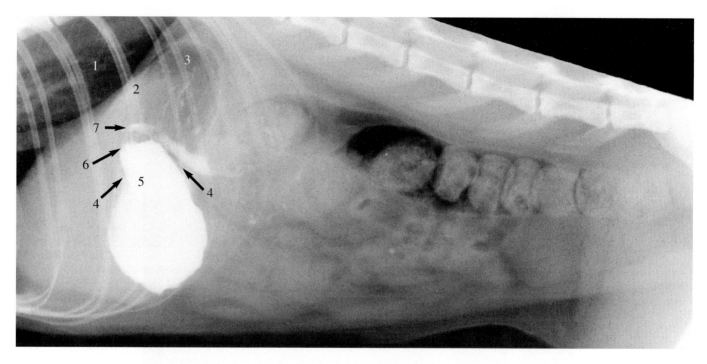

Figure 783   Right lateral recumbent projection of abdomen. Immediately after barium administration.

Very little barium is left in the oesophagus and it is just beginning to pass down the descending portion of the duodenum.

1   Oesophagus
2   Cardia of the stomach
3   Fundus of the stomach
4   Body of the fundus
5   Pyloric antrum
6   Pyloric canal
7   Cranial flexure of the duodenum

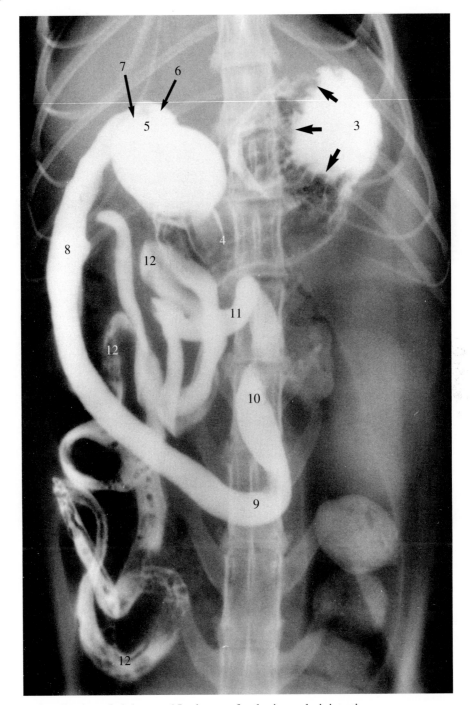

Figure 784   Ventrodorsal projection of abdomen. 15 minutes after barium administration.

Rugal folds of the stomach wall are seen in cross-section (arrows) around the fundic pool of barium, with streaking of barium along their length.

Note that the cat stomach is more 'J' shaped in this projection than is the dog, with the pylorus closer to the midline.

Bubbles of gas are present within the jejunal loops and gas appears to be collecting within the colon, highlighting the faecal boluses.

3   Fundus of the stomach
4   Body of the stomach
5   Pyloric antrum
6   Pyloric canal
7   Cranial flexure of the duodenum
8   Descending portion of the duodenum
9   Caudal flexure of the duodenum
10   Ascending portion of the duodenum
11   Duodenojejunal flexure
12   Loops of jejunum and ileum

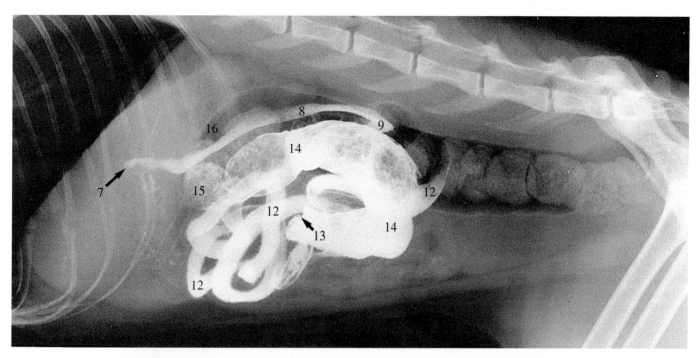

Figure 785   Right lateral recumbent projection of abdomen. 75 minutes after barium administration.

Only a trace of barium remains in the stomach and it is already collecting in the colon, coating the faecal boluses.

  7 Cranial flexure of the duodenum
  8 Descending portion of the duodenum
  9 Caudal flexure of the duodenum
12 Loops of jejunum and ileum
13 Ileocolic junction
14 Ascending colon
15 Right colic flexure
16 Transverse colon

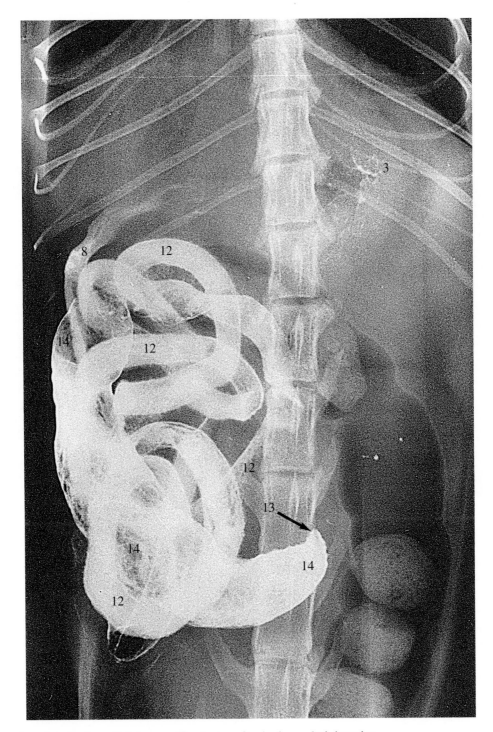

Figure 786 Ventrodorsal projection of abdomen. 75 minutes after barium administration.

 3 Fundus of the stomach
 8 Descending portion of the duodenum
12 Loops of jejunum and ileum
13 Ileocolic junction
14 Ascending colon

See right lateral recumbent projection of abdomen, Figure 785, also at 75 minutes.

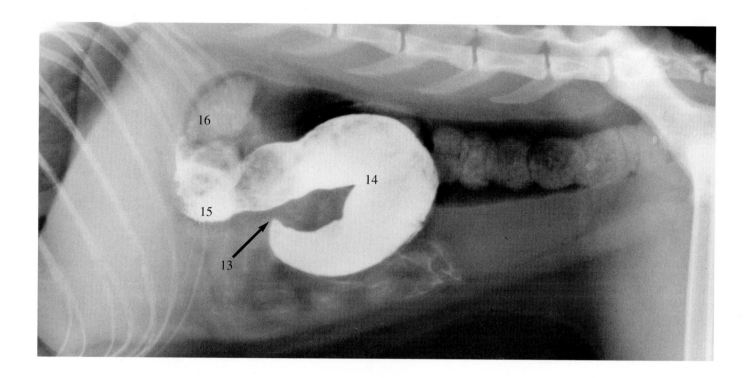

Figure 787   Right lateral recumbent projection of abdomen. 3 hours after barium administration.

The barium is almost totally in the colon although transit has stopped at a similar level as in the 75 minute film. It is probably being held up by the faecal boluses and the accumulation of gas which has occurred.

13 Ileocolic junction
14 Ascending colon
15 Right colic flexure
16 Transverse colon

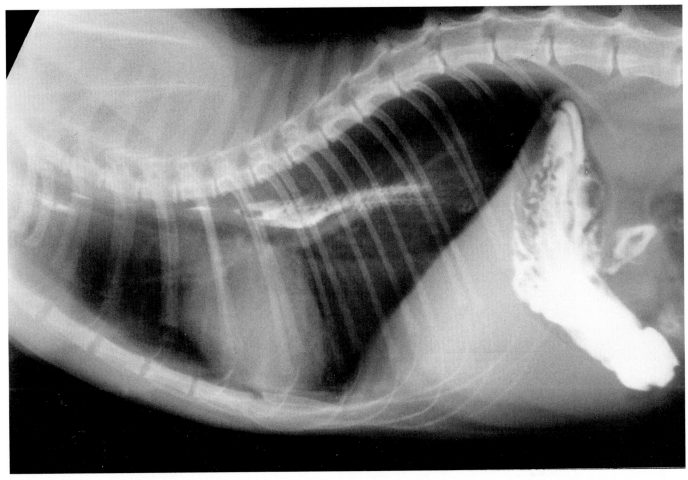

Figure 788   Right lateral recumbent projection of thorax. Normal appearance of liquid barium within the thoracic oesophagus of the cat. Radiograph taken during restraint with sandbags immediately following oral administration of liquid barium sulphate as part of a barium meal investigation. British domestic short haired cat adult.

Caudal to the base of the heart longitudinal striations, up to this point similar to the dog, give way to a 'herring bone' pattern reflecting the obliquely directed folds of mucosa. The latter corresponds to the change to smooth muscle in the wall of this segment of the cat's oesophagus.

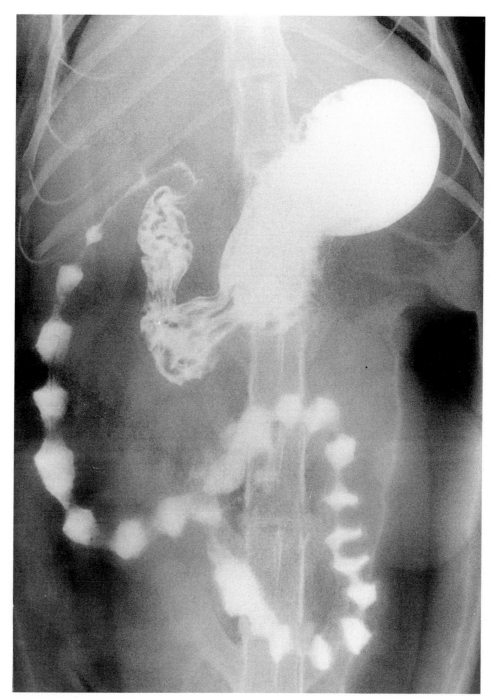

Figure 789   Ventrodorsal projection of abdomen. Duodenal beading and pseudostringing in the cat. Radiograph taken during restraint with sandbags 5 minutes after oral administration of liquid barium sulphate as part of a barium meal investigation. British domestic short haired cat adult.

Short but strong segmental peristalsis may occur along the proximal duodenum, resulting in regularly spaced, rather globular expansions, 'beads', of the barium column.

Linear filling defects within the intervening contracted segments represent mucosal folds indenting the narrowed bowel lumen and are described as 'pseudostringing'.

Note that the contracted portions of the bowel are symmetrically central to the expanded portions, in comparison with the asymmetric pattern seen in the presence of a linear foreign body.

A roundworm is highlighted by the contrast in the descending portion of the duodenum.

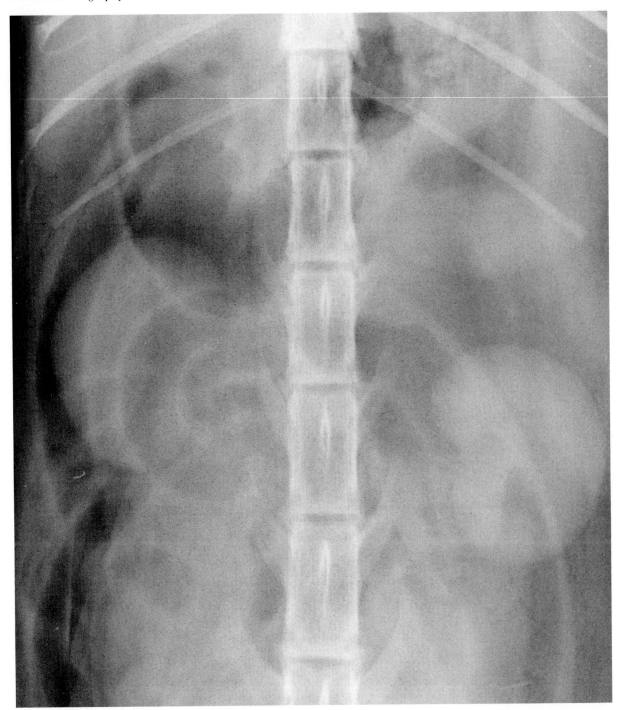

Figure 790 Ventrodorsal projection of abdomen. Intravenous urography (I.V.U.) with pneumocystography. Radiograph taken during general anaesthesia immediately after injection of an iodine-based, water-soluble contrast medium with prior insertion of air into urinary bladder. British domestic short haired cat young adult, neutered male (same cat as in Figures 791 and 792).

Nephrogram phase of I.V.U.
Sufficient contrast has reached the kidneys to show their size, shape, and position.

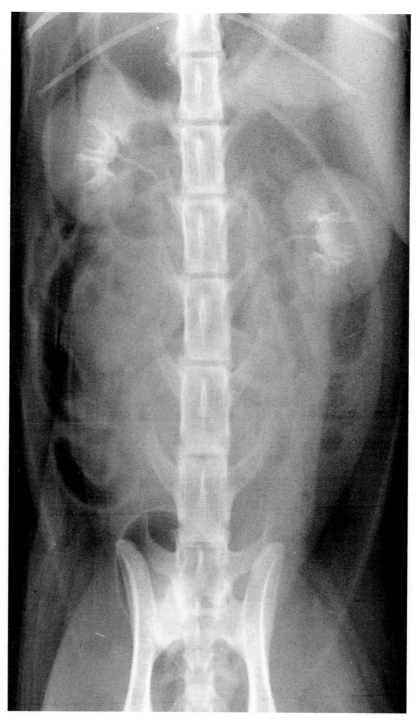

Figure 791 Ventrodorsal projection of abdomen. Intravenous urography (I.V.U.) with pneumocystography. Radiograph taken during general anaesthesia 5 minutes after injection of an iodine-based, water-soluble contrast medium with prior insertion of air into the urinary bladder. British domestic short haired cat young adult, neutered male (same cat as in Figures 790 and 792).

Pyelogram phase of I.V.U.

The renal pelves and their recesses are delineated and contrast is already beginning to collect in the urinary bladder, although this is not clearly seen because of superimposition of the right sacral wing.

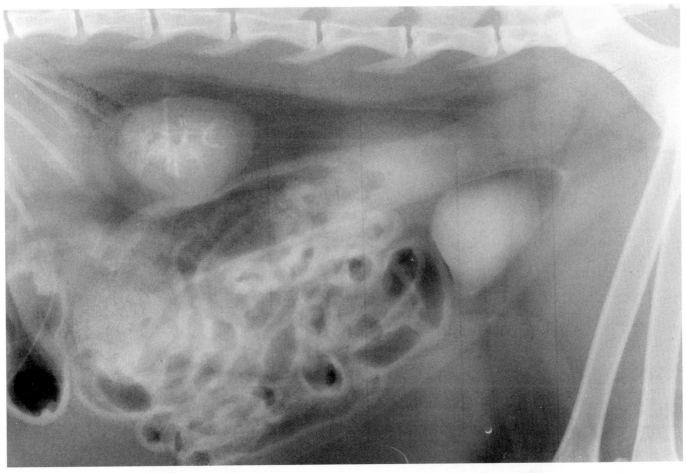

Figure 792 Lateral recumbent projection of abdomen. Intravenous urography (I.V.U.) with pneumocystography. Radiograph taken during general anaesthesia 10 minutes after injection of an iodine-based, water-soluble contrast medium with prior insertion of air into the urinary bladder. British domestic short haired cat young adult, neutered male (same cat as in Figures 790 and 791).

Pyelogram phase of I.V.U.
The bladder and the ureterovesical junctions are more easily seen in this projection. Clarity is enhanced by pneumocystography.

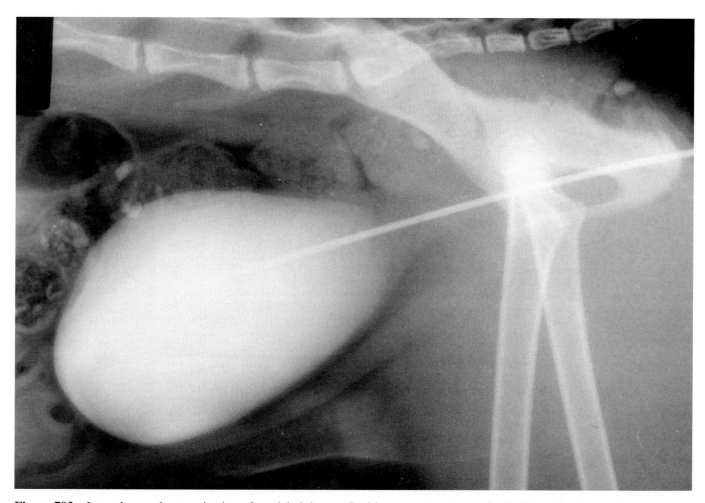

Figure 793   Lateral recumbent projection of caudal abdomen. Positive contrast cystography. Radiograph taken during general anaesthesia after insertion of an iodine-based, water-soluble contrast medium into the urinary bladder until full distension was reached, catheter still *in situ*. British domestic short haired cat young adult, neutered female (same cat as in Figure 794).

Note the position of the bladder and the presence of faecal boluses in the colon and rectum compared to Figure 794 of a pneumocystogram in the same cat, taken 48 hours later.

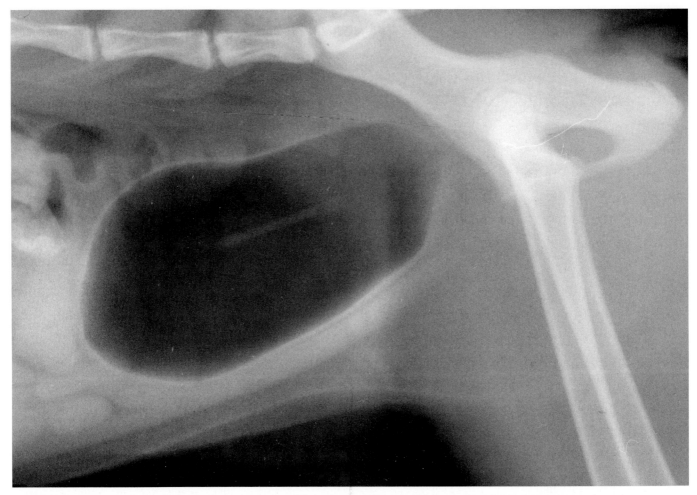

Figure 794 Lateral recumbent projection of caudal abdomen. Negative contrast cystography; pneumocystography. Radiograph taken during general anaesthesia after insertion of air into the urinary bladder until full distension was reached, catheter still *in situ*. British domestic short haired cat young adult, neutered female (same cat as in Figure 793).

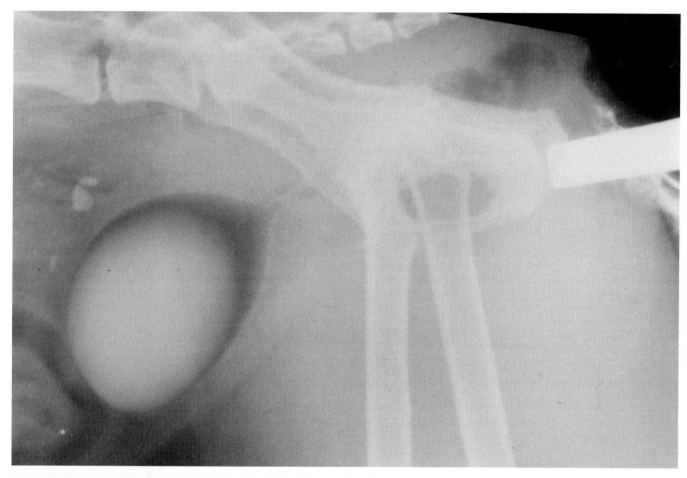

Figure 795 Lateral recumbent projection of caudal abdomen. Double contrast cystography. Radiograph taken during general anaesthesia after insertion of an iodine-based, water-soluble contrast medium followed by air into the urinary bladder until distension was reached. Burmese cat 7.5 years old, neutered female.

The bladder is moderately distended and the catheter has been removed.

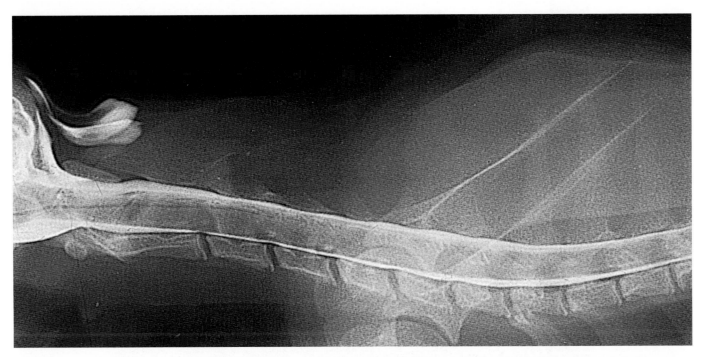

Figure 796 Right lateral recumbent projection of cervical and upper thoracic vertebrae (1st. cervical vertebra to 3rd. thoracic vertebra). Myelography in the cat. Radiograph taken during general anaesthesia immediately following the injection of water-soluble contrast medium into the cisterna magna. British domestic short haired cat 10 months old (same cat in all figures for myelography).

The subarachnoid space filled with contrast is at its widest at the 1st. and 2nd. cervical vertebrae. Thinning and slight indentation of the ventral contrast column occur over each cervical intervertebral disc space.

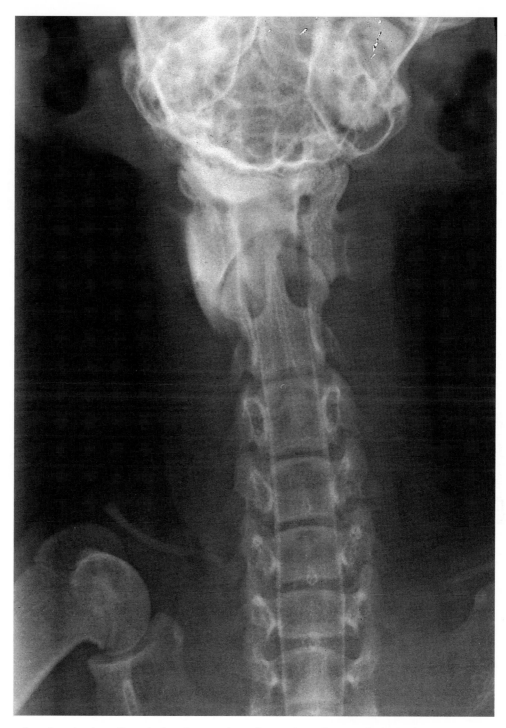

Figure 797 Ventrodorsal projection of cervical and upper thoracic vertebrae (1st. cervical vertebra to 2nd. thoracic vertebra). Myelography in the cat. Radiograph taken during general anaesthesia immediately following the injection of water-soluble contrast medium into the cisterna magna. British domestic short haired cat 10 months old (same cat in all figures for myelography).

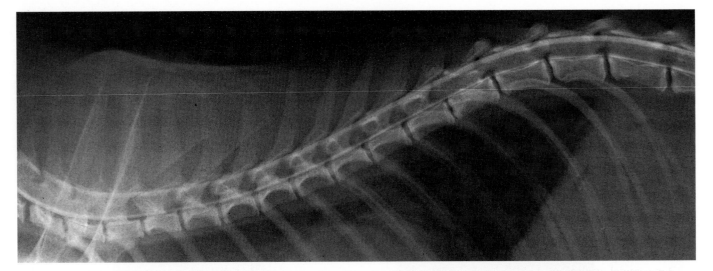

Figure 798 Right lateral recumbent projection of thoracic vertebrae (7th. cervical vertebra to 1st. lumbar vertebra). Myelography in the cat. Radiography taken during general anaesthesia following the injection of water-soluble contrast medium into the cisterna magna. British domestic short haired cat 10 months old (same cat in all figures for myelography).

Thinning and slight indentation of the ventral column over the intervertebral disc spaces can occur, as in the cervical vertebrae.

In the caudal thoracic region the ventral contrast column becomes narrower and the dorsal column broader, as in the dog.

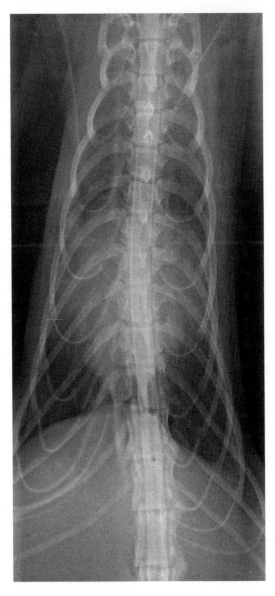

Figure 799 Ventrodorsal projection of thoracic vertebrae (1st. thoracic vertebra to 1st. lumbar vertebra). Myelography in the cat. Radiograph taken during general anaesthesia following the injection of water-soluble contrast medium into the cisterna magna. British domestic short haired cat 10 months old (same cat in all figures for myelography).

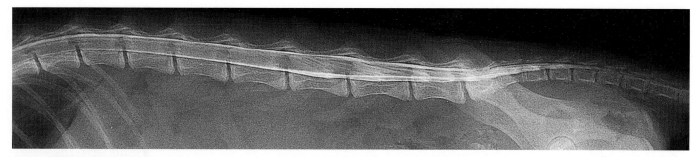

Figure 800   Right lateral recumbent projection of lumbar, sacral and cranial coccygeal vertebrae (13th. thoracic vertebra to 5th. coccygeal vertebra). Myelography in the cat. Radiograph taken during general anaesthesia following the injection of water-soluble contrast medium into the cisterna magna. British domestic short haired cat 10 months old (same cat in all figures for myelography).

The dorsal and ventral contrast columns start to converge through the 6th. lumbar vertebra, caudal to the lumbar enlargement of the cord, to taper around the cauda equina and finish in a fine point beyond the sacrum, much further caudal than in the dog.

Dorsocranial–ventrocaudal oblique radiolucent striations crossing the cord from the 4th. lumbar vertebra caudally indicate the roots of the spinal nerves.

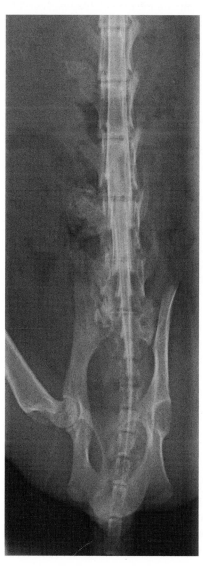

Figure 801   Ventrodorsal projection of lumbar, sacral and coccygeal vertebrae (13th thoracic vertebra to 6th. coccygeal vertebra). Myelography in the cat. Radiograph taken during general anaesthesia following the injection of water-soluble contrast medium into the cisterna magna. British domestic short haired cat 10 months old (same cat in all figures for myelography).

Bibliography

Ackerman, N. (1983) *Radiology of urogenital diseases in dogs and cats*. Iowa State University Press, Ames, IA.

Allen, W.E. and France, C. (1985) A contrast radiographic study of the vagina and ureters in the dog. *J. Small Anim. Pract.* **26**, 153–166.

Arnbjerg, J. and Heje, N.I. (1993) Fabellae and popliteal sesamoid bones in cats. *J. Small Anim. Pract.* **34**, 95–98.

Barrett, R.E., Delahunta, A., Roenigk, W.J., Hoffer, R.E. and Coons, F.H. (1976) Four cases of congenital portocaval shunt in the dog. *J. Small Anim. Pract.* **17**, 71–85.

Bennett, D. and Kelly, D.F. (1985) Sesamoid disease as a cause of lameness in young dogs. *J. Small Anim. Pract.* **26**, 567–579.

Dennis, R. (1992) Barium meal techniques in dogs and cats. *In Practice* **14**, 237–248.

Done, S.H., Goody, P.C., Evans, S.A. and Stickland, N.C. (1996) *Color atlas of veterinary anatomy*. Volume 3. *The dog and cat*. Mosby. London.

Evans, H.E. and Christensen, G.C. (1993) *Miller's anatomy of the dog*, 3rd. edn. W.B. Saunders, Philadelphia, PA.

Field, E.J. and Harrison, R.J. (1968) *Anatomical terms*, 3rd edn. Heffers. Cambridge.

Gaskell, C.J. (1974) The radiographic anatomy of the pharynx and larynx of the dog. *J. Small Anim. Pract.* **15**, 89–100.

Geary, J.C., Oliver, J.E. and Hoelein, B.F. (1967) Atlanto-axial sub-luxation in the canine. *J. Small Anim. Pract.* **8**, 577–582.

Getty, R. (1975) *Sisson and Grossman's The anatomy of the domestic animals*, 5th edn. W.B. Saunders, Philadelphia, PA.

Gibbs, C. (1986) Radiographic examination of the pharynx, larynx and soft-tissue structures of the neck in dogs and cats. *The 26th veterinary annual*. Scientechnia. Bristol.

Gilbert, S.G. (1968) *Pictorial anatomy of the cat*. University of Washington Press, Seattle, WA.

Grandage, J. (1974) The radiology of the dog's diaphragm. *J. Small Anim. Pract.* **15**, 1–17.

Grandage, J. (1974) The appearance of stomach gas in the dog. *Aust. Vet. J.* **50**, 529–532.

Grandage, J. (1975) Some effects of posture on the radiographic appearance of the kidneys of the dog. *J. Am. Vet. Med. Ass.* **166**, 165–166.

Hare, W.C.D. (1959) Radiographic anatomy of the canine. Pectoral limb. Part II. Developing limb. *J. Am. Vet. Med. Ass.* **135**, 305–310.

Hare, W.C.D. (1960) Radiographic anatomy of the canine. Pelvic limb. Part II. Developing limb. *J. Am. Vet. Med. Ass.* **136**, 603–611.

Hare, W.C.D. (1961) Radiographic anatomy of the cervical region of the canine vertebral column. Part II. Developing vertebrae. *J. Am. Vet. Med. Ass.* **139**, 217–220.

Holt, P.E., Gibbs, C. and Latham, J. (1984) An evaluation of positive contrast vagino-urethrography as a diagnostic aid in the bitch. *J. Small Anim. Pract.* **25**, 531–549.

Kealy, J.K. (1979) *Diagnostic radiology of the dog and cat*. W.B. Saunders, Philadelphia, PA.

McClure, R.C., Dallman, M.J. and Garret, P.G. (1973) *Cat anatomy*. Lea & Febiger. Philadelphia, PA.

Moon, M.L., Keene, B.W., Lessard, P. and Lee, J. (1993) Age related changes in the feline cardiac silhouette. *Vet. Radiol. Ultrasound* **34**, 315–320.

Morgan, J.P. (1981) *Radiology of skeletal disease – principles of diagnosis in the dog*. Iowa State University Press, Ames, IA.

Morgan, J.P. and Miyabayshi, T. (1991) Dental radiology: ageing changes in permanent teeth of beagle dogs. *J. Small Anim. Pract.* **32**, 11–18.

Nomina Anatomica Veterinaria – Nomina Histologica (1983) Published by the International Committee on Veterinary Gross Anatomy. *Nomenclature of the World Association of Veterinary Anatomy*, 3rd edn. Ithaca, NY.

Nomina Anatomica Veterinaria – Nomina Histologica (1992) Published by the International Committee on Veterinary Gross Anatomy. *Nomenclature of the World Association of Veterinary Anatomy*, 4th edn. Zurich.

O'Brien, T.R. (1978) *Radiographic diagnosis of abdominal disorders in the dog and cat*. W.B. Saunders, Philadelphia, PA.

Olsson, S.E. and Audell, L. (1978) Development and pathology of the canine acetabular rim. *Symposium on osteoarthritis and canine hip dysplasia*. Proceedings. Aurasen Kirjapaino, Forssa.

Poogird, W. and Wood, A.K.W. (1986) Radiologic study of the canine urethra. *Am. J. Vet. Res.* **47**, 2491–2497

Read, R.A., Black, A.P., Armstrong, S.J. *et al.* (1992) Incidence and clinical significance of sesamoid disease in Rottweilers. *Vet. Rec.* **130**, 533–535.

Root, C.R. (1974) Interpretation of abdominal survey radiographs. *Vet. Clin. North America* **4**, 768–786.

Rutgers, C. (1993) Diagnosis and management of portosystemic shunts. *In Practice.* **15**, 175–181.

Schebitz, H. and Wilkens, H. (1989) *Atlas of radiographic anatomy of the dog and cat.* 5th edn. Parey, Berlin.

Smallwood, J.E., Shively, M.J., Rendano, V.T. and Habel, R.E. (1985) A standardized nomenclature for radiographic projections used in veterinary medicine. *Vet. Radiol.* **26**, 2–9.

Smith, R.N. (1960) Radiological observations on the limbs of young greyhounds. *J. Small Anim. Pract.* **1** 84–90.

Smith, R.N. (1962) The normal and radiological anatomy of the hip joint of the dog. *J. Small Anim. Pract.* **4**, 1–9.

Smith, R.N. (1968) Appearance of ossification centres in the kitten. *J. Small Anim. Pract.* **9**, 497–511.

Smith, R.N. (1969) Fusion of ossification centres in the cat. *J. Small Anim. Pract.* **10**, 523–530.

Suter, P.F. (1982) Radiographic diagnosis of liver disease in dogs and cats. *Vet. Clin. North America Small Anim. Pract.* **12**, 153–173.

Suter, P.F. (1984) *Thoracic radiography. Thoracic diseases of the dog and cat.* Suter. Switzerland.

Thrall, D.E. (1994) *Textbook of veterinary diagnostic imaging.* 2nd edn. W.B. Saunders, Philadelphia, PA.

Vaananen, M. and Skutnabb, K. (1978) Elbow lameness in the young dog caused by a sesamoidal fragment. *J. Small Anim. Pract.* **19**, 363–371.

Vaughan, L.C. and France, C. (1986) Abnormalities of the volar and plantar sesamoid bones in Rottweilers. *J. Small Anim. Pract.* **27**, 551–558.

Webbon, P.M. and Clayton Jones, D.G. (1976) Radiological refresher–6. The elbow. *J. Small Anim. Pract.* **17**, 395–401.

Weber, W.J. and Berry, C.R. (1994) Determining the location of contrast medium in the canine lumbar myelogram. *Vet. Radiol. and Ultrasound.* **35**, 430–432.

Wheeler, S.J., Clayton Jones, D.G. and Wright, J.A. (1985) Myelography in the cat. *J. Small Anim. Pract.* **26**, 143–152.

Wright, J.A. (1977) A study of the radiographic anatomy of the cervical spine in the dog. *J. Small Anim. Pract.* **18**, 333–357.

Wright, J.A. (1979) The use of sagittal diameter measurement in the diagnosis of cervical spinal stenosis. *J. Small Anim. Pract.* **20**, 331–334.

Wright, J.A. (1979) A study of the radiographic anatomy of the foramen magnum in dogs. *J. Small Anim. Pract.* **20**, 501–508.

Wright, J.A. (1984) Myelography in the dog. *In Practice.* **6**, 25–27.